Empowering Women through better Healthcare and Nutrition in Developing Countries

Empowering Women through better Healthcare and Nutrition in Developing Countries

— *Editors* —
Sheel Sharma
Angella Atwaru Atero

CENTRE FOR SCIENCE & TECHNOLOGY OF THE NON-ALIGNED AND OTHER DEVELOPING COUNTRIES (NAM S&T CENTRE)

2012
REGENCY PUBLICATIONS
New Delhi - 110 002

ISBN 978-81-89233-75-4

Centre for Science and Technology of the Non-Aligned and Other Developing Countries (NAM S&T Centre)
Core-6A, 2nd Floor, India Habitat Centre, Lodhi Road,
New Delhi-110 003 (India)
Phone: +91-11-24644974, 24645134, Fax: +91-11-24644973
E-mail: namstct@gmail.com
Website: www.namstct.org

Published by : **REGENCY PUBLICATIONS**
(*Division of Daya Publishing House*)
4760-61/23, Ansari Road, Darya Ganj,
New Delhi - 110 002
Phone: 23245578, 23244987
Fax: (011) 23260116
e-mail : info@regency-books.com
website : www.dayabooks.com
website : www.regencybooks.com

Laser Typesetting : **Classic Computer Services**
Delhi - 110 035

Printed at : **Chawla Offset Printers**
Delhi - 110 052

PRINTED IN INDIA

Foreword

While writing this Foreword to this compilation of the papers presented by the experts and delegates from various countries in the three days International conference on "Empowering Women in Developing Countries through Better Care and Nutrition" held during 22-24th April, 2010 at BITS Pilani, Rajasthan, India gives me both jubilation and satisfaction that Centre for Science and Technology of the Non-Aligned and Other Developing Countries (NAM S&T Centre) has come forward to make experts from these countries deliberate on the issue as important as women empowerment through health and nutrition. The Centre for Science and Technology of the Non-Aligned and Other Developing Countries (NAM S&T Centre), as I have come to know, is an inter-governmental organization with a membership of 44 countries spread over Asia, Africa, Middle East and Latin America and it is doing a yeoman's job for these countries to catch up in the developmental race. The editor duo, Dr. Sheel Sharma, Professor and Head, Food Science and Nutrition, Banasthali University, India and Dr Atero Angella, S&T Communication Officer, UNCST, Uganda seemed to have worked overtime to give the compilation a coherence and continuity. I wish they take up many more such tasks and contribute tangibly towards the upliftment of the vulnerable and marginalized in developing countries. Above all, I applaud Prof. Arun P. Kulshrestha, Director, NAM S&T for his alacrity, acumen and aplomb with which he has been taking forward the causes of NAM contents. I am also appreciative Prof Nirupma Prakash, Chief, Women Studies and Societal Developmental Unit (WSSDU) for joining hands with NAM S&T Center to provide the academic ambience of an illustrious Institution; BITS, Pilani, India. Another key member, Dr V.P Kharbanda, editorial advisor to the NAM S&T, has played no less role in bringing this volume into its present shape.

I firmly believe that in order to bridge the hiatus of inequities between rich and the poor, men and women; access to nutritional and healthcare and education should become the foremost pertinent point in the movement for equality of the human race.

As a matter of fact, all development programmes need to address the rights of the underprivileged to welfare, equity and poverty alleviation; be they men, women or children.

To make women, especially from developing countries, contribute progressively towards the well being of planet earth and its inhabitants, their concern ought to be integrated with mainstream activities.

Aruna Roy

(Magsaysay award for community leadership and international understanding)
Mazdoor Kisan Shakti Sangathan (MKSS)
Devdoongri, Rajsamand
Rajasthan, India

Preface

State of health and nutrition of the common people of a country or region reflects its level of development, for socio-economic standing of a population influences its own availability of food resources and accessibility to health services of the population on one hand and shapes up the attitudes and behaviors of the people affecting the utilization of resources on the other. This applies even more aptly to the disadvantaged or unprivileged sections within the population. Women, especially in the developing countries, are invariably in an awful state of health, nutrition, education, economy and, above all, dignified existence. A plethora of menial jobs, ranging from household chores, agricultural activity, fire-wood gathering, water carrying from long distances; keep rural, undernourished women overworked and stressed. Exigencies of procreation and nurturing imposed on them by nature further aggravate their state of ill health and nourishment throughout life in general and in the states of expectant and nursing mothers in particular.

Adequate nutrition, healthcare, shelter, education, gainful employment and clean environment; the major factors that nurture life, are scarcely available to women. The basic duo, good health and optimum nutrition; the hallmarks of well nourished and healthy human hood, are also meagerly accessible to the common women. Name an arena; social, economic, political or educational and find inequalities galore and the dice loaded against women. As the women confined to lead a life of lopsidedness and inequity even in this era of changed awareness and advancing aspirations, tables need to be turned against all those forces that tend to undermine the existence, identity and progress of women.

While looking into the whole gamut of women subservience, subordination and subsistence, especially in the context of rural woman folk, two factors of prime importance emerge; poverty and gender discrimination. Poverty; a phenomenon that stares the developing countries straight in the face, is defined in its most basic terms as the inability to afford food worth a person's daily caloric needs. Adding to it, like fat adding to fire, is the weaker feminine gender of the woman. The ominous combine goes to erode the status of the woman making her *less equal* than her male counterparts. By being a part of this stifling set up, the female voice becomes feeble and identity diminutive.

Healthy women are the real wealth of societies. The survival and well being of women are not only important in their own right, but are also central to solving much broader economic, social and developmental challenges. When women die or are sick, their families, communities and nations suffer as well. Improving the nutrition and well being of women will not only nurture the health of societies, it will also decrease inequity and poverty.

In a welcome move, The Centre for Science and Technology of the Non-Aligned and Other Developing Countries (NAM S&T Centre) came forward to organize an International Conference on "Empowering Women in Developing Countries through Better Healthcare and Nutrition" at Birla Institute of Technology and Science (BITS), Pilani, Rajasthan, India; which was well attended and a real representative of the third world countries. Whereas, the sum and substance of the presentations pointed towards the grim realities that exist in relation to healthcare and nutrition of women in various countries, there were silver linings in the dark clouds in the form of information about identification of various critical control points and the road maps for acting and mending them. The conference acted as an eye opener as would become evident by going through compilation of the proceedings in the form of this volume.

The *saga of woman*, or as this *tale of travails, trials and tribulation* is euphemistically known – from an innocent child with dreamy eyes, an adolescent half-girl half-women on the threshold of marriage, a young woman endeavoring to invent her sense of worth in conjugal bliss and ensuing motherhood; to eventually becoming a disillusioned individual, discovering that life holds compromises and no promises – must change into being a human being, 'evenly equal' to man, in fighting odds and obstacles and in getting all good things that life can offer.

Let us all who believe in human dignity and equality, generate light and exhort action on all issues concerning *healthcare and nutrition* of the women with the avowed aim of garnering equality status and empowerment for them.

Prof. Sheel Sharma
Banasthali University,
Rajasthan, India

Ms. Angella Atwaru Atero
Science and Technology Communications Officer,
Uganda National Council for Science and Technology (UNCST),
Uganda

Introduction

The Millennium Development Goals provide a shared vision of a much improved world by 2015, where extreme poverty is cut in half; child mortality is greatly reduced; gender disparities in primary and secondary education are eliminated; women are more empowered; and health and environment indicators are improved.

Women are a great human resource in all countries and the role of women in society is critical for its development. However, the women force as yet comprises only a small percentage of the scientific and academic community barring teachers at the school and pre-school levels. In fact, they have an attitude to work with sincerity and loyalty while keeping pace with the required timings. Given proper own space, women can play an increasingly important role in social, industrial and economic development of the country and they should be encouraged to bring their vision and leadership, knowledge and skills, views and aspirations into the development agenda from the grassroots to international levels. To empower women is to increase their control over the decisions that affect their lives both within and outside the household. Through their empowerment women gain greater share of control over resources - material, human and intellectual, such as knowledge, information, ideas - and financial resources involving access to money and control over decision making in the home, community, society and nation.

In this context, women's health is of crucial importance, which is greatly affected by the ways in which they are treated and the status they are given by society as a whole. Proper nutrition is a key determinant of health, both in childhood and beyond. The nutritional status of girls is particularly important due to their future potential reproductive role and the intergenerational repercussions of poor female nutrition. Good nutrition plays an important role in maintaining the health of women. Adequate nutrition is essential to maintain the immune system and sustain healthy levels of physical activity, as also for the quality of life.

In many countries, food scarcity and poverty make adequate nutrition nearly impossible. Two sections of the population most vulnerable to malnutrition due to food scarcity are children, especially infants, and women. The under-nourishment in women that results in lack of breastfeeding exposes the infants to increasing risk of malnutrition and life-threatening infectious diseases. Women's health is therefore relevant not only to women themselves, but also has an impact on the health and development of the next generation. Many of the main causes of women's morbidity and mortality – in both rich and poor countries – have their origins in societies' attitudes to women, which are reflected in the structures and systems that set policies, determine services and create opportunities.

Investments in women's health can be argued on several grounds such as equity and human rights; existing gender disparity; multiple benefits of women's improved health such as the impact of the mother's health on her offspring and cost-effectiveness of reproductive health interventions. It is essential to view the health of women in a holistic way within the social, economic and political context of their lives. The health of a country's female population ensures health and education of the next generation and economic well being of households. The interface between health, technology and wider society can play a pivotal role in enhancing the quality of life of people. The relationship between health and development has undergone renewed scrutiny. There is search for new models to deal with global threats, soaring medical costs, technological costs, poverty and disease. Technological innovation offers unique opportunity for partnership between health and development sectors to change the pattern of work and enhance health-promoting habits. Broader strategies, such as poverty reduction, increased access to literacy, training and education, and increased opportunities for women to participate in economic activities, will also contribute to making sustainable progress in women's health.

Many health interventions directed specifically at women are among the most cost-effective healthcare measures available today with ripple effects that benefit children and increase household productivity as well. By addressing key health problems affecting women at all stages of their lives, governments can improve human welfare and national economic efficiency. Because women's health problems often begin in childhood and adolescence, efforts are needed to reach women at the earliest stage. Interventions during adolescence can help break the cycle of poverty, unwanted pregnancy and limited educational and economic opportunity. Efforts to enhance women's low social status and discourage gender-based discrimination are also vital because of the damaging effects these factors have on women's health. Governments in the developing countries must help establish essential services for women and ensure access to them by financing health programmes for the poor. International assistance agencies can do their part by sharing their expertise and influencing policy and funding priorities. Special attention to girls needs to be given, since adolescence is the stage at which the intergenerational cycle of early pregnancy, poor health and nutrition, and poverty can be broken. Also efforts to improve women's low social status and involve women more fully in development projects need to be emphasized.

In order to deliberate on the importance of the subject, the Centre for Science and Technology of the Non-Aligned and Other Developing Countries (NAM S&T Centre) organised a 3 days international conference on 'Empowering Women in Developing

Countries through Better Healthcare and Nutrition' from 22-24 April 2010 jointly with the Women Studies and Societal Development Unit (WSSDU) of the Birla Institute of Technology and Science (BITS), Pilani (Rajasthan), India. The Conference held at the BITS Campus was supported by the United Nations Children's Fund (UNICEF), Rajasthan, India.

The Inaugural Session was started with the Opening Remarks by Prof. Nirupama Prakash, Convenor and Chief of WSSDU followed by an introduction to the Conference by the Director, NAM S&T Centre with a brief mention about the role being played by the Centre in promoting South-South cooperation in various scientific areas, particularly on the issues related to women empowerment. Prof. L. K. Maheshwari, Vice Chancellor of BITS, Pilani welcomed the delegates and dignitaries. After the traditional 'Lighting of the Lamps' Ceremony, the Chief Guest, Dr. Padmanaban, Advisor (Public Health Administration), National Health System Resource Centre, National Rural Health Mission, Ministry of Health and Family Welfare, Government of India delivered the Inaugural Address on 'Social and Health Determinants of Maternal Mortality - Plan of Action for A Developing State' followed by an Address by the Distinguished Guest, Mr. Samuel Mawunganidze, Chief, UNICEF (Rajasthan).

The Conference was attended by 54 delegates from 18 countries, including 25 overseas participants, 4 representatives of the UNICEF (Rajasthan), 19 participants from the host country India, and 6 from the NAM S&T Centre. The overseas participants were from Cambodia [Dr. Chea Mary, IYCFP (Infant and Young Child Feeding Program) Program Coordinator, National Maternal and Child Health Center, Ministry of Health]; Egypt [Prof. Safaa EL Baz, Director, Regional Center for Training in Family Planning and Reproductive Health, Faculty of Medicine, Ain Shams University, Abassia, Cairo; and Dr. Taghreed Kamal Omar and Dr. Nagwa Ahmed Zein El Dein, Lecturer; Faculty of Nursing, Menoufiya University, Shebin El-Koom]; Indonesia [Ms. Sri Setiawati, Assistant Deputy to Minister for Ethics and Harmonization of S&T, Ministry of Research and Technology]; Iran [Dr. (Ms.) Ziba Nikaeen, Scientific Member, Iranian Research Organization for Science and Technology (IROST); Mrs. Tahmineh Shaverdi, Assistant Professor, Iranian Academy for Culture, Education and Research; Dr. (Ms.) Akram Ghadimi, National Research Institute for Science Policy (NRISP), Tehran; and Dr. (Ms.) Maryam Ghadimi, General Physician, Tehran]; Kenya [Mrs. Catherine Wachuka Mutie, Assistant Director of Research, Ministry of Higher Education, Science and Technology, Directorate of Research Management and Development, Nairobi and Ms. Kimani Lydia Wambui, Nutrition Officer, Ministry of Public Health and Sanitation, Provincial General Hospital, Nakuru]; Malaysia [Dr. Nayandeep Singh Kanwal, Executive Editor, Research Management Centre, University Putra Malaysia, Selangor]; Mauritius [Mrs. Aryamah Kumaree Doomun, Principal Nutritionist, Ministry of Health and Quality of Life and Mr. Vijaysingh Vishwamitra Doomun]; Mexico [Ms. Yesica del Moral, Researcher on Graphic Communication]; Myanmar [Dr. Mya Thandar Kyu, Lecturer, Department of Technical and Vocational Education, Ministry of Science and Technology, Nay Pyi Taw]; Nigeria [Mrs. Obi Maria Nwanyibuife, Chief Scientific Officer and Mrs. Edith Chibuzor Chima, Assistant Chief Int. Auditor, Raw Materials Research and Development Council (RMRDC), Abuja]; Oman [Dr. Asya Al-Riyami,

Director of Research and Studies, Ministry of Health, Muscat]; Russia [Ms. Lobach Vitalina, Researcher, Philosophy Department, Moscow State University, Moscow]; South Africa [Mrs. Sedibe Modiehi Heather, Researcher, University of the Witwatersrand, Johannesburg]; Sri Lanka [Dr. Nalika Gunawardena, Senior Lecturer, Department of Community Medicine, Faculty of Medicine, University of Colombo]; Syria [Prof. Imad Al-Din Al-Tanukhi, New Material Hospital, Baramke Faculty of Medicine, Damascus University]; Tanzania [Ms. Judith Francis Kadage, Research Officer (IPR),Tanzania Commission for Science and Technology, Dar-es-Salaam; and Uganda [Ms. Atero Angella Atwaru, Science and Technology Communication Officer, Uganda National Council for Science and Technology (UNCST), Kampala].

39 scientific papers were presented in the Inaugural and four Technical Sessions, which were co-chaired respectively by Dr. Sunita Saxena, Director, Institute of Pathology, Indian Council of Medical Research (ICMR), New Delhi, India and Mrs. Maria Obi of Nigeria; Prof. A.K. Sarkar, Dean ID and FD-1 of BITS, Pilani and Mrs. Catherine Wachuka Mutie of Kenya; Prof. R.N. Saha, Deputy Director, BITS, Pilani and Mrs. Aryamah Kumaree Doomun of Mauritius; and Prof. Ravi Prakash, Dean (Research), BITS, Pilani, India and Prof. Safaa El Baz of Egypt.

The present publication is a follow up of the above Conference on 'Empowering Women in Developing Countries through Better Healthcare and Nutrition' and is aimed at widely disseminating the knowledge and information generated at the above Conference among the scientific community and the public at large.

I gratefully acknowledge the dynamic involvement and untiring efforts of Ms. Angella Atwaru Atero, Science and Technology Communication Officer at the Uganda National Council for Science and Technology (UNCST) and Prof. Sheel Sharma from Banasthali University, Rajasthan, India for technical editing of this publication. I am indebted to Ms Aruna Roy, Mazdoor Kisan Shakti Sangathan (MKSS) of India for sparing her valuable time in writing a 'Foreword' for this book. Last but not the least, the valuable services provided by the entire team of the NAM S&T Centre, in particular, Mr. M. Bandyopadhyay, Dr. V. P. Kharbanda, Ms. Apeksha Yadav and Mr. Pankaj Buttan in compiling the papers and giving shape to this volume is greatly appreciated. I hope that the publication will serve as a valuable reference material on women's nutrition and healthcare particularly in developing countries for policy makers, the scientific community and the public at large.

Prof. Arun P. Kulshreshtha

Director and Executive Head,

NAM S&T Centre

Contents

Foreword *v*
Aruna Roy

Preface *vii*
Sheel Sharma and Angella Atwaru Atero

Introduction *ix*
Arun P. Kulshreshtha

1. **Health and Nutrition for Women and Children in Cambodia** 1
Mary Chea

2. **Impact of Health Education on Mothers and Nurses to Prevent Shaken Baby Syndrome Among High Risk Infants** 26
Nagwa Ahmed Zein El Dein and Aida Abd. El-Razek

3. **Quality of Care Provided to Thalassemic Children at Menoufia University Hospital** 39
Taghreed Kamal, Maha Khalifa and Hanaa Ibrahim

4. **Herbals in Promoting Nutrition among Children and Women** 61
Aarati Saxena

5. **Empowering Women in India through better Reproductive Healthcare** 68
Devendra Kothari

6. **The Role of Awareness, Comprehension and Attitude Constructs in Behaviour Adoption towards Alleviation of Nutritional Anaemia: A Before-and-After Study of Adolescent School Girls** 87
Sanjana R. Bhat and Nirupama Prakash

7. **Health and Nutrition Concerns of Women in Reproductive and Post-Reproductive Years in Developing Countries** 99
Sheel Sharma

8. **Assessment of the Prevalence of Under-nutrition and Anaemia in Adolescents Residing in Villages around Pilani Area of Rajasthan State in India** 111
Nirupma Prakash, Suman Kapur, Devinder Kumar, Urvashi Kaushik, R.P. Pareek and Taniya Mozumder

9. **The Impact of Decentralization Health Authority on Safe Motherhood Program in Indonesia** 120
Sri Setiawati

10. **The Role of Employment on Women's Mental Health** 133
Akram Ghadimi and Ghazaleh Nazifkar

11. **The Effect of Hygiene and Nutrition on Women's Empowerment** 139
Maryam Ghadimi and Kobra Ghadimi

12. **Health of Women in Iran** 146
Ziba Nikaeen and Zinat Nikaien

13. **Empowering Women through Better Healthcare and Nutrition: The Case of Kenya** 151
Catherine W. Mutie and Florence M. Kyallo

14. **HIV/AIDS and Low Births Weight in Kenya: Experiences, Challenges and Effective Interventions** 161
Wambui Lydia Kimani

15. **Women in Politics and Public Life (Modern Russia)** 176
Vitalina Lobach

16. **Maternal Health and Low Birth Weight Problems in Tanzania: Possible Reasons and Potential Remedies** 189
Judith Francis

17. **Healthcare and Nutrition in Myanmar** 201
Mya Thandar Kyu and Aye Aye Thaw

18. **Women Economic Empowerment through Value Addition to Local Raw Materials: The Role of Raw Materials Research and Development Council, Abuja, Nigeria** 214
Maria N. Obi

19. **Nutrition Knowledge, Beliefs and Dietary Habits and their Gender Association amongst Omani Elderly in Nizwa Wilayat: An Input For Policy Implications** 230
Asya Al Riyami and Saleh Al Hadabi

20. **A Method for Effectively Employing Graphic Communication Campaigns in the Prevention and Resolution of Health and Nutritional Problems** 243
Yésica A. del Moral Zamudio

21. **Narratives Around Dietary and Exercise Practices of Young Urban Females** 263
M.H. Sedibe and Shane Norris

22. **Prevalence of Under-nutrition and Associated Factors Among Females Aged 13–16 Years in Plantation Sector Medical Officer of Health (MOH) Area in Sri Lanka** 274
A.M.S. Niranjala and N. Gunawardena

23. **Role of Elected Women in Panchayati Raj and their Knowledge Level in Reproductive and Child Healthcare** 291
Geeta Malhotra and Kailash Kumar Mishra

24. **Traditional Leafy Vegetables as a Source of Pro-Vitamin A Carotenoids for Under Five Year Olds in Uganda** 301
A. Atero Angella, Agnes Namutebi and Margaret Kabahenda

25. **Maternal and Child Health** 314
Doomun Aryamah Kumaree

Chapter 1

Health and Nutrition for Women and Children in Cambodia

Mary Chea

National Nutrition Programme, National Maternal and Child Health Centre,
Ministry of Health, Cambodia
E-mail: marychea13@yahoo.com, chea.mary50@gmail.com

ABSTRACT

Cambodia has made significant improvements in child health and survival in recent years; however, there are still problems with maternal health and nutrition status. Under-five and Infant mortality rates declined by 33 per cent and 31 per cent respectively over the period 2000 to 2005. Maternal mortality is still high accounting for 437 per 100,000 live births in 2000 and 472 per 100,000 live births in 2005. There was no significant improvement in anemia among children, and CAS 2008 showed that wasting and underweight did no significantly decline from 2005 to 2008. Some nutritional indicators have improved substantially over the same period, but remained unacceptably high. The main objective of the paper is to share experiences on the current women and child nutritional status and the implementation of the National Nutrition Programme in Cambodia. The paper concludes that improved IYCF (Infant and Young Child Feeding) practices in combination with micronutrient interventions are partially credited to the significant improvement of Cambodian child and women health and survival. These successes also rely on a combination of interventions and a supportive political, legal, and community environment.

Keywords: *Nutrition, Mother, Child, Micronutrients, Infant and young child feeding, Pregnant women, Women in reproductive age, Postpartum women.*

Materials and Methods

Comprehensive integrated approaches have been used, including:

1. Highlighting Current Policies, Strategies, and Interventions Addressing Nutrition
2. Implementation of Infant and Young Child Feeding (IYCF)
   - Policy/legal environment: Sub-decree on Marketing of Products for IYCF and National Policy on IYCF
   - Facility-based provision of quality IYCF services: establishment of Baby Friendly Hospital Initiative, management of malnutrition and IYCF counseling through pre and in-service training
   - Community-based activities: establishment of Baby Friendly Community Initiative
   - Advocacy/communication strategy: use of behavior change communications and mass media campaign
3. Micronutrient Intervention

   (*a*) Micronutrient Supplementation
   - Vitamin A Supplementation for children 6-59 months and post partum mothers within 6 weeks of delivery
   - Iron/Folate Supplementation for pregnant and post partum women
   - A study on Multi-micronutrient Supplementation for children < 2 years of age
   - Weekly Iron/Folate Supplementation

   (*b*) Fortification
   - Universal Iodization
   - Small-scale fish sauce and soy sauce fortification with iron
   - Small-scale noodle and wheat flour fortified with multi-micronutrients

   (*c*) Food-based Implementation
   - Homestead food production
   - Food security and nutrition

   (*d*) De-worming
   - For children 1-5 years
   - For pregnant and post partum women

Introduction

Geodemography

Cambodia is located in Southeast Asia and bordered by Thailand to the west, Laos and Thailand to the north, the gulf of Thailand to the south and Viet Nam to the east. It covers a total land area of 181,035 square km^2 (CDHS 2005). Cambodia has 24 provinces, 159 districts, 8 khans, 26 cities, 1,417 communes, 204 sangkats, and 14,073 villages (NIS, 2009).

According to the 2008 Census, total population is 13, 4 comprising 6,516,054 males (48.64 percent) and 6,879, 628 females (51.36 percent) with annual growth rate of 1.54 per cent and population density of 75 per km^2 (National Institute of Statistics, 2009).

Health

Cambodia has significant improvement in child health and survival recently, but still has problems with maternal health and nutrition status. It is one of 36 high burden countries in the world for maternal and child under-nutrition, with 44 per cent of children below the age of five years chronically malnourished, 28 per cent underweight and 8 per cent acutely malnourished. Cambodia Anemia rates are also high with 62 percent children below the age of five years anemic. Twenty percent of women are chronically energy deficient (thin), and 44 per cent of women of reproductive age and 57 of pregnant women are anemic. The under-five mortality rate has declined from 124 in 2000 to 83 in 2005 and the infant mortality rate from 95 to 66 in 2005 in the same period. Maternal mortality is one of the highest in the region accounted for 437 per 100,000 live births in 2000 and 472 per 100,000 live births in 2005 (CDHS,2000 and CDHS, 2005). Life expectancy at birth is 64 for females and 61 for males (NIS, 2009).

Health and Nutrition Status of Women and Children

Anaemia among Children

Anemia is the most common nutritional deficiency in the world and it is also a serious problem in Cambodia, affecting children; especially under-5 year year olds, women in reproductive age, pregnant women and post-partum women. There was no a significant reduction of anemia rate among under 5 year old children, women in reproductive age and pregnant women in Cambodia within the 5 year periods.

The 2000-2005 Cambodia Demographic and Health Survey showed that there was no decline in overall anemia rate among fewer than 5 children which is accounted for 63 per cent to 62 per cent respectively (Figure 1.2). According to their ages, the anemia prevalence of children aged 6-8, 9-11, 12-17 month olds is much higher compared to other age groups of under than 5 children (Figure 1.1). This can be translated that the lack of breastfeeding practices, appropriate complementary practices and other micronutrient supplementation lead to rapid increase of anemia rate during this rapid growth in the first year of life. However, iron deficiency anemia is not only a cause of child anemia in Cambodia as estimated by WHO which is accounted for 50 per cent globally. The causes of child anemia in Cambodia is estimated to be 30 per cent of iron deficiency; 30 per cent of hemoglobinopathies or inherited conditions that affect the red blood cell; 30 per cent of other micronutrient deficiencies including Folate, vitamin B12, vitamin C and vitamin A; 15 per cent of intestinal parasites and 10 per cent of malarias.

Anemia among WRA and PW

According to WHO cut-off point of 40 per cent to describe a severe public health problem, anemia among women in Cambodia is the most common serious nutritional

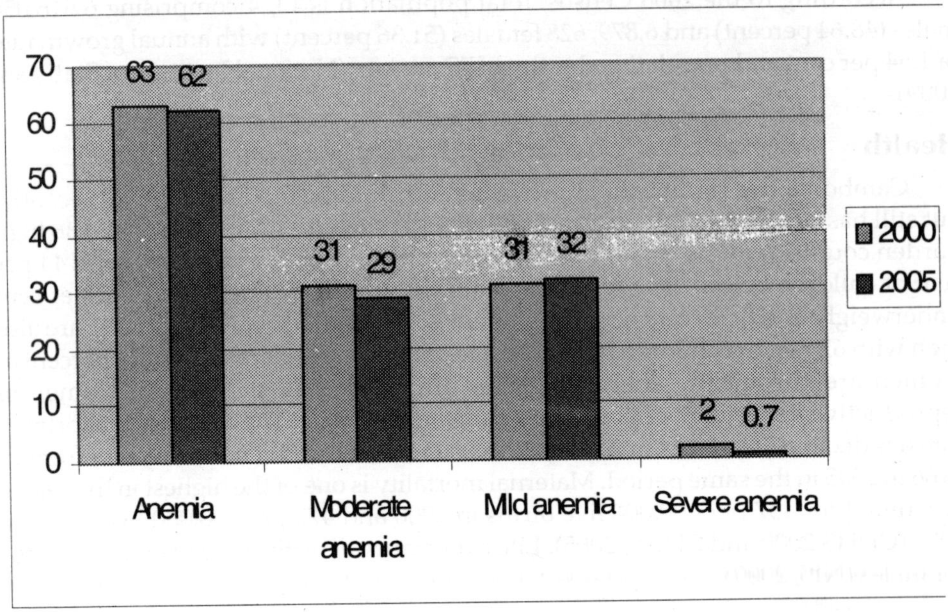

Figure 1.1: Prevalence of Anemia among Children 6-59 months

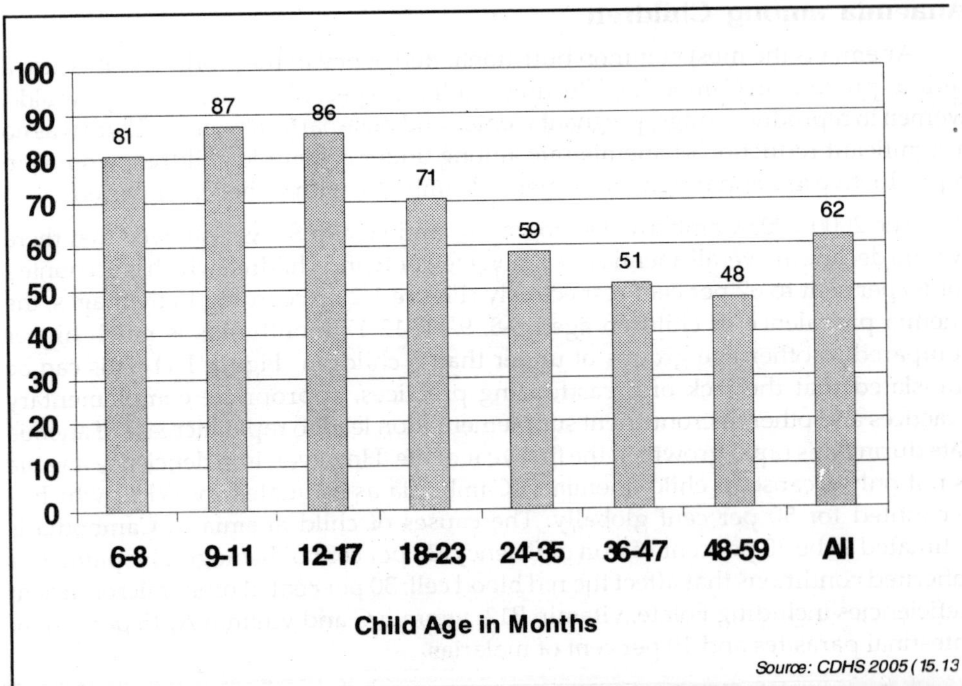

Source: CDHS 2005 (15.13

Figure 1.2: Prevalence of Anaemia in Children Below 5 Years by Age (Hb < 11 g/dl) CDHS 2005

deficiency, affecting all age groups that lead to increased risk of infection, preterm delivery, and prenatal and maternal mortality and the reduction of productivity and economic development. It was seen the small reduction of anemia prevalence among WRA and PW. As seen from Figures 1.3 and 1.4, prevalence of anemia among WRA was slightly declined from 57.8 per cent to 46.6 per cent and the prevalence of anemia among pregnant women was slightly declined from 66.4 to 57.1 in 5 year periods (CDHS 2000-2005).

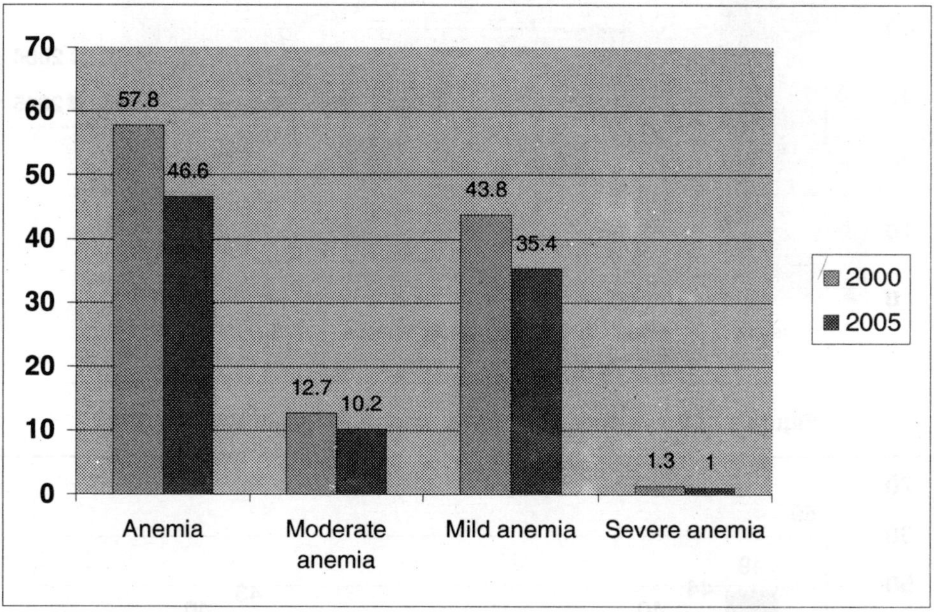

Figure 1.3: Prevalence of Anemia among Women in Reproductive Age (WRA)

It is likely to be seen that, iron deficiency anemia is the main cause of anemia in Cambodia. This is due to the lack of iron-rich food intake, iron absorption, iron Folate tablets, especially during delivery and post partum period. This is the urgent need for the iron supplementation for WRA, PW and Post partum women (PPW) for Cambodia.

Child Malnutrition

Child malnutrition remains a serious problem in Cambodia, effecting especially children below the age of 5 years. Child malnutrition resulted in the reduction of cognitive development that leads to the less productivity in adulthood, high morbidity and mortality. Although, there has been reduced in the prevalence of malnutrition, this will not be enough to reach the Millennium Development Goal in 2015. This needs to be called for urgent action.

As seen from Figure 1.5, the prevalence of child malnutrition among three main indicators, the rate of chronic malnutrition (stunting) was gradually reduced from 59 per cent to 40 per cent in the period of 12 years; however, it has stagnated and possibly started to reversed in acute malnutrition (wasting) and underweight (WHO Global Database on Child Growth and Malnutrition 2007 and CAS 2008).

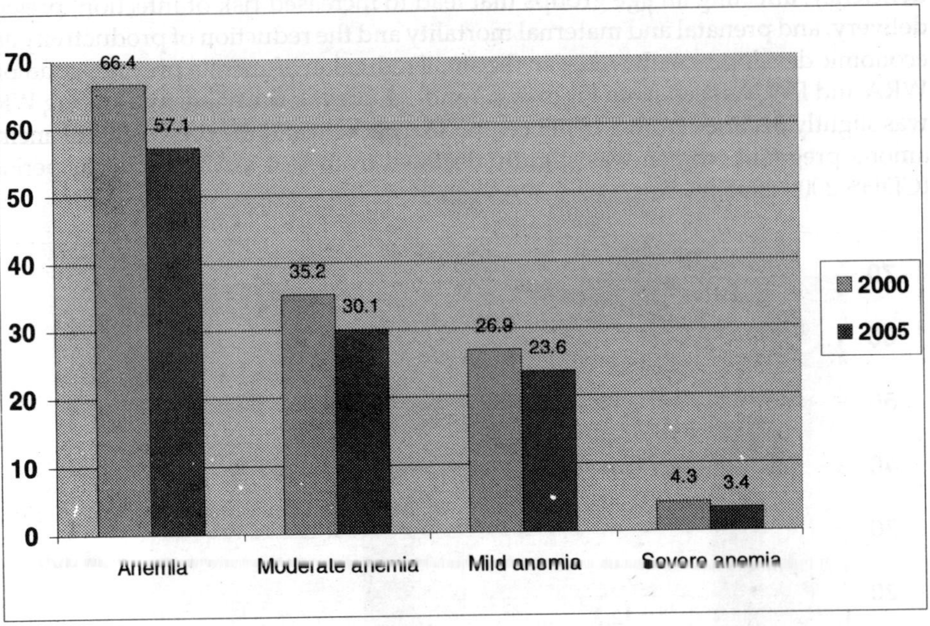

Figure 1.4: Prevalence of Anemia among Pregnant Women (PW)

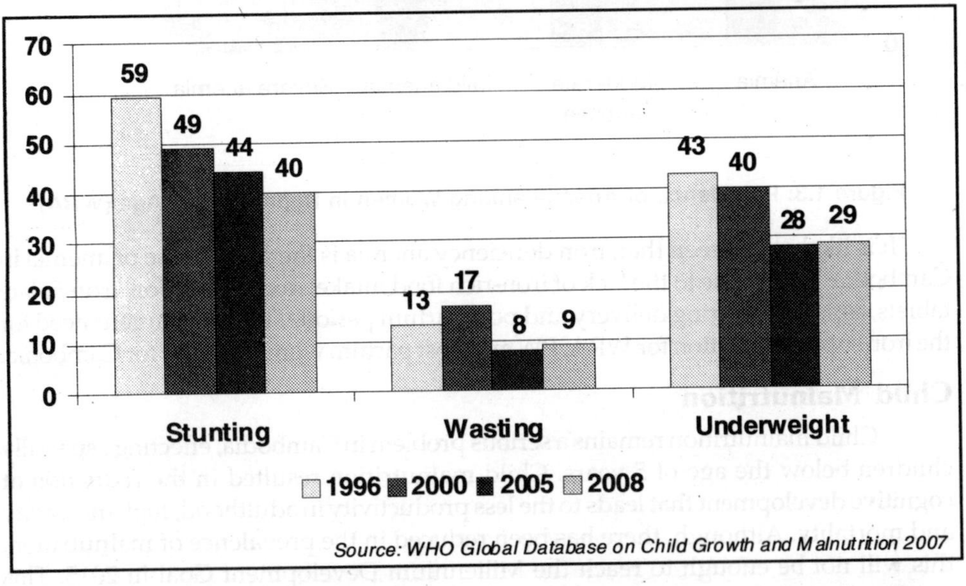

Figure 1.5: Trends in the Prevalence of Child Malnutrition Cambodia 1996-2008

It is obviously seen in Figure 1.6 that urban poor are most vulnerable to the increase in wasted children rate almost double in three-year period from 2005 to 2008 in urban poor which is likely to be related to the increase of food prices (CDHS 2005 and CAS 2008).

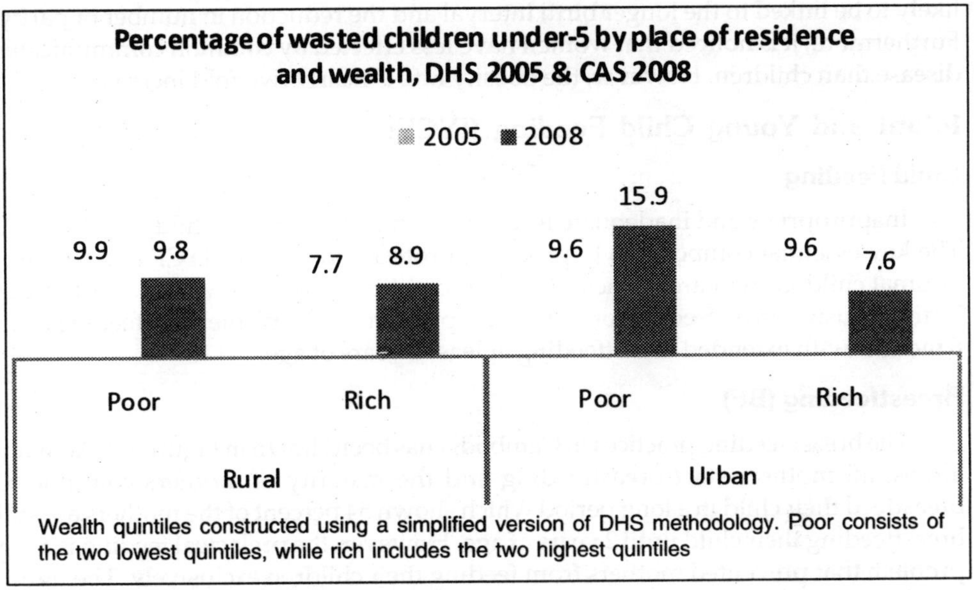

Figure 1.6: Prevalence of Wasted Children Under 5, 2005-2008

Breaking down by provinces, 6 provinces have wasting rate > 10 per cent and 9 provinces have wasting rate from 10 per cent and more.

Women Malnutrition

It is seen that the both chronic and acute malnutrition has significant improvement in three- year period. The improvement in women nutrition status is

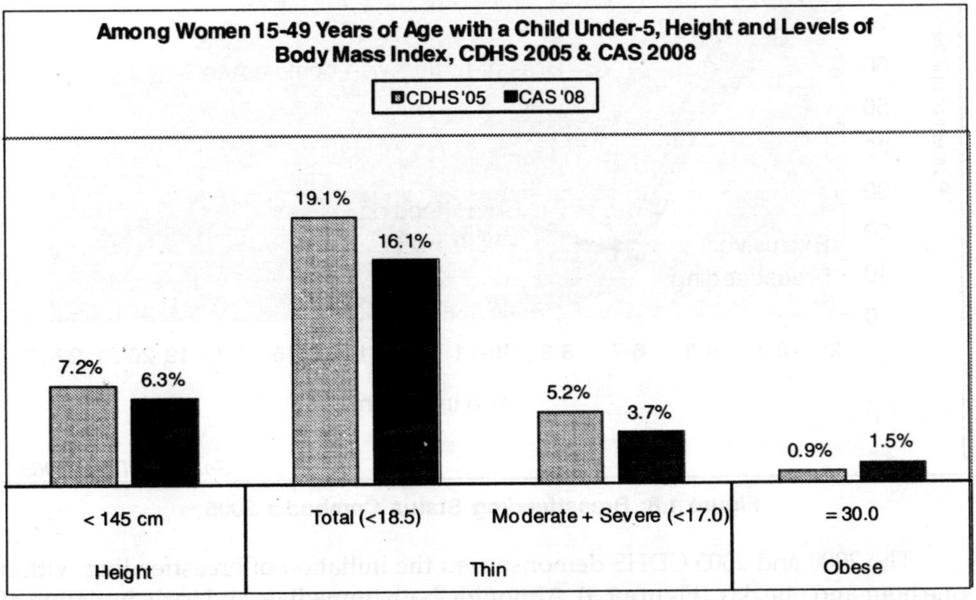

Figure 1.7: Women Malnutrition

likely to be linked to the longer birth interval and the reduction in number of parity. Furthermore, it is noticed that women have less effected by common communicable disease than children. However, the obesity rate is nearly two fold increase.

Infant and Young Child Feeding (IYCF)

Child Feeding

Inappropriate and inadequate feeding practices leads to the child malnutrition. The key essential components to promote, protect and support IYCF and enhance optimal child growth are immediate initiation of breastfeeding within one hour of birth, exclusive breastfeeding for 6 months, appropriate complementary feeding from 6 months with extended breastfeeding at least 2 years of age.

Breastfeeding (BF)

The breast feeding practices in Cambodia has been shown in Figure 1.8. Actually almost all mothers start breastfeeding and the majority of mothers continue to breastfeed their child in a long period which shown 54 percent of the mothers are still breastfeeding their child until 2 years of age. However, the prelacteal feeding is a big problem that prevented mothers from feeding their children exclusively. The figure illustrated that mothers still introduced water in a very early age group. This initiation of water and other food beside breast milk is not only preventing child from getting colostrums, but also put children at risk of infection which contributed to malnutrition.

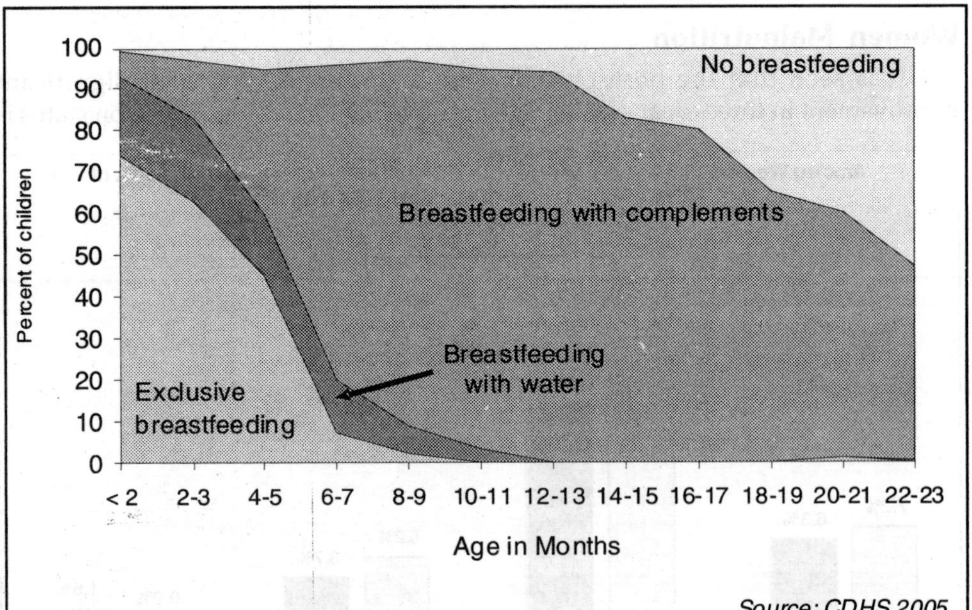

Figure 1.8: Breastfeeding Status Cambodia 2005

The 2000 and 2005 CDHS demonstrated the initiation of breastfeeding within one hour and one day (Figure 1.9). Although, both immediate and early initiation of

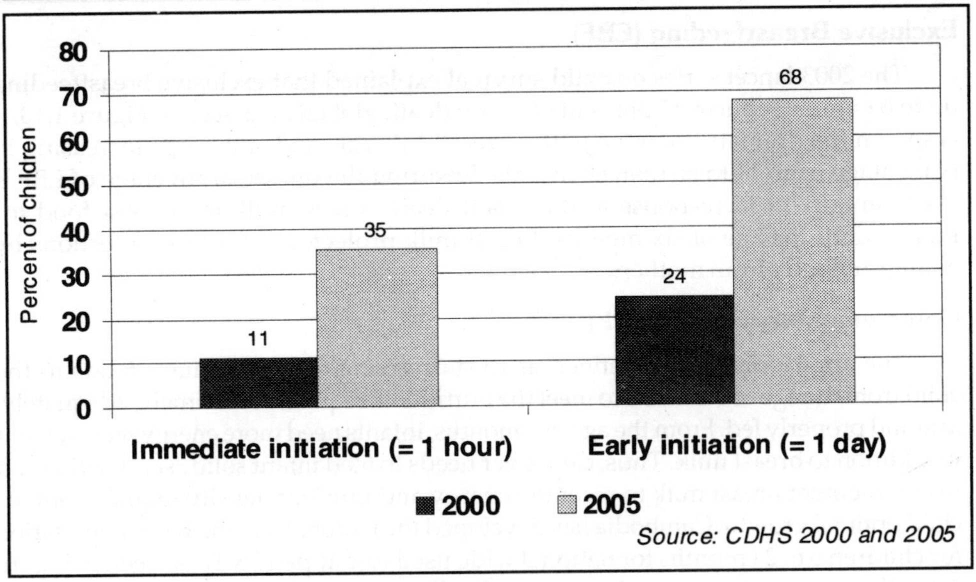

Figure 1.9: Early Breastfeeding Rates Cambodia 2000 and 2005

breastfeeding were significant increase about two fold increase, the rate is still low which is 35 per cent and 68 per cent respectively. The consequences of late initiation do harm children that lead to the child malnutrition, morbidity and mortality.

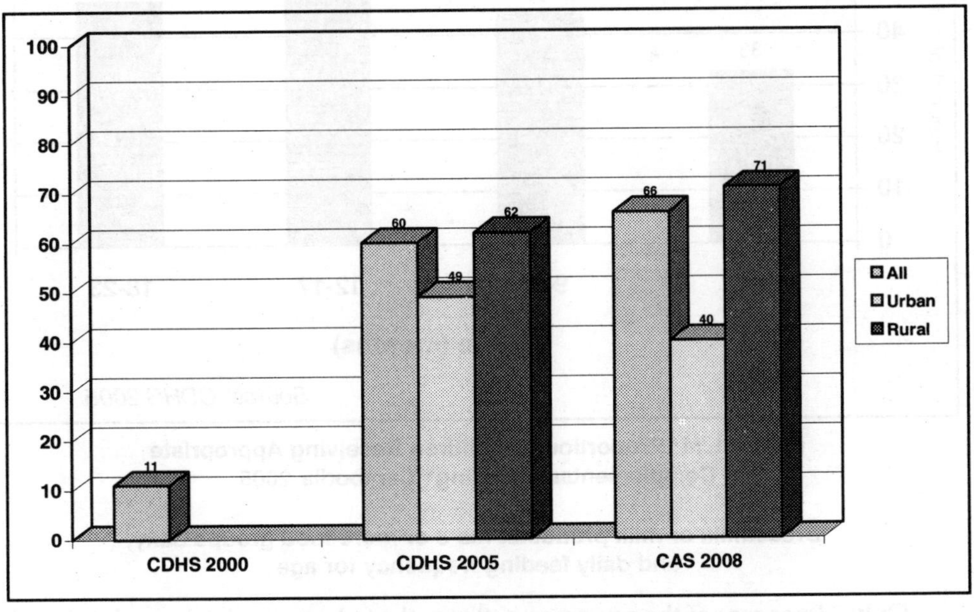

Figure 1.10: Trend of Exclusive Breastfeeding

Exclusive Breastfeeding (EBF)

The 2003 lancet series on child survival explained that exclusive breastfeeding up to 6 months reduces 13 per cent of infant death globally. As seen in Figure 1.10, it is shown the dramatic increase in the overall EBF rate and still keeps increasing in percentage from 11 to 60 than 66 in 2008. Ensuring the universal coverage of EBF is really important in response to the infant death. Breast milk is the best food for infants until the age of six months. Breast milk protected child from infections by getting antibody from mothers.

Complementary Feeding (CF)

The appropriate CF is defined as to start giving complementary foods to the child from the age of 6 months to meet the nutritional requirements timely, adequately, safe and properly fed. From the age of 6 months, infants need more energy requirement in addition to breast milk. Thus, care giver needs to feed infant solid/semi-solid food to complement breast milk to meet the energy and nutrient density requirement for child optimal growth. Cambodia has developed the national feeding recommendation for children 6 to 24 months for national wide used (see appendix 1). As seen in Figure 1.11, the appropriate complementary feeding in Cambodia was not adequate according to the above definition.

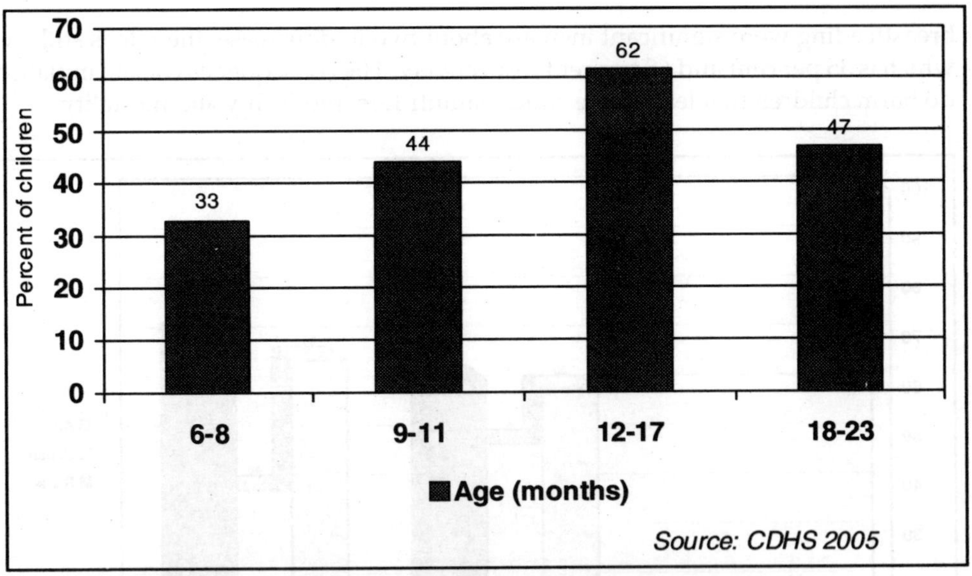

Figure 1.11: Proportion of Children Receiving Appropriate Complementary Feeding* Cambodia 2005

***Breastmilk or milk products, fed 3 or more food groups daily, and daily feeding frequency for age**

Only 33 per cent of the age group 6-8 months fed appropriately, and it slightly increased up to 62 per cent among the age group 12-17 months. Then it declined to 47 per cent among the age group 18-23 months. The 2005 Cambodia Demographic and

Health Survey clearly stated that the complementary feeding practices may get worse than the above mentioned as seen that there was lack of quantity of each meals, energy and nutrient-density of the meals being fed.

Trends in Postpartum Vitamin A Supplementation

The revised 2007 National Vitamin A Policy Guidelines stated that high dose of Vitamin a (200,000 IU) should be provided to all postpartum women within 6 weeks after delivery. The delivery system mostly through monthly out reaches activities rather than institutional deliveries.

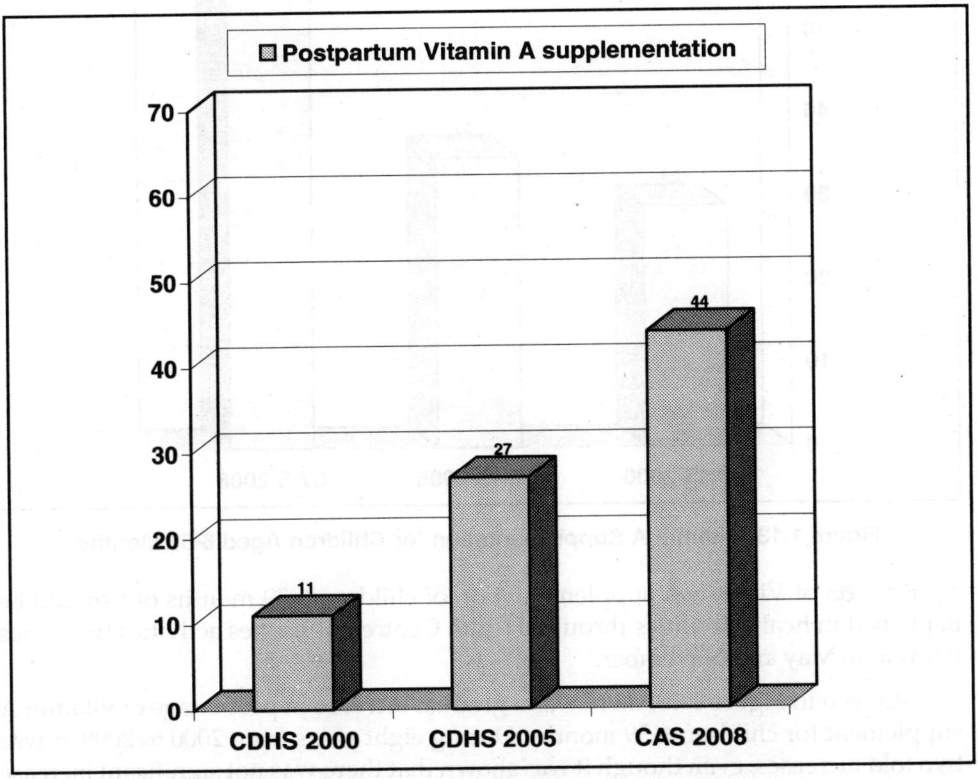

Figure 1.12: Postpartum Vitamin A Supplementation

As seen in Figure 1.12, the trends of Vitamin A supplementation among post partum women has four folds increase in percentage from 11 per cent to 44 per cent in 8 years (CDHA 2000 and CAS 2008). However, most mothers was not benefit from that as the higher coverage seen in rural than in urban areas.

Trends in Vitamin A Supplementation

In Cambodia, the initiation of Vitamin A supplementation was started in 1994 when it was integrated into the immunization programme by Ministry of Health. Then in 1996, the supplementation was fully included into the National Immunization Days. The 2007 National Vitamin A Policy Guidelines clearly stated that the

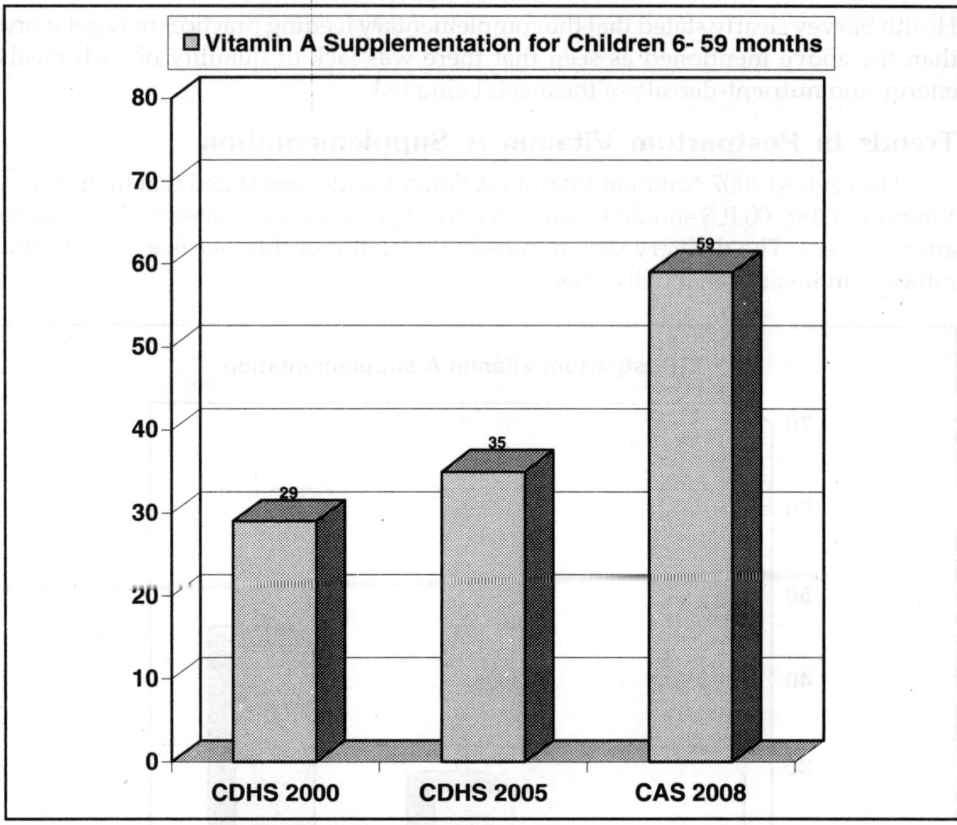

Figure 1.13: Vitamin A Supplementation for Children Aged 6-59 Months

distribution of Vitamin A supplementation of children 6-59 months old should be happened in health facilities through Health Centre outreaches activities two times per year in May and November.

As seen in Figure 1.13, there was a gradual increase in percentage of vitamin A supplement for children 6-59 months. During eight years from 2000 to 2008, it was two fold increases, even though it was shown that there was not significant increase in 5 years according to 2000 and 2005 Cambodia Demographic and Health Survey.

Trends in Iron Supplementation

Cambodia has established the system for supplementation of iron to pregnant and post partum women. The National Guidelines for the use of Iron Folate Supplementation to pregnant and post partum women recommend that women should take at least 90 tablets of iron/folic acid (60 mg of iron and 400 µg folic acid) and 42 tablets during post partum period at first post partum contact. The tablets will be available from hospitals, health centres, or outreach activities.

Figure 1.14 showed the percentage of women receiving iron/Folate supplementation 90, 60-89 and <60 tablets during pregnancy by duration period.

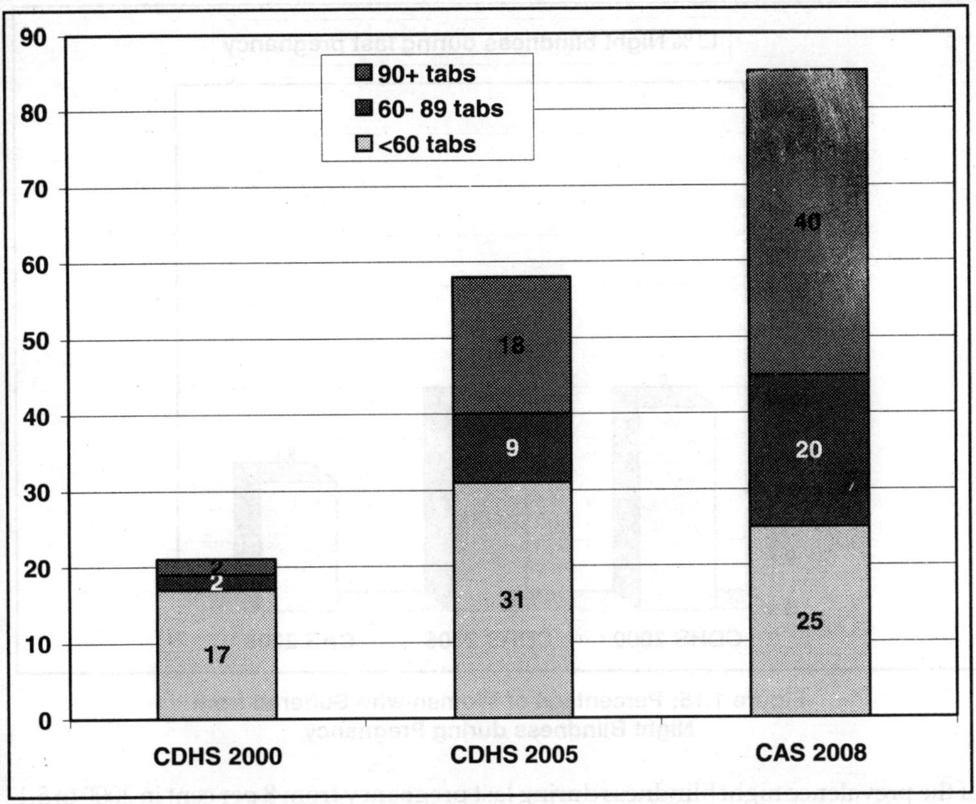

Figure 1.14: Iron/Folate Supplementation during Pregnancy by Duration Period

Only 2 per cent of pregnant women received 90 tablets and 17 per cent of them received <60 tablets in 2000. The trend is much better as seen in the figures from 2005 to 2008. There was nearly double increase in percentage of women received 90 tablets of more during pregnancy in three years period. Also, the percentage of pregnant women received <60 tablets was reduced from 31 per cent to 26 per cent (CHDS 2000, CAS 2008).Even the consumption of iron/Folate tablets will not be entirely treated anaemia, it will prevent from getting worse. Other causes of anaemia among pregnant should be identified to fully solved the problem.

Maternal Vitamin A Deficiency

Vitamin A deficiency has an adverse effect on both women and children in Cambodia. The deficiency of vitamin A damages immune system leading to the increase of infection. In addition, the vitamin A deficiency also cause and effect of iron metabolism and hemoglobin production. For pregnant women, night blindness that is the clinical manifestation of vitamin. A deficiency made pregnant women suffers from pregnancy related complications such as nausea and can become preeclampsia (CDHS 2000, 2005). According to cut off recommended by WHO to determine vitamin A deficiency as public health problem is night blindness rate > 5 per cent in last pregnancy. As seen in the Figure 1.15, there has been a slight reduction

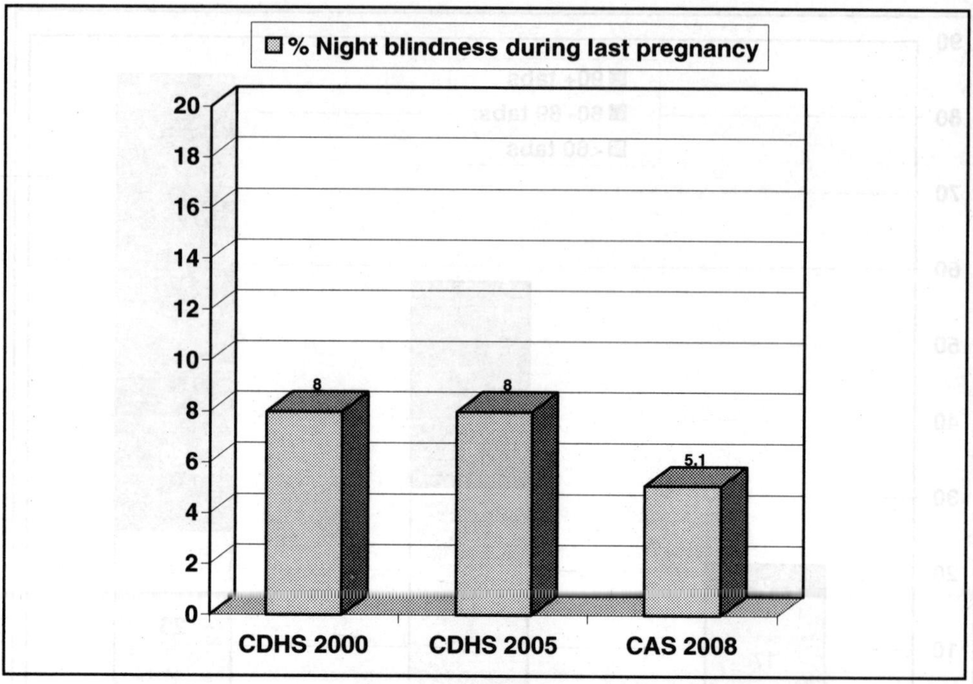

Figure 1.15: Percentage of Women who Suffered from Night Blindness during Pregnancy

of the prevalence night blindness during last pregnancy from 8 per cent in 2000 to 5.1 per cent in 2008, but this still a public health problem.

To improve the health and nutrition status of Cambodian women and children, the National Nutrition Programme, Ministry of Health developed the first National Nutrition Strategy aimed to provide a clear focus and long term direction for addressing maternal and child under nutrition Cambodia. The overall goal of the National Nutrition Strategy is to contribute to reduce maternal and child morbidity and mortality by improving the nutritional status of women and children in Cambodia. Thus, the strategy will contribute to the achievement of the national strategic development goals as articulated in various national strategic frameworks, including the Cambodia Millennium Goals, the Health Strategic Plan for 2008-2015, the Rectangular Strategy, the National Strategic Development Plan 2006-2010, the Strategic Framework for Food Security and Nutrition in Cambodia 2008-2012, the Cambodia Nutrition Investment Plan 2008-2015, and the Food Security and Support Program.

The strategy focuses specifically on what the Ministry of Health can do to address maternal and young child under nutrition. It is therefore limited in scope to address the full spectrum of causes of under nutrition, which requires a broad coalition of multi-sect oral interventions. Every effort has been made to link the strategy to other policy and strategic frameworks in the area of nutrition, which are currently under development such as: the Strategic Framework for Food Security and Nutrition in

Cambodia 2008-2010, the Cambodia Nutrition Investment Plan 2008-2012, and the Food Security Support Program. In addition, the strategy outlines the importance of reaching-out to other sectors beyond health via advocacy and development partnerships in areas relevant to nutrition. A National Nutrition Strategy costing exercise will need to be conducted, and adequate funds need to be allocated for the strategy's implementation.

The three key results to be achieved are:

- ✰ **Key result 1:** Reduction in protein-energy malnutrition and micronutrient deficiencies in young children
- ✰ **Key result 2:** Reduction in protein-energy malnutrition and micronutrient deficiencies in women
- ✰ **Key result 3:** Strengthened national leadership, cross-sectoral collaboration and increased allocation of resources in the area of food security and nutrition.

In line with the key results, objectives and specific targets have been developed.

Five strategic approaches have been developed to reach the key results and objectives:

1. Increase the coverage of proven and cost effective maternal and young child nutrition interventions through health system strengthening, advancing progress in decentralization of health service delivery and mainstreaming of nutrition into all health programs.
2. Increase the coverage of proven and cost effective maternal and young child nutrition interventions through strengthening community involvement in nutrition activities and improving individual and family practices on maternal, infant and young child feeding and general nutrition.
3. Strengthen multi-sector linkages, improve the collaboration with concerned government structures/civil society and enhance the consideration of nutrition in overall national strategies and sector plans and programs.
4. Develop effective leadership and technical nutrition capacity of government and non government development partners for the implementation of the National Nutrition Strategy
5. Increase availability of information for policy makers and program planners through improved monitoring, evaluation and research

Current Policies, Strategies, and Interventions Addressing Nutrition

Goal of National Nutrition Programme (NNP)

The goal of NNP is to reduce maternal and child morbidity and mortality by improving the nutritional status of women and children in Cambodia.

Nutrition Areas of Focus of the NNP

NNP focuses on three main areas includes protecting, promoting and supporting infant and young child feeding practices (breastfeeding and complementary feeding), preventing and controlling malnutrition and micronutrient deficiencies; Vitamin A, Iron, Zinc and Iodine, and policy and strategic development and planning, implementation, monitoring and evaluation.

Current Policies, Strategies, and Interventions Addressing Nutrition

- ☆ Cambodia Millennium Development Goals 1, 4, and 5
- ☆ National Strategic Development Plan 2006-2010
- ☆ National Strategy for Poverty Reduction 2003-2007
- ☆ Health Strategic Plan (HSP) 2003 -2007 and HSP2 2008-2015
- ☆ Cambodia Nutrition Investment Plan (CNIP) 2003-2007, 2nd plan (2009-2015) to be developed in 2009
- ☆ Strategic Frame Work for Food Security and Nutrition in Cambodia 2008-2012
- ☆ Child Survival Strategy (CSS), 2006
- ☆ National Strategy for Reproductive and Sexual Health in Cambodia 2006-2010
- ☆ National Nutrition Strategy 2009-2015

Implementation of Infant and Young Child Feeding (IYCF)

Goal of Infant and Young Child Feeding Program is to improve the survival and well being of infants and young children by improving their nutritional status, growth, and development through optimal feeding. There are four main objectives of the programme.

1. To increase early initiation of breastfeeding within 1 hour of delivery
2. To increase exclusive breastfeeding of infants < 6 months old
3. To Improve appropriate complementary feeding starting at 6 months of age with continued breastfeeding for at least two years or beyond
4. To support the provision of appropriate care for sick and malnourished children

Four main strategies to improve IYCF practices include Policy / legal environment, Facility-based provision of quality IYCF services, Community-based activities and Advocacy / communication strategy.

Policy/Legal Environment

To protect promote and support optimal infant and young child feeding, Cambodia has developed materials and system putting in place for the successful implementation includes Sub-decree on Marketing of Products for IYCF adopted in 2005 and the revised National Policy on IYCF 2008.

Facility-Based Provision of Quality IYCF Services

Cambodia has changed in hospital policies/actions through the establishment of Baby Friendly Hospital Initiative (BFHI), management of severe malnutrition and IYCF counseling at health facilities through in-service and pre-service training. The implement of BFHI has stared since 2004 and 16 hospitals has accredited as BFHI in 5 years (2004-2009). To response to the problems severely acute malnutrition, 20 hospitals has provided the services of management of severe malnutrition from 2003-2009. IYCF counseling Course has been introduced through in-service training since 2004 national wide.

Community-Based Activities

Baby friendly Community Initiative has established since 2004 under the main technical and financial supported from WHO and UNICEF. The total 3.547 villages are declared as BFCI villages which is about 25 per cent of the total village in Cambodia (2004-2009). Nutrition Education and Food Demonstration are main strategies to improve IYCF practices at the community.

Advocacy/Communication Strategy

The use of communication strategy through mass media campaign and behavior change communications has been carried out since 2005. World Breastfeeding Week celebration, in particular, has set up since 2001. Currently, National Nutrition Programme (NNP) is cooperating with National Center for Health Promotion to develop Communication strategy for Complementary Feeding that will be launched in 2010 in some selected provinces.

Micronutrient Intervention

Micronutrient Supplementation

Vitamin A Supplementation to Children 6-59 Months and Post Partum Women

The universal Vitamin A Supplementation Strategy for Children usually is distributed two times a year in May and November for children 6-59 months in the recommended doses (MoH 2007a).

Children 6–11 months are given a capsule of 100,000 IU (blue capsule) and children 12 - 59 months are given 200,000 IU (red capsule). All post partum women are given a capsule of 200,000 IU within 6 weeks after delivery at the health centres, referral hospitals or during monthly outreach services (See Appendix 2).

Iron/Folate Supplementation to Pregnant and Post Partum Women

In Cambodia, the universal supplementation of Iron/Folate stated that women should take at least 90 tablets during pregnancy and 42 tablets during post partum period.

A Study on Multi-Micronutrient Supplementation (GFC)

A three year study on Good Food for Children (Combating anemia and micronutrient deficiencies among young children in rural Cambodia through in-home fortification and nutrition education) has been started since 2007 in Svay Rieng OD with support from the A2Z Micronutrient Project, Helen Keller International, Health Sector Support Project (HSSP), WHO and UNICEF. The study completed in February 2010 and will disseminate the result by June 2010. Plan for scaling up micronutrients supplementation (Sprinkles) is developed and is being implemented in some selected provinces in Cambodia.

Weekly Iron/Folate Supplementation

Weekly Iron/Folate Supplementation Program for Women of Reproductive Age in Secondary Schools in 5 provinces (Kampot, Kep, Kampong Speu, Pursat, and Kompong Thom) and in communities in one OD in Kampong Thom (Baray Santouk OD) stared started in December 2008 and finished in December 2009. Guideline for the supplementation will be developed for the distribution in school ad in the community.

Fortification

Food fortification in Cambodia is a very early stage of development. The vitamin A fortified of Wheat flour and noodles fortified with vitamin A have been done and consumed in small population. Presently, some small enterprises have stopped duc to the limited or stop-go funding. However, being recognized that this is the most important way to introduce the fortification that should be reached to the vulnerable groups such as pregnant women, post-partum women and children 6-59months. A public private partnership is one possible way to make the fortification work. Learning from the experiences from Africa, Latin America, the Middle East and other part of Asia, SAFO aims to "upgrade the availability of Vitamin A fortified staple foods (like palm oil, sugar, fish sauce, wheat flour, instant noodles) at an affordable price for poor people (especially women and children) in Cambodia".

Iodized salt is universal use in Cambodia. The 2005 Cambodia Demographic and Health Survey reported that 73 per cent of all Cambodian household use iodized salt. It has been that fish sauce and soy sauce fortification with iron and noodle and wheat flour fortified with multi-micronutrients have been implemented in small-scale only by some local NGOs and small enterprises. The currently, the Sub-national Committee on Food Fortification under the Ministry of Planning is looking at the possibilities for food fortification.

Food-based Implementation

Homestead Food Production

Homestead food production which consisted of home gardening (vegetables and fruits) and animal husbandry combined with targeted nutrition education is a strategy aims to improve the intake of micronutrient reach food among women and young children (Nancy Haselow and Akoto Osei, 2010). In Cambodia, HKI is the main body who is implementing the activities which really help to improve nutritional status of mother and child.

Food Security and Nutrition

Food security and nutrition is under the leadership of Council for Agricultural and Rural Development (CARD). Food security and nutrition is recognised as the priority intervention for Cambodian Government in response to the Cambodian Millennium Development Goal. To achieve the goal, CARD in collaboration with Technical working group on Food security and nutrition (TWG-FSN) developed the strategic Framework for Food Security and Nutrition in Cambodia 2008-2012 (SFFSN). The goal of SFFSN is to "focus on the achievement of substantial progress towards improved FSN in Cambodia." (CARD, 2008).

De-worming

Interventions aimed at reducing parasitic infections, are also likely to reduce anemia. The World Health Organization recommends regular deforming of children in countries with high prevalence of intestinal worms. In Cambodia, deforming of children 1-5 years has been integrated with biannual vitamin A in desupplementation.

In early 2000 more than 70 per cent of Cambodian children were infected with intestinal worms. In July 2004 Cambodia became the first country to protect three out of four school-age children (nearly three million) with regular anthelminthic treatment against intestinal worms and reach WHO's 2010 target six years ahead of schedule. Cambodia has made it happen. Drugs are distributed across 24 Provinces by thousands of teachers. The campaigns were conducted by the Cambodian Ministry of Health, Education and Sport, with the support of WHO (World Health Organization), together with UNICEF, the Japanese Government and the Sasakawa Memorial Health Foundation. The success demonstrates what can be achieved when the political will is there together with financial support from donors and partners.

Deworming in Cambodian schools is promoted by the production and distribution of a school kit, a package that includes deforming pills, health education posters and pamphlets for teachers, games and attractive pictures for children giving simple messages on how to prevent infection.

Proposed Response

Key Principles of Response

The overall response to the current situation should be nationwide and a comprehensive and intersect oral approach. Most urgent in need are the urban poor and provinces with high levels of acute malnutrition (6 provinces: Bantey Meanchey, .andal, Pursat, Kg. Speu, Kg. Chhnang, and Svay Rieng). A combination of *short-*, *nedium-* and *long-term* actions should be promoted for achieving sustainable impact. Continuous monitoring of Nutrition and Food Security Monitoring data is required in order to assess potential impact of economic crisis and high food prices and the effectiveness of nutrition (and food security) interventions.

Health Sector

Immediate/Short-Term

In-short term solution, acute malnutrition for children under 5 years of age should be identified and managed as the following:

- ✩ Establishing a simple system for screening (using MUAC – Mid-upper Arm Circumference) and referral for malnutrition starting with the most affected areas
- ✩ Strengthening current hospital-based management of severe malnutrition
- ✩ Developing community based models of management of children with acute malnutrition, including food supplementation

In addition to this, it should be scaled up the high-impact interventions include Vitamin A, deforming, diarrhoea treatment with ORS/zinc and in-home fortification using multi-micronutrient powders (Sprinkles).

Medium/Long-Term

To achieve medium and long term goal, improving Infant and Young Child Feeding (IYCF) practices and maternal nutrition should be mainly focussed on.

IYCF practices should be carried out as the following:

- ✩ Rolling-out of IYCF interventions at health facility and community
- ✩ Behaviour Change Communication for IYCF (breastfeeding and complementary feeding)
- ✩ Enforcement of the Sub-decree on Marketing of Products for IYCF

Improving maternal nutrition need to be carried out by providing antenatal/ postnatal care services, giving Iron/Folate supplementation and deforming. Main strategies to improve women's health is setting up a programme of Weekly iron/ Folate supplementation for women of reproductive age both in school and in the community and strengthening current family planning programme.

Other Sectors

Other strategies set up by other sectors beside actually health help to improve women and child nutritional status. These include targeted food-related interventions: food aid, food for work, subsidized food (short-term to mitigate the impact of the current situation). Addressing low purchasing power of poor families to ensure food security through:

- ✩ Social protection and safety nets; expansion of Health Equity Funds, exploring the introduction of cash transfers, and etc.
- ✩ Homestead production (home gardening and animal husbandry) intervention on increasing availability, accessibility of quality food and combined with Nutrition Intervention

Improving hygiene and access to improved water and sanitation and fortification of staple foods with multiple micronutrients are two main activities that carried out outside health sector to promote health and nutrition of women and children in Cambodia.

Future Considerations

There is not yet evidence that food prices are going to drop to pre-crisis levels. If prices stay high, the nutrition situation will likely worsen. The global recession is likely to make it more difficult for many families in Cambodia. As the recession deepens the impact on nutrition will be felt more and more, especially in combination with high food prices.

Conclusions

Improvements in maternal nutrition are giving kids a better start, but this improvement is not carrying on through the first 5 years. The malnutrition-infection cycle for children under 5 is worsening and this is likely to have been caused by the increases in food prices. Infection has increased in both urban and rural areas, but levels are much higher in rural areas. Consumption of quality food is decreasing in both urban and rural areas, but the decrease is larger in urban areas. Poor urban areas have been affected the most by increased food prices and it can be considered an emergency situation in those areas. Many rural areas and entire provinces are facing crisis levels of acute malnutrition.

List of Acronyms and Abbreviations

BFCI: Baby Friendly Community Initiative
BFHI: Baby Friendly Hospital Initiative
CAS: Cambodia Anthropometric Survey
CDHS: Cambodia Demographic and Health Survey
CMDG: Cambodia Millennium Development Goals
CNIP: Cambodia Nutrition Investment Plan
CSS: Child Survival Strategy
GPSC 08: General Population Census of Cambodia 2008
HC: Health Center
HSP: Health Strategic Plan
HSSP: Health Sector Support Project
IMCI: Integrated Management of Childhood Illness
IYCF: Infant and Young Child Feeding
MUAC: Mid-upper Arm Circumference
NMCHC: National Maternal and Child Health Center
NIS: National Institute of Statistics
NNP: National Nutrition Programme
NNS: National Nutrition Strategy

OD: Operational District
PHD: Provincial Health Department
PW: Pregnant Women
WBW: World Breastfeeding Week
WRA: Women in Reproductive Age

References

1. CAS 2008 (Cambodia Anthropometric Survey 2008), National Institute of Statistics, Ministry of Planning, Cambodia
2. CARD, 2008. Strategic Framework for Food Security and Nutrition in Cambodia 2008-2012 (SFFSN), Kingdom of Cambodia
3. CDHS, 2000 (National Institute of Public Health and National Institute of Statistics, Phnom Penh, ORC Macro, 2006). Cambodia Demographic and Health Survey 2000, Phnom Penh, Cambodia and Calverton, Maryland, USA: National Institute of Public Health, National Institute of Statistics and ORC Macro.
4. CDHS, 2005 (National Institute of Public Health and National Institute of Statistics, Phnom Penh, ORC Macro, 2006). Cambodia Demographic and Health Survey 2005, Phnom Penh, Cambodia and Calverton, Maryland, USA: National Institute of Public Health, National Institute of Statistics and ORC Macro.
5. General Population Census 2008, National Institute of Statistics, Ministry of Planning
6. Lancet series 2003
7. MoH, 2008. National Policy on Infant and Young Child Feeding revised 2008, National Nutrition Programme, National Maternal and Child Health Center, Phnom Penh, Cambodia
8. MoH, 2007a. National Vitamin A Policy Guidelines revised 2007, National Nutrition Programme, National Maternal and Child Health Center, Phnom Penh, Cambodia
9. MoH, 2007b. National Guidelines for the Use of Iron Folate Supplementation to Prevent and treat Anemia in Pregnant and Post partum Women 2007, National Nutrition Programme, National Maternal and Child Health Center, Phnom Penh, Cambodia
10. MoH, 2008. Nutrition in Cambodia 2008, An Analysis of Nutritional Status, Trends and Responses, National Nutrition Programme, Phnom Penh, Cambodia
11. Nancy Haselow and Akoto Osei, Paper presentation on Homestead Food Production Program an integrated (agriculture and nutrition) model for addressing under nutrition during the Asia-Pacific.
12. Regional Workshop : reduction of stunting through Improving of Complementary Feeding and Maternal Nutrition, Bangkok, Thailand 25-27 March 2010.

13. Strategic framework for Food Security and Nutrition in Cambodia 2008-2012, Council for Agricultural and Rural Development in consultation with the Technical Working Group on Food Security and Nutrition, Phnom Penh, 2008
14. WHO Global Database on Child Growth and Malnutrition, 30 November 2007.

Appendix 1
Recommended Complementary Feeding Guidelines for Cambodia

RECOMMENDATIONS ON COMPLEMENTARY FEEDING			
Age	**Texture**	**Frequency**	**Amount at each meal** [a]
6 month	Start with thick enriched Borbor, well mashed foods, e.g. mashed cooked banana, sweet potato, pumpkin, etc.	Start foods 2 times per day plus frequent breastfeeds at least 8 times per day	Start with 2-3 tablespoonfuls per feed
7-8 months	Thick enriched Borbor, well mashed foods,	Increasing to 3 times per day plus frequent breastfeeds at least 8 times per day	Increasing gradually to 1/2 of Chan Chang Koeh at each meal
9-11 months	Thick enriched Borbor, finely chopped or mashed foods, and foods that baby can pick up	3 meals plus 1 snack between meals plus breastfeeds at least 6 times per day	Increasing gradually to 1 Chan Chang Koeh
12-24 months	Family foods, chopped or mashed if necessary, thick enriched Borbor	3 meals plus 2 snacks between meals plus breastfeeds as the child wants, at least 3 times per day	1 Chan Chang Koeh
[a] If baby is not breastfed, give in addition 1-2 extra meals per day.			

Thick enriched Borbor that cannot fall/drip off spoon as base add:

- Fish, egg, blood, chopped meat, tofu, and beans
- *Vegetables: morning glory leaves, amaranth leaves, pumpkin, yellow sweet potato, and other vegetables*
- Cooking oil
- Iodized salt

Snacks: ripe fruits (banana, mango, papaya), fried banana/sweet potato, Angsom, bean/pumpkin sweet soup, etc.

Source: National Policy on Infant and Young Child Feeding, 2008.

Appendix 2
Protocol for Universal Vitamin A Capsule Supplementation

Screen all children and mothers coming for any reason to health centers or referral hospitals.		
Give vitamin A to children (6-59 months) that have not received a dose in the previous four months.	Children 6-11 months Children 12-59 months	100,000 IU 200,000 IU
Give vitamin A capsule once to mothers, irrespective of their mode of infant feeding, within six weeks after delivery - if they did not receive vitamin A at delivery.		200,000 IU
For all children during outreach services around May and November		
Give vitamin A capsule to children (6-59 months) that have not received a dose in the previous four months	Children 6-11 months Children 12-59 months	100,000 IU 200,000 IU
For all post-partum women within 6 weeks after delivery during any outreach services every month throughout the whole year		
Give vitamin A capsule once to mothers, irrespective of their mode of infant feeding, within six weeks after delivery - if they did not receive vitamin A at delivery.		200,000 IU

Source: National Vitamin A Policy Guidelines 2007.

Chapter 2

Impact of Health Education on Mothers and Nurses to Prevent Shaken Baby Syndrome Among High Risk Infants

Nagwa Ahmed Zein El Dein[1] and Aida Abd. El-Razek[2]*

[1]Lecturer of Pediatric Nursing, Faculty of Nursing, Menoufya University
[2]Assistant Professor, Faculty of Nursing Menoufya University, Egypt
**E-mail: nagwa_ahmedzin@ymail.com*

ABSTRACT

Shaken Baby Syndrome (SBS) is a violent act of abused without intention that can causes myriad neurological, cognitive, and other functional deficits which may leads to infant's death. Childcare providers, and parents must be ducted on the risk factors, signs and symptoms, as well as strategies to prevent frustration from infant crying[(16)] *So, the aim of this study is to* (1) Assess risk factors for (SBS) among infants (2) provide effective knowledge, skills and teaching materials as well as preventive strategies for both mothers of high risk infants and nurses about (SBS). Health Beliefs Model and Social Cognitive Theory (SCT) was applied as the theoretical framework for this study.

Setting: The study was conducted at 2 MCH (El- Garbi and Kebly) as well as Teaching Hospital at Shebin El Kom. *Sample*: Nurses working at the previous settings from obstetric, pediatric, premature and pediatric surgical units (35 nurses) at Teaching Hospital and convenient mothers with high risk infants elicited from all infants 2 days/week. Mothers attending the 2 MCH for vaccinating their infants (50) were attending the health education sessions and appointed at the forth vaccination schedule for retention test. *Aquasi experimental study was conducted* which health education session was used as intervention. Pretest-Posttest and retention (follow up test questionnaire) were completed by study participants. Data was collected from the sample and categorized as wrong answer, I don't know, incomplete and complete answer for each test then analyzed with appropriate statistical tests.

Results: revealed that, after attending health education sessions mothers and nurses knowledge related to SBS were improved and they perceived the risk factors attributed to shaken aggravation as well as they develop strategies for preventing frustration from infant crying. Further studies are recommended on large sector of population to include all risk factors and health education for this subject should be a part of health education provided at MCH and hospitals.

Keywords: *Shaken baby syndrome, Inconsolable crying, Risk factors.*

Introduction

Shaken Baby Syndrome is a traumatic brain injury that happens when a baby is violently shaken [10]. A baby has weak neck muscles and a large heavy head. Shaken makes the fragile brain bounce back and forth inside the skull and causes bruising, swelling, and bleeding which can leads to permanent severe brain damage or death. The characteristics injuries of shaken baby syndrome are subdural hemorrhages, retinal hemorrhage, damage to the spinal cord and neck as well as fractures of ribs and bones. These injuries may not be immediately noticeable. Identifying risk factors among infants are an important first step in preventing SBS. A combination of infant, caregiver, social, and environmental risks interact and play a role [7].

It was estimated that 10 per cent to 12 per cent of all infant deaths from child abuse were a result of SBS. There are approximately 50, 000 cases of SBS in the United States yearly, and statistically, 1 of 4 cases results in death as well as approximately, 7 per cent to 30 per cent of shaken infants die, 30 per cent to 50 per cent have significant cognitive or neurological deficits, and up to 30 per cent will experience no long-term effects. A range of injuries may result from SBS such as permanent brain injury, paralysis, blindness, seizures, cerebral palsy, delay normal development, behavioral difficulties, or permanent vegetative state. [8]. Most of parents aren't prepared for the fact that they may have to cope with a crying baby for two or three hours a/day.So, head injuries occur from rapid and repetitive flexion, extension and rotation of the head and neck around a relatively stable torso with or without impact injury[8].

Small infants and children are at high risk for (SBS) due to their small size in comparison to the adult perpetrator. Shaken generally is attributed to perpetrator's level of tension and frustration which is often aggravated by an infant crying or irritability [5] Risk factors leads to (SBS) are numerous which includes parent's age, unstable family environment, low socioeconomic status, premature infant or disability, unrealistic child- rearing expectations, rigid attitude, or impulsive parents which lead to feeling of inadequacy, maternal depression, isolation, child abuse, and/or domestic violence [14]

Clinical presentation of (SBS) includes a wide variety of symptoms ranging from the very mild to the most critical of states. The infant may presented with the history of poor feeding, vomiting, lethargy or irritability, hypothermia or chills, failure to thrive, increase sleeping and failure to smile or be verbal. These symptoms may persist for days or weeks. Physicians may reveals these signs to other illness or viral infection and may resolved with out the route cause being discovered. In more severe cases the infant may exhibit more life threatening signs and symptoms of neurological impairment following violence shaken. The care taker may put the infant to bed anticipating the child will be recover, which may leads to a missed opportunity for early intervention, in these cases the child will be presented with respiratory failure including apnea, decreased level of consciousness, seizures, breadycardia, bulging fontanels, rib fractures, retinal hemorrhage, or produce evidence of cardiac collapse requiring cardiopulmonary resuscitation. This is in addition to lack of external injury which leads to falsely minimized healthcare provider's suspicions of possible maltreatment [10] [12].

Inconsolable crying is the leading reason a baby is shaken, as a results stress and discouragement be obvious among parents. So, parents should be educated about better coping with their infant's crying. There are different types of crying. Child development professionals have determined that babies don't cry the same exact way every time. The clue that determined the causes of crying should be interpreted by parents through the situations surround the cry as hunger, tiredness, discomfort, pain, colic, frustration, loneness, over stimulation, worry / fears, or boredom. So, parents should be able to analyze every type of crying and provide the child's with appropriate strategies to accommodate with the situation without shaken. Those strategies includes, changing diaper, holding infants, providing motions as rocking, swinging, let him suck, turn of some noise, massage the infant, distract infant attention or let other one to care after[1].

Two theories are widely used in providing healthy behavior have served as the theoretical framework of this study. Health Belief Model (HBM)[3] and Social Cognitive Theory (SCT)[2]. The concept of HBM related to providing healthy behavior through participation in health education session which includes: (1) Persons perceived susceptibility of their infants at high risk for (SBS) (2) Perceived severity and consequences of the disease (3) Perceived benefits from a wariness sessions (4) Taking action cues (5) Self efficacy to their abilities to perform preventive strategies in which the person learn new behavior. The Social Cognitive Theory define human behavior as a dynamic and reciprocal interaction of personal factors, actions and environment [2] people are more likely to engage in a certain behavior when they believe that they are capable of executing the behavior successfully and this is know as self efficacy. Therefore, healthcare providers involved in the care of infants are in an ideal position to identify and educate families, public and other healthcare professional about the risk factors, dangers and consequences of infant shaken. *So, the aim* of this study is to assess risk factors among infants and provide mothers of high risk infants and nurses with health education about (SBS) as well as appropriate preventive strategies to avoid frustrations from infant crying.

Subject and Methods

Setting

The study was conducted at 2 MCH (El- Garbi and Kebly) as well as Teaching Hospital at Shebin El Kom. (Pediatric Medicine, Pediatric Surgery, Premature, and Obstetric Department)

Sample

Nurses working at Shebin El Kom Educational Hospital from Obstetric, Pediatric, Premature and Pediatric Outpatient Units (25 nurse) as well as (10) nurses from the two maternal MCH were invited to attend the sessions after the pretest was collected from them and mothers of high risk infants recruited from all mothers attending the 2 MCH for vaccinating their infants for one month 2 days/week (50 mothers) were attending the health education sessions and appointed at the forth vaccination schedule for retention test.

Inclusion Criteria: including

1. Mothers eligible for this study with high risk infants for (SBS).
2. A convenient nurses present at the time of the session which they are in an optimal position to address the risk factors and long term consequences from SBS with parents before discharge or when they vaccinate the infants.

Design

A quasi experimental design was use to apply in this study in a form of pretest, posttest and retention test.

Tools

Tool I

Two questioner sheets was developed by the researchers one for mothers and the other for nurses including the following partitions.

Part I

Includes biosocial characteristics for nurses as, age, level of education, years of experience, and their department. Also, biosocial data for mothers and their infants were collected as age, parity, level of education, occupation, as well as presence of an accidental, history of previous trauma due to shaken as well as presence of risk factors among infants as prematurity, low birth weight, colic, and numbers of hrs of crying.

Part II

Includes knowledge about definition of shaken, causes risk factors, signs and symptoms of shaken, and how to prevent it. These questions were asked for mothers and nurses with the edition of pathology and methods of diagnosis for nurses.

Part III

Ask about knowledge related to the types of infant crying and the different methods used to overcome and accommodate with infant frustrations.

Part IV

Assessment part for children to identify risk factors depends on observation, measurement and physical examination for head and neck.

Tool II

Video – Tapes representing and explain Shaken Baby Syndrome prevention from www.Shakenbaby.ca Educational Resources Kit (DVD/CD ROM)[18].

Tool III

Brochures contains the meaning of (SBS) signs and symptoms, causes, types of infant crying and methods used to deal with frustration as well as a pictures of Shaken Baby provided to mothers and nurses at the end of session.

Methods

To provide healthcare providers and mothers with the appropriate knowledge and skills related to prevention of SBS. The researchers require an informed consent from the authorized personnel about the procedures and methods of data collections to provide us with appropriate class for sessions which occupied with data show to present the topic with video-tape from the lab top which representing the Shaken Baby and consequences results from shaken.

Procedure

After eliciting the risk factors among infants through physical examination a pretest questionnaire was collected from both their mothers and nurses through interview before the session for both of them. After that a post test questionnaire was collected immediately.Every session take about 45 minutes including video presentation takes about 15 minutes and the lecture discussion takes about 30 minutes, every session including 5-7 audience (mothers or nurses) 2 days/week after that, mothers at MCH were appointed after 3 months for retention test to be implemented. Data collection was beginning from June 2009 to December 2009.

Data Analysis

The collected data were categorized as I don't know, wrong answer, incomplete answer, and complete answer after that analyzed with appropriate statistical tests.

Results

Table 2.1 showed socio-demographic characteristics of mothers which representing that more than thirty percent (36 per cent) for mothers age were less than 25 years and (30 per cent) were between 25-35 years and the other third (43 per cent) were more than 35 years respectively. As regards to the educational levels (36 per cent) were gain preparatory schools and (20 per cent) of the mothers were had higher education. Majority of mothers were house wives (70 per cent) and have 3 children (28 per cent) or more (36 per cent).

Table 2.2 showed the biosocial characteristics of healthcare providers which represents that (42, 8 per cent) of healthcare provider age were ranged between 25-35 years, about half of them (48,5 per cent) were diploma nurses and (57 per cent) had 5-10 years of experience.

Table 2.3 represented the identified risk factors among the studied sample which constitutes inconsumable crying (56 per cent), depressed fontanels (10 per cent), large ratio of the head (8 per cent), weak neck muscle, lack of head control. Premature infants constitute (6 per cent) while unfused sutures and low birth weight constitutes (4 per cent and 2 per cent) respectively.

Table 2.1: Distribution of Studied Mother's by their Socio-Demographic Characteristics

Socio-Demographic Characteristics	*Participants Mothers*	
	NO = 50	*Per cent*
Age		
> 25	18	36
25-35	15	30
<35	17	34
Educational level		
Read and Write	12	24
Preparatory	18	36
Secondary	10	20
University	10	20
Occupation		
House wife	35	70
Working	15	30
Gravidity		
1	8	16
2	18	36
3 or more	24	48
No. of living children		
1	8	16
2	10	20
3	14	28
4 or more	18	36
Previous of accidental trauma from Shaken		
Yes	0	0
No	50	100

Table 2.4 showed distribution of mothers knowledge about SBS there were a significance difference P< 0.05 in mothers knowledge post test, retention test than in pretest regards to the definition of SBS, causes, risk factor, signs and symptoms, prevention, and strategies used to overcome frustration.

Table 2.5 showed distribution of nurse's knowledge about Shaken Baby Syndrome. There were a significance difference (P<0.05)in nurses knowledge regards to the definition, causes, risk factor, signs and symptoms, pathophysiology, methods of diagnosis, and prevention, as well as strategies used to overcome frustration in posttest, retention test than pretest. While nurses knowledge not different significantly (P>0.05) in relation to the methods of diagnosis.

Table 2.2: Distribution of the Studied Healthcare Providers According to Socio-Demographic Data

Socio-Demographic Characteristics	*Participants Healthcare Providers*	
	NO = 50	*Per cent*
Age		
> 25	7	20
25 -35	15	42,8
< 35	13	37,2
Qualifications		
Professional nurse	12	34,2
Diploma nurse	17	48,5
Midwifes nurse	6	17,2
Experience/years		
>5	8	22,8
10-May	20	57,1
< 10	7	20,1

Table 2.3: Identified Risk Factors among Infants of Studied Sample

Risk Factors	*NO*	*Per cent*
1. Inconsolable crying (Colic)	28	56.0
2. Depressed fontanels	5	10.0
3. Large ratio of the head to body	4	8.0
4. Weak neck muscles	3	6.0
5. Lack of head control	3	6.0
6. Unfused sutures	2	4.0
7. Premature infants	3	6.0
8. Low birth weight	1	2.0

Table 2.6 showed distribution of mother response about the type of infants crying and related strategies to overcome frustrations. There was a significance difference regarding nurse's knowledge in relation to the different types of infant crying as well as different strategies used to overcome frustration in post test, retention test than pretest. In relation to the mothers benefits from different methods of presentation nearly equal percentage of mother's responses (67,3 per cent and62 per cent) (87 per cent -85 per cent) benefits from videos and presentation at post test and retention test. While all of them were benefits from brochure at retention test.

Table 2.4: Distribution of Studied Mother's by their Knowledge About SBS in Pre/Post and Retention Test

Knowledge About SBS	*Pre Test*		*Post Test*		*Retention*		X^2
	N0= 50	*%*	*N0= 49*	*%*	*N0=40*	*%*	*P. Value*
Definition of SBS							X^2
I don't know	18	36	0	0	5	12,5	41.38**
Wrong answer	8	16	0	0	5	12,5	P<0.05
Incomplete answer	13	26	14	28.5	7	17,5	
Complete answer	11	22	35	71,5	23	57.5	
Causes of SBS							X^2
I don't know	22	44	2	4,08	3	7,5	73.28**
Wrong answer	18	36	2	4,08	4	10	P<0.05
Incomplete answer	5	10	6	12,2	12	30	
Complete answer	5	10	39	79.5	21	52.5	
Risk factors of SBS							X^2
I don't know	15	30	1	2.04	5	12,5	35.68**
Wrong answer	13	26	4	8,16	6	15	P<0.05
Incomplete answer	12	24	7	14,2	9	22,5	
Complete answer	10	20	37	75,5	20	50	

Table 2.5: Knowledge of Healthcare Providers about Shaken Baby Syndrome

Knowledge About SBS	*Pre Test*		*Post Test*		*Retention*		X^2
	N0= 50	*%*	*N0= 49*	*%*	*N0=40*	*%*	*P. Value*
Signs & Symptoms of SBS							X^2
I don't know	10	20	3	6,12	5	12,2	44.89**
Wrong answer	13	26	5	10,2	3	7,5	P<0.05
Incomplete	15	30	3	6,12	7	17,5	
Complete	12	24	38	77,55	25	62,5	
Can SBS prevented?							X^2
I don't know	23	46	0	0	2	5	67.16**
Wrong answer	9	18	2	4,08	4	2,5	P<0.05
Incomplete	11	22	2	4,08	5	12,5	
Complete	7	14	45	91,8	29	72,5	
Strategies used to overcome Shaken							X^2
I don't know	25	50	1	2,04	4	10	74.15**
Wrong answer	12	24	1	2,04	3	7,5	P<0.05
Incomplete	4	8	3	6,12	9	22,5	
Complete	9	18	44	89,7	24	60	

Table 2.6: Distribution of Mothers Responses about the Types of Infants Crying and Related Strategies to Overcome Frustrations

Mothers Responses	*Pre Test*		*Post Test*		*Retention*		X^2
	NO= 50	*%*	*NO= 49*	*%*	*NO=40*	*%*	*P. Value*
Type of crying							X^2
I don't know	15	30	1	2.04	6	15	29.07*
Wrong answer	10	20	0	0	4	10	P<0.05
Incomplete answer	11	22	3	6,12	6	15	
Complete answer	14	28	36	73,4	24	60	
Strategies used to overcome frustration							X^2
I don't know	16	32	2	4,8	4	10	46.41**
Wrong answer	18	36	2	4,8	4	10	P<0.05
Incomplete answer	8	16	14	28,5	13	32,5	
Complete answer	8	16	31	62,3	19	47,5	
Benefits from methods of presentation							X^2
Discussion and presentation	0	0	33	67.3	25	62	66.95**
Video	0	0	35	87.5	34	85	P< 0.05
Brochure	0	0	28	57.1	40	100	

Table 2.7 showed distribution of nurses knowledge about types of infant crying and different strategies to overcome frustration.There were a significance difference (P<0.05) regarding nurses distribution at posttest, retention test than pretest for their knowledge about infant crying and their strategies to overcome frustration.

Table 2.7: Distribution of Nurse's Knowledge about Types of Infant Crying and Different Strategies to Overcome Frustration

Knowledge about Type of Infant Crying and its Preventions	*Pre Test*		*Post Test*		*Retention*		X^2
	NO= 35	*%*	*NO= 30*	*%*	*NO=25*	*%*	*P. Value*
Knowledge about type of infant crying							X^2
I don't know	8	22,8	0	0	2	8	24.22*
Wrong answer	2	5,7	1	3,3	1	4	P<0.05
Incomplete answer	10	28,5	4	13,3	3	12	
Complete answer	15	42,8	25	83,3	19	76	
Strategies used to overcome frustrations							X^2
I don't know	10	28,5	1	3,3	4	16	25.53*
Wrong answer	2	5,7	1	3,3	4	16	P<0.05
Incomplete answer	7	20	3	10	7	28	
Complete answer	16	45,7	25	83,3	10	40	

Discussion

Shaken Baby Syndrome usually results from a parent or care givers shake a baby because the baby would not stop crying. Since crying was the primary reason that the infants were shaken, it is important to inform parents how to deal with frustration of crying baby as well as to equip them with sufficient knowledge and skills required to cope with the situation. Also, it is important to encourage this information shared by healthcare providers [13]

Risk factors identified among those infants represented by more than half of the sample (56 per cent) have colicky crying and the infants normally spend approximately 1.5 to 3 hours or more a day crying which places those infants at risk; many studies supported that the incidence of SBS correlates with the incidence of early infant crying. Inconsolable, "colicky," require more attention, to prevent feelings of mother's helplessness and frustration as well as result in decreased confidence in parenting ability. This can lead to further feelings of inadequacy, guilt, anger, withdrawal, and an altered perception of the infant. [8] The study also revealed to many others risk factors as depressed fontanels (10 per cent), large head proportion (8 per cent), weak neck muscles, lack of head control, premature birth (6 per cent), and unfused sutures. Critical risk factors assessment, and physical findings associated with SBS provide strategies for intervention and prevention of SBS, the information provided and skills to cope with both crying and the stress that it provokes, should also reviewed by health professional to help care taker adapt with crying of their infants especially when the parents are unaware of the potentially fatal effects of SBS.

The National Center on Shaken Baby Syndrome [16] estimated that approximately 20 per cent of victim of (SBS) die from their injuries, while one third suffer from severe disabilities. So, it is important to aware mothers and healthcare providers about the danger of (SBS) meanwhile, that the sample emphasizes on care takers 50 mothers and the available healthcare providers (35) nurses. The mother's age ranged between 20 to more than 35 years which is the target group to be concerned with the topic of the research. Also, more than one third of them (36 per cent) passed the preparatory education which means that they can read the brochures instructional strategies and be benefits from it when needed. Also, about half of them (48 per cent) have 4 or more children which burden them with a lot of tension and stressors and make them liable for more frustrations which provoke them with Shaken Baby.

Educational programs have been shown to raise awareness about the danger of Shaken Baby Syndrome to care givers, day care centers, healthcare providers, legal representative as well as provide health strategies to deal with crying infants which can bring about a significant reduction in the number of cases of Shaken Baby Syndrome. [6] In our study nearly half of nurses (48,2 per cent) were diploma nurses which they were the most contacted nurses with mothers and the other half of nurses were professional nurses (34,2 per cent) and midwives nurses constitutes (17,2 per cent). Which mean that they need to understand the effect of Shaken on the infants as well as strategies to cope with it to transfer those knowledge to care givers. The study revealed that healthcare providers had deficiency in their knowledge regarding the term of shaken, causes, risk factors, signs and symptoms, and methods of prevention in pretest interview compared with a posttest which represented a significance increased in their knowledge (P< 0.05) Also, mothers knowledge regarding Shaken Baby Syndrome definition, causes, signs and symptoms, methods of preventions and strategies used to overcome frustrations shown a significance increase in their knowledge posttest compared to pretest and retention test. This result concede with results of [(6)] held from 1998- 2004 and suggested that adults learned best when information helped them to cope with life changing events. Also, they comparing the rate of Shaken Baby Syndrome following the introduction of the program to the rate of Shaken Baby Syndrome in the 6 years period to the program and they found that the rate drop from average of 8,2 cases/year to 3,8 cases/year a 53 per cent reduction in the rate of Shaken Baby Syndrome consequences. This percentage represented a decreased of 22,2 cases per 100,000 live birth a 47 per cent reduction. Also, program held by (Rottmond, 2004)[(13)] at Pennsylvania Baby Shaken Syndrome Prevention and awareness shown a reduction in the incidence of (SBS) by 50 per cent. So that, parents and nurses should be provided with appropriate knowledge and skills frequently to avoid unexpected consequences of Shaken Baby Syndrome.

Although there are a considerable percentage of mothers (28 per cent) have a complete knowledge about the type of infant crying but they have a lack on skills about how to deal with that frustrations provoked from crying in pretest compared to post test (73,4 per cent). So, it is important to acquire care takers about that knowledge to prevent consequences from (SBS). Ronald and their colleagues [(14)] examine the relationship between infant crying and the incidence of Shaken. After 4 years the reported hospital cases showed that the number of (SBS) increased around 2-3 weeks of infant age peak at 12-14 weeks and decreased after which is related to the normal crying curve. So, it is very important for care givers to be aware of this connection between the frustration over early infant crying and Shaken Baby. Moreover, care giver need to understand that the crying is a normal, temporary and infant crying not their fault but the fault is the Shaken.

Nurses also showed increase in their knowledge about types of infant crying and strategies used to overcome frustration in pretest (45,7 per cent) rather than post test (83 per cent) respectively, this results conceded with Barr *et al.* (2008)[(4)] which found a statistically significance increased in the caregiver and parents knowledge about infant crying and understanding the danger and strategies to overcome frustration from Shaken Baby Syndrome.

In this study mothers and nurses asked about how much they benefited from presentation, video- tapes and brochure, the majority of the mothers responses were around video presentation (46,9 per cent) this percentage decreased to 32 per cent at post test may be due to drop in the size of the sample at post test. In contrast to the use of brochures which represents an increase in the percentage from (16,3 per cent to 35 per cent) which means that the brochures still remain with mother and they were read it when needed. In addition the brochure gives parents something they were in immediate need when they have a crying baby which it can give them accurate and supportive advice. So, they can not get so frustrated. On the other hand, more than half of nurses (51 per cent and 54,2 per cent) benefited from Video- Tapes rather than other methods of presentation at posttest and retention test respectively this means that nurses may be willing to administer materials that are positive and education but they are reluctant to listen to presentation or reading a brochure. In contrast Dias study (2005) [(6)] shows only two third of parents viewed the Video- Tapes and subsequently only 23 per cent of them remember viewing it when asked after a 7 months follow up. Overall, all mothers and nurses appreciate the usefulness of the information provided and believed that knowledge and skills were satisfactory and highly relevant to them.

Conclusion

To prevent Shakerism among mothers you should identify risk factors among infants and parents, provide health education to care taker and health professionals and train them about SBS to reduce morbidity and mortality. Also, this information should be a part of health education provided at MCH and hospitals.

References

1. Barr, R.,Sandberg, M., and Coleman, K., Understanding Infant Crying to Prevent Shaken Baby a Prevention Institute (2002), (801) 627- 399
2. Bandura, A. Social Foundation of Thought and Actions, Asocial Cognitive Theory, Englewood Cliffst Prentice Hill (1986)
3. Backer M.H; The Health Belief Model and Personal Health Behavior. Health Education Monography, SOPHE. California. (1974) (2) No 4
4. Barr, R.G., Rivora F.P., Barr, M., Cummings. P., Taylor J., Lengual and Mereadeth E. Effectiveness of Educational Materials Design to Change Knowledge and Behaviors Regarding Crying and Shaken Baby Syndrome in Mothers of Newborn Infant, a Randomized Trial, Medical Association Journal. (2008)
5. Duhaime, A.C., Christian C. W., Rocke L.B.,& Zimmerman, R.N: Non accidental Head Injury in Infants – (SBS) The New England Journal of Medicine.,(1998); 338-(25):1822-1830
6. Dias, M., Preventing Abusive Head Trauma among Infants and Young Children, A hospital Based Parents Education Programs Preventing Shaken Baby Syndrome, Period of Purple crying British, Colombia. (2005): available from USA SBS (dontshake.org) 23/1/2008, 08:16pm
7. Franklin, S); Understanding Shaken Baby Syndrome and Neonatal Care. W.B Sunders Company. (2004) 4(2); 105-116
8. Leslie A. (2008): Shaken Baby Syndrome Journal of Perinatal and Neonatal Nursing January/March (2008) Volume 22 Number 1 Pages 68 - 76
9. Ludwing, S., and Warman, M., Shaken Baby Syndrome: A review of 20 Cases (1984); Annex13:104-107
10. Michl, N: Baby Shaken Syndrome, International Association of Forensic Nurses, (2005); (1)3:111-117
11. National Institute of Health. NINDS Shaken Baby Syndrome Information, What is Shaken Baby Syndrome (SBS) http//:www.ninds.n.h.gov/jobs and training/ index.htm up date.htm (2007); 14

12. University of British Colombia. Parents Helping Infants Study: Educational Intervention to Change the Knowledge, Attitude, and Behavior of New Parents about Early Infant Crying (2008(mailto:cnicole@cw.bc.ca?subject=NCT00175422, B04-0785, Parents Helping Infants Study: Educational Intervention to Change the Knowledge, Attitudes and Behavior of New Parents About Early Infant Crying

13. Rottmond, C. RN. Pennsylvania's Shaken Baby Syndrome Prevention and Awareness Programs, Saving Babies Lives one Family at a Time, Penn State Milton S, Hershey Medical Center (2004) July 24/2008, 01:31am

14. Ronald, G and Colleagues: Infant Crying, How is Crying Link to Shaken Baby Syndrome, Preventing Baby Shaken Syndrome, British, Colombia, (2006) 4480 k120.

15. Thomas, D., Leiche, C., Hughes, C., Madgian, A., and Doweli,K., Emerging Practices to Prevention of Child Abuse and Neglect. Department of Health and Human Services (DHHS): Administration on Children, Youth, and Families (ACF): Washangton, (DC) government Print Office. (2003):

16. The National Center on Shaken Baby Syndrome http://www.don'tshake.org/ (2004).

17. Wyszynski. M.E. Shaken Baby Syndrome: Identification and Intervention, Neonatal Intensive Care Unite, St Elizabeth's Medical Center, Boston, Massachusetts, U.S.A. (1999); Sep, 3(5):262-18.www.babyshaken.ca. A baby Shaken, infant crying and the Alberto Shaken Baby Syndrome Prevention Campaign, What Professionals Needs To Know,SBS press National Prof, A.B Jun (2007) Web _Slid 5/1/007, 6,30 Am.

Chapter 3

Quality of Care Provided to Thalassemic Children at Menoufia University Hospital

*Taghreed Kamal**, *Maha Khalifa and Hanaa Ibrahim*

Pediatric Nursing, Faculty of Nursing,
Menoufia University, Egypt
**E-mail: taghreedson@yahoo.com*

ABSTRACT

Aims of this study were to assess parent's quality of care provided to thalassemic children and to assess nurse's quality of care provided to thalassemic children at specified setting. A convenient sample of 100 children with thalassemia and 26 nurses was selected to carry out this study. Quality of care questionnaire sheet was used to assess parents and nurses knowledge about thalassemia and observational checklist to assess nurses' practices provided to thalassemic children. Nursing practice was assessed by observing the nursing intervention for thalassemic children during blood transfusion according to his/or her needs with total number of seventy two observations. The study was conducted at the pediatric department, Menoufiya University Hospital (Suzan Mubarak Hospital). The *results* of this study showed that approximately all thalassemic children had thalassemia major, majority of them were males (63 per cent) and don't follow dietary regimen (43 per cent). The study *concluded* that the majority of parents had incomplete knowledge about thalassemia and its management. Also, there were shortage in nurses' knowledge and practice in some aspects of thalassemia management. Therefore, this study *recommended* that in-service education programs are needed to upgrade parents and nurses knowledge as well as their level of performance. Community services should be established in the form of societies to provide public awareness, financial support, companies and health education coverage for thalassemic children and their parents.

Keywords: *Thalassemia, Quality of care.*

Introduction

β-thalassemia is the most common genetically determined, chronic hemolytic anemia in Egyptian children (Hussein *et al.*, 2007). Mahmoud (2009) identified that there are 10,000 registered thalassemia cases and more than 20,000 non registered cases in Pediatric Hematology Unit at Cairo University. He also added that 95 per cent are beta thalassemia major and 5 per cent are thalassemia intermedia or hemoglobin H disease. However, carrier rates range between 5.5 per cent to 9.5 per cent.There are estimated 60 - 80 million people in the world who carry beta thalassemia trait alone (Davidson, 2008).

Moreover, severe thalassemia affected babies are likely to die before reaching two years of age. At least, 41,500 deaths probably occur each year in low- and middle-income countries. Also, 0.3 per cent of all deaths are children under five years (Weaheral *et al.*, 2006).

Thalassemic patients suffer from serious impairments in quality of life that impose persistent threat on them due to other associated health problems such as heart failure, liver dysfunction and susceptibility to infection (Deepika *et al.*, 2007 and Davidson, 2008). For this reason, thalassemia imposes further burden on care givers especially for those who suffer from persistent stress that causes anxiety and mood disorder. These problems reduce parent's physical and psychological abilities to carry up their responsibilities (Davidson, 2008). Therefore, quality of care provided by parents might not meet many healthcare needs of their children.

Above all, thalassemic children needed intensive care due to their continuous need for regular blood transfusion, subcutaneous infusion of iron chelating agents, regular investigations, supportive management and healthy life style (Wong's, 2007). However, inadequate quality of care could cause increased likelihood of physical and mental retardation. It also might increase the risk of deadly hemosiderosis due to iron over load.

For this reason, nursing role is pivotal to the comprehensive care of individuals with thalassemia. It centers on providing ongoing education about the disease, ensuring a system of preventive health management, recognition and management of acute illnesses, timely coordination and integration of subspecialty care to manage personal care at home (Krepia *et al.*, 2006).

Also, nurses play a central role in developmental and emotional anticipatory guidance as well as empowerment of patients and their families for their own advocacy. Pediatric nurses should seek to broaden the range of their interventions through incorporating recent advances of knowledge and technology related to thalassemia care into their practice (Truong and Ferguson, 2003). For this reason, this study aims to assess parent's quality of care provided to thalassemic children and to assess nurse's quality of care provided to thalassemic children at specified setting.

Aim of the study

Aims of this study were:

1. To assess parent's quality of care provided to thalassemic children.
2. To assess nurse's quality of care provided to thalassemic children at specified setting.

Research Questions

1. Do parents provide adequate care for their children with thalassemia?
2. Are nurses caring for thalassemic children providing standardized care?

Materials and Method

Materials

Research Design

A descriptive design was selected.

Setting

The study was conducted at the pediatric department, Menoufia University Hospital (Suzan Mubarak Hospital).

Sample

All available children (100) with thalassemia and their parents were selected from the previously mentioned setting. As well a number of 26 nurses were observed and interviewed.

Tools

Three tools were utilized for the study.

Tool One

Quality of care questionnaire sheet. It was adopted from Hashem (2006) and Salem (2007) then modified by researchers. It assesses parent's quality of care provided to thalassemic children. It included the following parts:

Part One

Biosocial characteristics of studied sample:

1. Patients' profile form which included patients' name, address, Telephone number, age, diagnosis and gender.
2. Biosocial data related to parents such as parents' age, level of Education and family history of the disease.

Part Two

Knowledge and reported care of parents about thalassemia.

It was divided into three main categories:

- ☆ *First*: Knowledge about thalassemia.

  It included multiple choice questions about definition, prevention, clinical manifestation, types, warning signs and causes of complications.

- ☆ *Second*: Care provided to thalassemic children.

  It included multiple choice questions about dietary regimen, dental care, diarrhoea, appetite, activity, medication, investigation and immunization.

- ☆ *Third*: Social services.

  It included multiple choice questions about social services.

Tool Two

Nurses' knowledge questionnaire sheet. It was adopted from Hashem (2006), Wong's (2007) and Kulger (2008). It assesses nurses Knowledge about thalassemia. It included:

1. Biosocial data related to nurses such as nurse's age, level of education, years of experience, previous training.
2. Nurses knowledge about thalassemia which was divided into five categories:

   - ☆ *First*: It included multiple choice questions about definition of Thalassemia, types, clinical manifestation, sex and hemoglobin level.
   - ☆ *Second*: It included multiple choice questions about management of Thalassemia, new trends, warning signs, complications and nurses' Role.
   - ☆ *Third*: It included multiple choice questions about purpose of Desferal, methods of injection, precaution, side effects, frequency of Administration and iron exertion.
   - ☆ *Fourth*: It included multiple choice questions about investigation.
   - ☆ *Fifth*: It included multiple choice questions about blood transfusions, Child weight, precautions, blood reactions and its management.

Scoring System for Each Question

Level of Knowledge	*Score*
Complete	2
Incomplete	1
Don't know	0

Total Scoring System for Level of Knowledge

Level of Knowledge	*Score*
Complete	> 66 per cent
Incomplete	33-66 per cent
Don't know	<33 per cent

Tool Three

Observational checklist of nursing care for thalassemic children. It was adopted from Hashem (2006) and modified by researchers. It assesses nurses' practices provided to thalassemic children.

It was divided into three main phases:

- ☆ *First phase*: Care provided before blood transfusion. It included assessment of growth and development and vital signs.
- ☆ *Second phase*: Care provided during blood transfusion.
- ☆ *Third phase*: Care provided after blood transfusion such as assessment of vital signs, observation of iron chelation side effects and health education.

Scoring System for Each Step

Level of Performance	*Score*
Complete	2
Incomplete	1
Not done	0

Total Scoring System for Performance

Level of Performance	*Score*
Complete	>66 per cent
Incomplete	33-66 per cent
Note done	<33 per cent

Methods

1. A review of the past and current literature, local and international related literature was done.
2. Tools were developed and submitted to two pediatric nursing experts and one pediatrician to check the validity of the tools.
3. An official permission for data collection was obtained from the administrator of Menoufiya University Hospital.
4. For ethical considerations, meetings were conducted with nurses and parents before starting data collection to explain the purpose of the study,

privacy of their information, confidentiality of their names and their acceptance to participate in the study.

5. A pilot study was carried out at the above mentioned setting on five nurses and ten parents to assess the reliability, clarity, consistency of the study tools, and the time needed to fill each tool. Sample of the pilot study was a part of the studied sample.
6. Data was collected two days/week at morning and afternoon shifts. The researcher started interviewing parents individually for ten minutes. Questionnaire sheet was submitted to each nurse. They took ten minutes to fill the required data. Nurse's performance was indirectly observed and recorded while providing blood transfusion (before, during and after). Each nurse was observed at least three times and the most common nursing performance was recorded.
7. Data was coded, tabulated and analyzed by using SPSS statistical package version 13 on IBM. Mean standard deviation, t-test and Chi-square (X^2) were used. Level of significance was set as P-value ‹ 0.05.

Limitations of the Study

1. There were only 26 nurses available at the unit who were caring for all thalassemic children.
2. There were only 24 nurses working during blood transfusion because the other 2 were supervisor.

Results

Figure 3.1 shows that children age varied between 4 months to 15 years old.

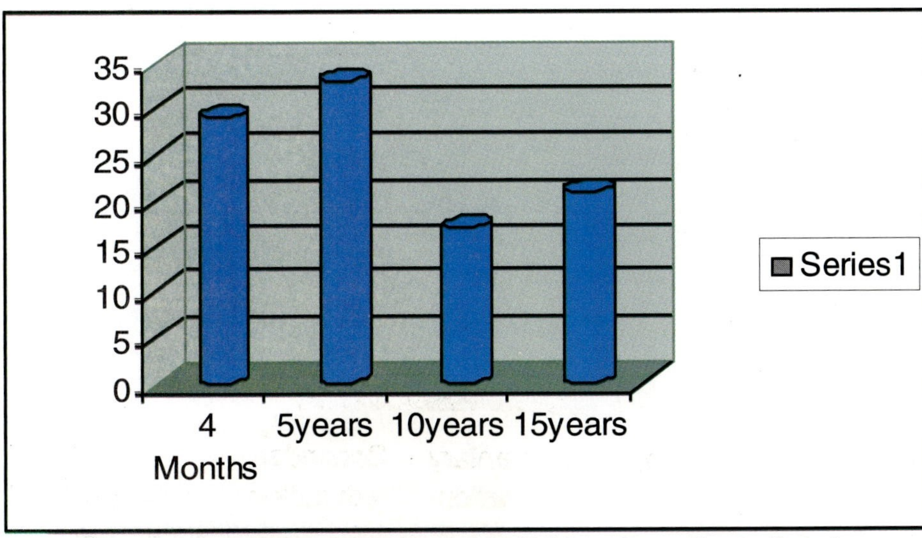

Figure 3.1: Distribution of Thalassemic Children According to their Age

Figure 3.2 illustrates that the majority of thalassemic children were males (63 per cent)

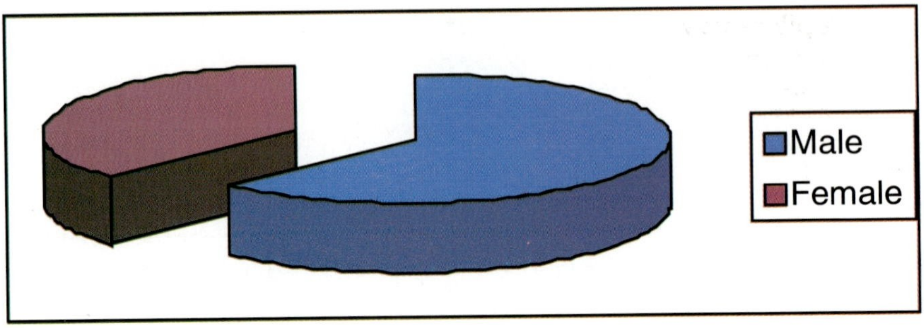

Figure 3.2: Distribution of Thalassemic Children According to their Sex

Figure 3.3 shows that the majority had thalassemia major.

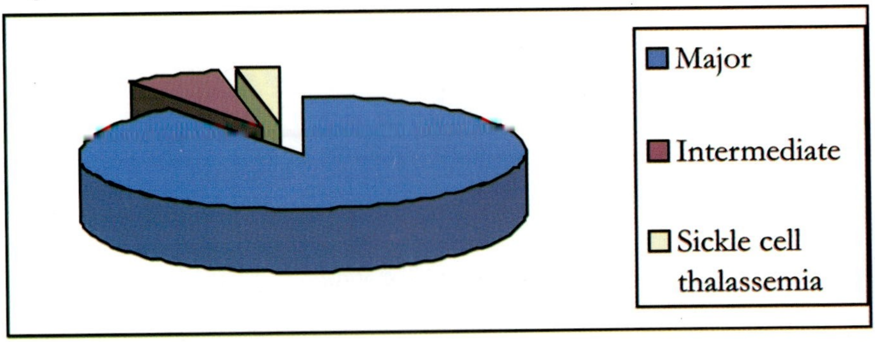

Figure 3.3: Distribution of Thalassemic Children According to their Diagnosis

Figure 3.4 shows that the majority of parents were either illiterate or had secondary education.

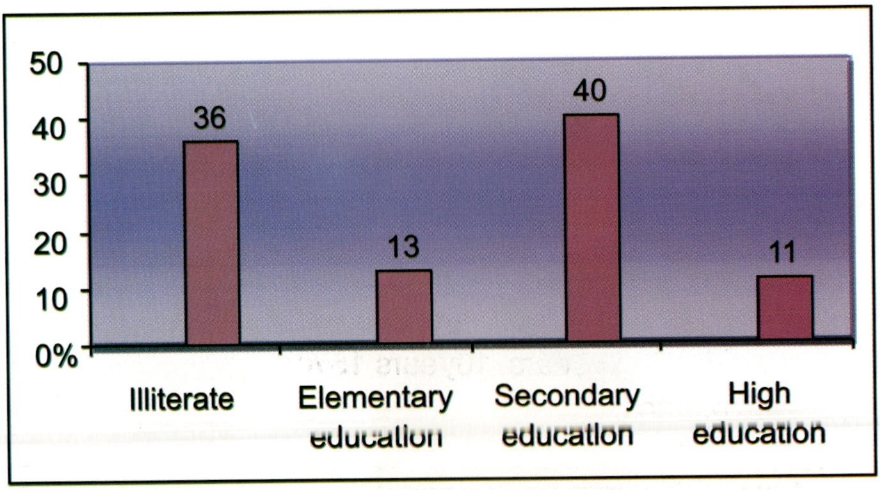

Figure 3.4: Distribution of Parents' According to their Level of Education

Figure 3.5 shows that the majority had 20 years old.

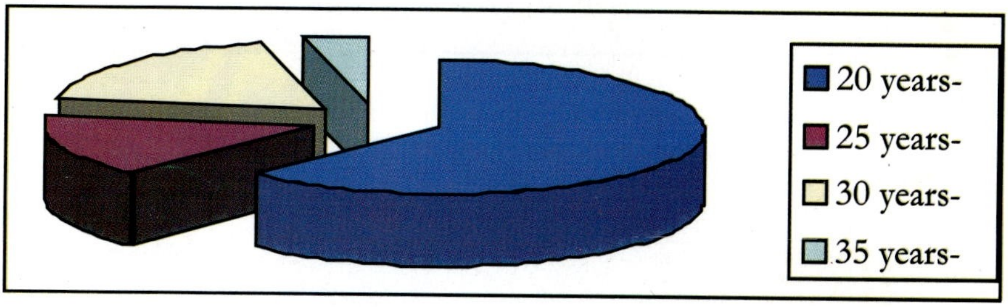

Figure 3.5: Distribution of Nurses According to their Age

Figure 3.6 shows that most of nurses had 5 years experience.

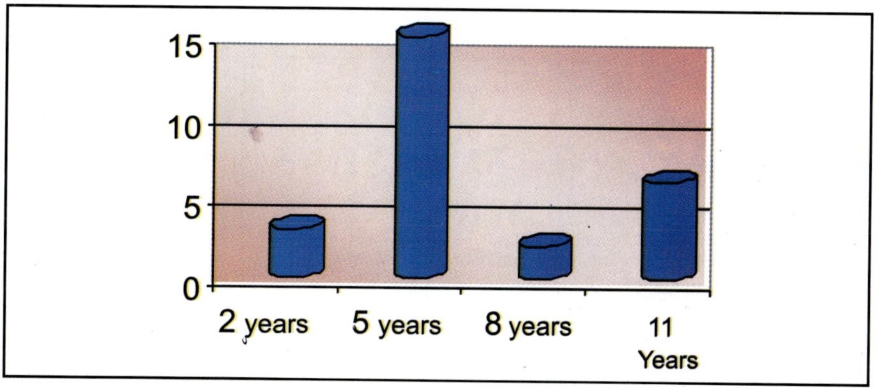

Figure 3.6: Distribution of Nurses According to their Years of Experience

Figure 3.7 shows that consanguinity is higher between relatives.

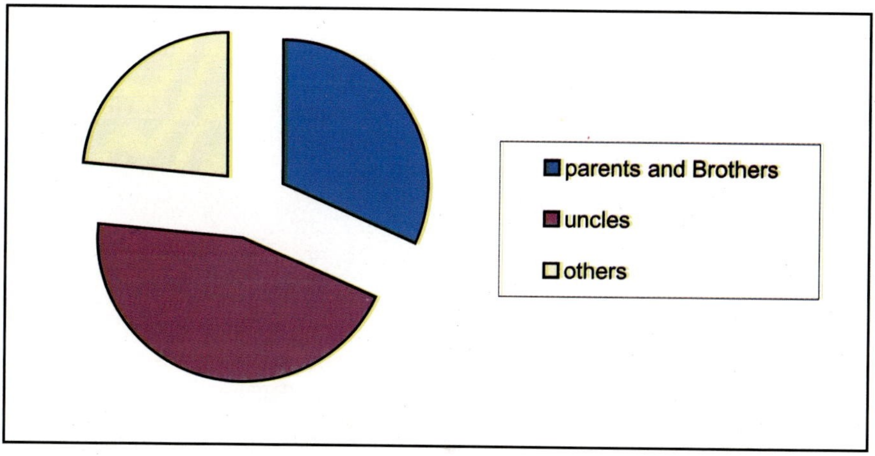

Figure 3.7: Illustrates the Consanguinity of Thalassemic Children

It was clear from Table 3.1 that there were knowledge deficit in relation to prevention, contributing factors, clinical manifestation, types and management among all parents' levels. Above all, there was only statistical significant difference at 5 per cent related to parents' knowledge about definition of thalassemia.

Table 3.1: Parents' General Knowledge about Thalassemia Distributed by their Level of Education

Knowledge of Parents	Illiterate (n=36)		Elementary Education (n=13)		Secondary Education (n=40)		High Education (n=11)		Total (n=100)		X^2
	No	%	No	%	No	%	No	%	No	%	
1. Definition											
Complete	15	41.7	7	53.8	23	57.5	11	100	56	56	11.71*
Don't know	21	58.3	6	46.2	17	42.5	0	0.0	44	44	
2. Prevention											
Complete	9	25	7	53.8	14	35	3	27.3	33	33	6.65^{ns}
Incomplete	5	13.9	1	7.7	9	22.5	1	9.1	16	16	
Don't Know	22	61.1	5	3 8.5	17	2.5	7	63. 6	51	51	
3. Contributing factors											
Complete	5	13.9	2	15.4	10	25	3	27.3	20	20	2.0^{ns}
Don't know	31	86.1	11	84.6	30	75	8	72.7	80	80	
4. Clinical manifestation											
Complete	7	19.4	5	38.5	11	27.5	6	54.5	29	29	5.69^{ns}
Incomplete	29	80.6	8	61.5	29	72.5	5	45.5	71	71	
5. Types											
Complete	4	11.1	2	15.4	10	25	1	9.1	17	17	5.08^{ns}
Incomplete	5	13.9	1	7.7	6	15	3	27.3	15	15	
Don't know	27	75	10	76.9	24	60	7	63. 6	68	68	
6. Management											
Complete	7	19.4	2	15.4	11	27,5	7	63. 6	27	27	0.11^{ns}
Incomplete	24	66.7	9	6 9.2	22	55	4	36.4	59	59	
Don't know	5	13.9	2	15.4	7	7.5	0	0.0	14	14	
7. Complications											
Complete	23	63.9	9	69.2	28	70	10	90.9	70	70	4.78^{ns}
Incomplete	4	11.1	0	0.0	3	7.5	0	0.0	7	7	
Don't know	9	25	4	30.8	9	22.5	1	9.1	23	23	
8. Alarming signs for hospitalization											
Complete	18	50	8	61.5	24	60	9	81.2	59	59	6.12^{ns}
Incomplete	9	25	1	7.7	7	7.5	2	18.2	19	19	
Don't know	9	25	4	0.8	9	2.5	0	0.0	22	22	

**: $P < 0.01$; ns: $P > 0.05$.

Table 3.2 shows that there were no statistical significant difference between general knowledge of nurses having different levels of education except for hemoglobin value at 1 per cent.

Table 3.2: General Knowledge of Studied Nurses about Thalassemia Distributed by their Level of Education

Knowledge of nurses	*Nursing Diploma (n=16)*		*Technical Nursing Diploma (n=8)*		*Bachelor Degree (n=2)*		*Total (n=26)*		*X^2*
	No	*%*	*No*	*%*	*No*	*%*	*No*	*%*	
1. Types									
Complete	9	56.3	5	62.5	2	100	16	61.5	0.49^{ns}
Don't know	7	43.7	3	37.5	0	0.0	10	38.5	
2. Clinical manifestation									
Complete	12	75	5	62.5	1	50	18	69.2	0.68^{ns}
Don't know	4	25	3	37.5	1	50	8	30.8	
0. Hemoglobin value									
Complete	14	87.5	8	100	0	0.0	22	84.6	12.56**
Don't know	2	12.5	0	0.0	2	100	4	15.4	
4. Warning signs for hospitalization									
Complete	13	81.3	8	100	2	100	23	88.5	0.71^{ns}
Incomplete	1	6.3	0	0.0	0	0.0	1	3.8	
Don't know	2	12.5	0	0.0	0	0.0	2	7.7	
5. Complications									
Complete	16	100	7	87.5	2	100	25	96.2	0.31^{ns}
Don't know	0	0.0	1	12.5	0	0.0	1	3.8	
6. Nurses role									
Complete	14	87.5	7	87.5	2	100	23	88.5	1.05^{ns}
Incomplete	2	12.5	1	12.5	0	0.0	3	11.6	

**: $P < 0.01$; ns: $P > 0.05$.

It was clear that nurses having technical nursing diploma had the best knowledge about methods of desferal administration. Above all, there were statistical significant differences between nurses having different levels of education in relation to times of administration and iron excretion at 5 per cent and 1 per cent levels.

Table 3.4 illustrates Knowledge of studied nurses' about blood transfusion process. The majority of nurses had complete knowledge about indications for blood transfusion, complications, and precautions during or after blood transfusion. Whereas, the only statistical difference that was found was at 5 per cent related to knowledge of nurses about vital signs.

Table 3.3: Knowledge of Studied Nurses' about Desferal Administration Distributed by their Level of Education

Knowledge of Desferal Administration	Nursing Diploma (n=16)		Technical Nursing Diploma (n=8)		Bachelor Degree (n=2)		Total (n=26)		X^2
	No	%	No	%	No	%	No	%	
1. Utilization of Desferal									
Complete	12	75	5	62.5	0	0.0	17	65.4	4.46^{ns}
Don't know	4	25	3	37.5	2	100	9	34.6	
2. Methods of administration									
Complete	14	87.5	8	100	1	50	23	88.5	3.96^{ns}
Don't know	2	12.5	0	0.0	1	50	3	11.5	
3. Precautions during administration									
Complete	12	75	6	75	1	50	19	73.1	0.59^{ns}
Don't know	4	25	2	25	1	50	7	26.9	
4. Side effects									
Complete	10	62.5	5	62.5	1	50	16	61.5	0.12^{ns}
Don't know	6	37.5	3	37.5	1	50	10	38.5	
5. Duration of administration									
Complete	12	75	5	62.5	2	100	19	73.1	1.22^{ns}
Don't know	4	25	3	37.5	0	0.0	7	26.9	
6. Times for administration/week									
Complete	5	31.3	7	87.5	1	50	13	50	5.63*
Don't know	11	68.7	1	12.5	1	50	13	50	
7. Iron excretion									
Complete	6	37.5	7	87.5	1	50	14	53.8	3.74*
Don't know	10	62.5	1	12.5	1	50	12	46.2	

*: $P < 0.05$; ns: $P > 0.05$.

Table 3.5 represents reported physical care provided by parents' for their thalassemic children. There were no statistical significant differences between reported cares provided by parents' having different levels of education except in having dietary regimen in favor for parents' having secondary education. A statistical significant difference was found at 5 per cent level of significance.

Table 3.6 illustrates that there were no statistical significant differences between reported care for medications, investigation and immunization provided by parents' having different levels of education. Meanwhile the more highly educated parents, the more frequent adherence to perform investigations every 3 months. For this reason, a statistical significant difference was found at 5 per cent level of significance.

Table 3.4: Knowledge of Studied Nurses' about Blood Transfusion Process for Thalassemic Children

Knowledge of Nurses	*Nursing Diploma (n=16)*		*Technical Nursing Diploma (n=8)*		*Bachelor Degree (n=2)*		*Total (n=26)*		*X²*
	No	*%*	*No*	*%*	*No*	*%*	*No*	*%*	
1. Indication for blood transfusion									
Complete	12	75	8	100	2	100	22	84.6	2.95^{ns}
Incomplete	3	18.8	0	0.0	0	0.0	3	11.5	
Don't know	1	6.2	0	0.0	0	0.0	1	3.8	
2. Complications									
Complete	11	68.8	5	62.5	2	100	18	69.2	0.94^{ns}
Don't know	5	31.2	3	37.5	0	0.0	8	30.8	
3. Complications of iron overload									
Complete	4	25	4	50	0	0.0	8	30.8	5.04^{ns}
Incomplete	6	37.5	2	25	2	100	10	38.5	
Don't know	6	37.5	2	25	0	0.0	8	30.8	
4. Vital signs during blood transfusion									
Complete	3	18.7	6	75	1	50	10	38.5	2.99*
Don't know	13	81.3	2	25	1	50	16	61.5	
5. Precautions before blood transfusion									
Complete	14	87.5	8	100	1	50	23	88.5	3.96^{ns}
Incomplete	2	12.5	0	0.0	1	50	3	11.5	
6. Precautions during blood transfusion									
Complete	15	93.8	5	62.5	2	100	22	84.6	4.39^{ns}
Incomplete	1	6.2	3	37.5	0	0.0	4	15.4	
7. Precautions after blood transfusion									
Complete	14	87.5	5	62.5	2	100	21	80.8	7.25^{ns}
Incomplete	2	12.5	3	37.5	0	0.0	5	19.2	

*: $P < 0.05$; ns: $P > 0.05$.

Table 3.7 illustrates the percent distribution of complete nursing performance. It was found that only 41.7 per cent of studied nurses assessing children's weight. Meanwhile, none of them assessing height, development and vital signs before blood transfusion. Also the table reveals that the majority of nurses provide required care during blood transfusion. At the same time, none of them assess or monitor patients' vital signs as well as the rate of blood transfusion as required during blood transfusion. It reveals also that more than three quarters of nurses (83.3 per cent) document amount of blood and types of reactions. At the same time, none of them assess vital signs, observe side effects of iron chelation, or provide health education after blood transfusion.

Table 3.5: Reported Physical Care Provided by Parents' for their Thalassemic Children According to their Levels of Education

Reported Physical Care	Illiterate (n=36)		Elementary Education (n=13)		Secondary Education (n=40)		High Education (n=11)		Total (n=100)		X^2
	No	%	No	%	No	%	No	%	No	%	
1. Dietary care											
a. Have dietary regimen											
Yes	19	52.8	4	30.8	29	72.5	5	45.5	57	57	8.43*
No	17	47.2	9	69.2	11	27.5	6	54.5	43	43	
2. Dental care											
a. Daily brushing teeth											
Yes	11	30.6	3	32.1	17	42.5	5	45.5	36	36	3.15^{ns}
Sometimes	20	55.5	9	69.2	19	47.5	5	45.5	53	53	
No	5	13.9	1	7.7	4	10	1	9	11	11	
Frequency of brushing											
Once	5	13.9	2	15.4	11	27.5	3	27.3	21	21	1.13^{ns}
Twice	6	16.7	1	7.7	6	15	2	18.2	15	15	
b. Dental check ups											
Yes	4	11.1	3	32.1	5	12.5	2	18.1	14	14	1.37^{ns}
No	32	88.9	10	76.9	35	87.5	9	81.9	86	86	
c. Frequency of dental check ups/year											
Once	3	8.3	0	0.0	2	5	1	9	6	6	4^{ns}
Twice	1	2.8	3	32.1	3	7.5	1	9	8	8	

*: $P < 0.05$; ns: $P > 0.05$.

Table 3.6: Reported Care for Medications, Investigations and Immunizations Provided to Thalassemic Children According to Parents' Level of Education

Items	Illiterate (n=36)		Elementary Education (n=13)		Secondary Education (n=40)		High Education (n=11)		Total (n=100)		X^2
	No	%	No	%	No	%	No	%	No	%	
1. Frequency of desferal administration											
5-7 items	18	50	3	23.1	24	60	6	5 4.5	51	51	5.42^{ns}
Don't know	18	50	10	76.9	16	40	5	45.5	49	49	
2. Purpose of desferal											
Complete	27	75	8	61.5	28	70	8	72.7	71	71	3.13^{ns}
Don't know	9	25	5	38.5	12	30	3	27.3	29	29	

Contd...

Table 3.6–Contd...

Items	*Illiterate (n=36)*		*Elementary Education (n=13)*		*Secondary Education (n=40)*		*High Education (n=11)*		*Total (n=100)*		*X²*
	No	*%*	*No*	*%*	*No*	*%*	*No*	*%*	*No*	*%*	
3. Time of administration											
Complete	18	50	3	23.1	24	60	6	54.6	51	51	0.1^{ns}
Don't know	18	50	10	76.9	16	40	5	45.4	49	49	
4. Other Medication											
Yes	15	41.7	2	15.4	17	42.5	7	63.6	41	41	0.52^{ns}
No	21	58.3	11	84.6	23	57.5	4	36.4	59	59	
5. Investigations											
a. Every 3/M											
Done	5	13.9	2	15.4	7	17.5	6	54.5	20	20	9.37^{*}
Not done	31	86.1	11	84.6	33	82.5	5	45.5	80	80	
b. Every/year											
Done	5	31	1	7.7	6	15	5	45.5	17	17	7.47^{ns}
Not done	31	86.1	12	92.3	34	85	6	54.5	83	83	
6. Immunization											
a. Obligatory											
Done	36	100	13	100	40	100	11	100	100	100	0.0^{ns}
b. Nonobligatory											
Done	2	5.6	0	0.0	9	22.5	2	18.2	13	13	7.16^{ns}
Not done	34	94.4	13	100	31	77.5	9	81.8	87	87	
c. Types of nonobligatory											
Hep A	1	50	0	0.0	7	77.8	2	100	10	76.9	2.74^{ns}
Hep B	1	50	0	0.0	1	11.1	0	0.0	2	15.4	
Influenza virus	0	0.0	0	0.0	1	11.1	0	0.0	1	7.7	

*: $P < 0.05$; ns: $P > 0.05$.

Table 3.8 illustrates correlation between knowledge and practice. There is significant positive correlation between knowledge of nurses and their practice.

Figure 3.8 represents that more than 85 per cent of thalassemic children go to physicians. Meanwhile, approximately all of them don't receive other services.

Discussion

In the present study, it was noted that the age of studied children ranged from 4 months to 15 years old. This could be related to the difficulty of diagnosing thalassemia before 4 months of age and their short life span due to shortage of care. Also, the majority of thalassemic children was males and had major type. These results were corresponding with Mitra and Mashayekhi (2004),Abou-Ella (2004) and Sadati *et al.* (2004).

Table 3.7: Care Provided by Nurses to Thalassemic Children Before, during and After Blood Transfusion

Provided Care	*Not Done*		*Incomplete*		*Complete*	
	No	*%*	*No*	*%*	*No*	*%*
A. Before blood transfusion						
1. Assessment of growth						
a. Weight (Infant and child)	4	16.6	10	41.7	10	41.7
b. Height	0	0.0	0	0.0	0	0.0
2. Assessment of development:						
a. Assess development	0	0.0	0	0.0	0	0.0
3. Vital signs:						
a. Assess vital signs	0	0.0	0	0.0	0	0.0
4. Assess for blood type and hemoglobin level.	0	0.0	0	0.0	24	100
B. During blood transfusion						
1. Wash hands and wear gloves	2	8.3	2	8.3	14	58.3
2. Prepare the necessary equipments	2	8.3	2	8.3	20	83.3
3. Explain the procedures to child/ parent	2	8.3	0	0.0	22	91.7
4. Assess vital signs	24	100	0	0.0	0	0.0
5. Check doctors order for blood type	0	0.0	0	0.0	24	100
6. Connect tube & start blood transfusion	2	8.3	0	0.0	22	91.7
7. Monitor the rate of blood transfusion	24	100	0	0.0	0	0.0
8. Monitor patient's vital signs	24	100	0	0.0	0	0.0
C. After blood transfusion						
1. Document blood amount and type of reaction	4	16.7	0	0.0	20	83.3
2. Assess vital signs	24	100	0	0.0	0	0.0
3. Observe side effect of iron chelation.	24	100	0	0.0	0	0.0
4. Provide health education about diet, medication and general care	24	100	0	0.0	0	0.0

0 means that action not done.

Results of this study further showed that parents of thalassemic children who were relatives represented 38 per cent of the study. These results were consistent with Abo-Salem (1999) and Hashem (2006). This could be explained as consanguinity which is a problematic social phenomenon in Egypt can lead to homozygousity of thalassemia trait. For this reason, Dale *et al.* (2005) asserted that nurses in all areas of practice will become involved in the provision of information about genetic testing and assisting individuals and families in decision making and adjustment to new genetic information.

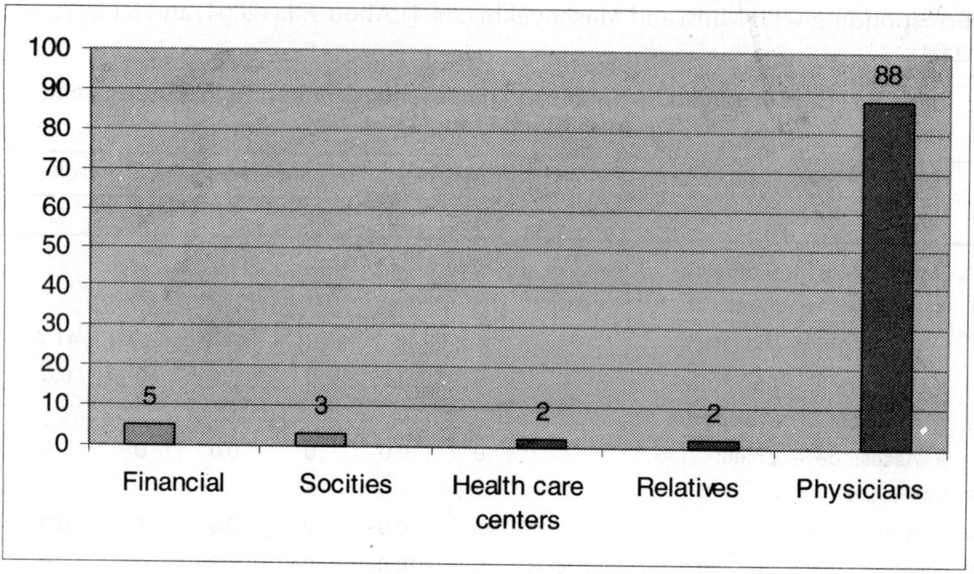

Figure 3.8: Services Provided by Community to Thalassemic Children

Table 3.8: Correlation Between Knowledge and Practices of Nurses in Relation to Care of Thalassemics

Parameter	*Knowledge*	
	r	*p*
Practice	0.92	‹0.001

Concerning the level of education, the present study also clarified that thirty six percent of parents were illiterate. This rendered children more liable to receive poor quality of care.

In the present study, it was illustrated that the majority of studied nurses had 20 years old and have five years experience. This could show that the majority of nurses have limited experience and education regarding providing care to thalassemic patients. Vahey *et al.* (2004) Indicated that the agency of healthcare research quality identified that in order to achieve quality, nurses should keep learning and conducting research rather than being stagnated in their educational background. For these reasons, these nurses needed to be provided with higher levels of education and training in order to be able to carry up their responsibilities and provide advanced quality of care.

Although parents had different levels of education, the majority of them had incomplete knowledge about prevention, contributing factor, clinical manifestations, types and management. These findings were consistent with Cappellini *et al.* (2000) Krepia *et al.* (2006). Insufficient knowledge of parents about thalassemia could be due to limited health education provided by healthcare providers for parents.

The study illustrated that majority of nurses had complete knowledge about clinical manifestations and hemoglobin value. On the other hand, more than three quarters of them had knowledge about warning signs for potential hospitalization, complications. However, nurses could have acquired this knowledge from physicians and working experience with patients.

Also, it was noted that bachelor degree nurses had better knowledge than technical nursing degree related to types of thalassemia, complications and nursing role. This could be related to their higher level of education which might provide them with scientific basis in order to provide better practice related to nursing care of thalassemia.

Above all, two thirds of included nurses had knowledge deficit about complications of iron overload. This rendered thalassemic children more liable to complications related to iron overload, liver damage, heart, and endocrine glands. However, iron overload predisposes to organ enlargement and dysfunction.

Also there was adequate knowledge about indications for blood transfusion, complications and precaution during or after blood transfusion. Such findings were in agreement with what was mentioned by Rosenthal (2007). In other words, Sazama *et al.* (1999) mentioned that although blood used for transfusion provides significant therapeutic benefits. Each blood component transfused carries a small risk of an acute or late adverse effect. Therefore, well-trained nursing must be conscientious in all stages of blood component administration, from sample collection through and beyond transfusion. Proper recognition and management of acute adverse effects may be lifesaving for some patient.

Regarding reported dietary care, approximately half of thalassemic children followed certain dietary regimen and the others didn't have any dietary restriction. The majority of children were sharing families in their normal diet this could be due to poor financial resources and parents were emotionally unable to deprive their children from certain foods. This finding was consistent with Dudek (2001).

Furthermore, this study revealed that children had poor dental care and limited dental check ups. These results agree with El-Awany (2002) and Tsiantis *et al.* (2004). It might be attributed to mothers' ignorance of the importance of dental care for their children.

Deepika *et al.* (2007) explained that lower educational attainment in parents might contribute to poor understanding of the nature of illness which in turn may attribute to more severe illness.

Concerning desferal utilization, the study showed that the majority of parents had good understanding of the purpose of desferal utilization and approximately half of them were able to identify its frequency properly. However, parents were unable to administer it regularly because it was expensive. These findings were in line with Olivieri (1999).

This rendered children liable to complications related to irregular administration of desferal. However, adequate administration of chelation therapy markedly improves the prognosis of disease, reduces iron accumulation and iron mediated organ damage which might reduce morbidity and mortality rate (Pignatti *et al.*, 2004).

Regarding the administration of medications, it was noted that only 40 per cent of thalassemic children received additional medications. These medications contained Diacan, L-Qarantine and Folic acid supplementation. Although all thalassemic children needed Folic acid supplementation to renew red blood cells, the majority of them did not receive it. This caused them to be more liable to receive blood transfusion due to lowered level of hemoglobin (Park, 2007). Folic acid is important for thalassemic children because low level of Folic acid can cause anemia through interfering with the normal division and maturation of red blood cells (Monson, 2007).

For reported compliance with investigations, the present study revealed that only one quarter of thalassemic children complied with required reported investigations and the majority of children did not comply with reported investigations due to poor financial resources and knowledge deficit about the importance of investigations. This finding agreed with Hashem (2006).

Regarding children's immunizations, it was found that all parents of thalassemic children provided obligatory immunization. Meanwhile, the minority of them (13 per cent) provided non obligatory immunization due to inadequate financial resources and knowledge deficit. Wong's (2007) mentioned that post splenoectomy thalassemic children could have overwhelming infections. Therefore, these children should receive the pneumococcal and meningococcal in addition to their regular obligatory immunizations.

In this study, the majority of nurses did not follow some internationally identified guidelines such as assessment of vital signs, weight, height or child's development. Vital signs should be monitored prior to transfusion, 15 to 20 minutes after starting transfusion and post transfusion as stated by Ministry of Health (2009). Such finding could be attributed to shortage of nurses' number and their lack of training.

All nurses performed blood test according to doctor's order to assess blood type and hemoglobin level. These findings were in line with Goodnough *et al.* (2003) and Ministry of Health (2009).

The present study revealed that majority of nurses provided all required items of care during blood transfusion except monitoring vital signs as required. However, Sazama *et al.* (1999) and Rosenthal (2007) ascertained that staying with the patient for the first few minutes of blood transfusion and monitoring signs and symptoms of its complications will help to early detect any reaction from blood transfusion.

In this study, the majority of nurses didn't determine the rate of blood during transfusion which could lead to volume overload. Ministry of Health (2009) mentioned that nurses should start blood transfusion slowly at rate 1ml/min for first 15 minutes. This will help to avoid volume overload and to detect any blood reaction such as hemolytic, allergic and febrile reactions.

Regarding nursing care after blood transfusion, it was observed that none of nurses assessed vital signs, observed side effects of iron chelation therapy or provided health education. Such findings were in agreement with Castledine (2006). These may be due to working over load and nurses/patient ratio was insufficient. This rendered patients to be more liable to hypotension, hypocalcaemia and cardiac arrest that might threaten patients' lives.

As regards documentation of nursing action, it was obvious that three quarters of nurses were documenting blood transfusion. At the same time, these results were consistent with Ahmed (1998) and Akhtar *et al.* (2003)

Good documentation practice also may facilitate quality improvement measures by aiding in the implementation of new clinical practice guidelines. Besides, structural measures of quality typically should include the documentation of nursing actions to deliver high quality of nursing care (Navuluri, 2001). However, to improve quality of care, reporting system must become more comprehensive, standardized and widely available.

Regarding services provided to thalassemic children, it was noted that the majority of them seeked medical care in the hospital and they did not receive any other community services at Shebin Elkom. These findings were consistent with Krepia *et al.* (2006).

In this study, the majority of nurses didn't educate parents about community services and support. Such findings were in line with Krepia *et al.* (2006). For these reason Health education programs were required to assist mothers in building more assertiveness in their behavior and helping them to pursue effective ways of asking for support from existing support systems.

Conclusion

The present research shows that majority of parents had incomplete knowledge about thalassemia and its management and most of studied nurses were inexperienced in providing nursing care for thalassemic children and did not follow many internationally identified guidelines.

Recommendations

The following recommendation could be inferred from the above mentioned conclusions.

1. In-service education programs are needed to upgrade parents and nurses knowledge as well as their level of performance.
2. Strict supervision for the application of nursing procedures such as blood transfusion and desferal administration must be imposed.
3. Scientific committees should be established from experts in the field both medical and nursing to plan strategies that enhance providing health education for parents.
4. Community services should be established in the form of societies to provide public awareness, financial support, companies and health education coverage for thalassemic children and their parents.

5. Further studies should be done to assess the impact of different strategies to upgrade parents and nurses' knowledge and practices related to thalassemia and its management.

References

1. Abou-Ella, S. (2004). Detection of alpha thalassemia among children with microcytic hypochromic anemia. Master degree. Menofia University.
2. Abo -Salem, L.Y. (1999).Self care program for children suffering from β-thalassemia major. Doctorate thesis, Alexandria University, Faculty of Nursing, PP 1-53.
3. Ahmed, M. (1998). Evaluation of the Quality of Nursing care utilizing a Retrospective Auditing Technique at Shebin El kom Teaching Hospital. Unpublished thesis, Faculty of nursing, Menofia University.
4. Akhtar, S., Weaver, J., Pierson, D and Rubenfeld, G. (2003).Practice Variation in Respiratory Therapy Documentation during Mechanical ventilation, American College of Chest Physicians.(124):2275-2282. Retrieved from http://chest journal. Org/misc/terms/shtml.
5. Cappellini, L., Robbiolo, B.M., Bottasso, R., Coppola, G. and Fiorelli, A. (2000). Venous thromboembolism and hypercoagulability in splenectomized patients with thalassaemia intermedia. page 467–473.
6. Cappellini, N., Cohen, A., Eleftherion, A., Piga, A., and Porter, J. (2000). Guidelines for the clinical management of thalassemia. In Cao, MD and Galanello, MD. (2007). Beta-Thalassemia [Cooley's a.nemia, Mediterranean Anemia. Includes: Thalassemia Major (Beta-Thalassemia Major), Thalassemia Intermedia, Thalassemia Minor (Beta-Thalassemia Minor, Heterozygous Beta-Thalassemia).
7. Castledine, G. (2006) Blood transfusion: poor technique, record keeping and communication. British Journal of Nursing; 15: 7, 369. in Abstract Thompson, C.L. *et al.* (2008) Blood transfusions 1: how to monitor for adverse reactions. Nursing Times; 104: 2, 32–33. http://www.nursingtimes.net/nursing-practice-clinical research.
8. Dale, M., Suzan P., William, S., Peter, P and Andreas, L. (2005). Projected Incidence of Mechanical Ventilation in Ontario to 2026: preparing for the aging baby boomers. Crit care Med.33 (3):574-579.
9. Davidson, A.M. Thalassemia. (2008). Retrieved from http://www. answers. com/topic/spleen.
10. Davidson, R.M., London, L.M and Ladewig, A.P. (2008). Maternal – Newborn Nursing Women's Health Across the life span. (8th ed) United State. Chapter 19. Page 464.
11. Deepika, S., Satish, J and Santosh, C. (2007). Quality of life issues in caregivers of youngsters with thalassemia. Retrieved from http://www.thalforum.ca/ forums/showthread.php?t=1142&goto=newpost

12. Dudeks, G. (2001). Nutrition Essentials for Nursing Practice. (4th ed). Lippincott Company, pp.68-82.

13. El-Awany, T. (2002): Nutritional Program for children with B thalassemia major and their mothers. Doctoral degree. Faculty of Nursing. Tanta University.

14. Goodnough, L.T. (2003). Transfusion medicine: Looking to the future. Lancet, 361(9352): 161–169.

15. Hashem, **S.** (2006). Thalassemic children and their mother's understanding: Effect on compliance to thalassemia management plan. Doctorate degree. Mansoura University.

16. Hussein,G., Fawzy, M., Serafi, T.E., Ismail. E,F., Metwally, D.E., Saber, M.A., Giansily, M., Schved, J.F., Pissard, S and Martinez, P.A.(2007). Rapid detection of beta-Thalassemia alleles in Egypt using naturally or amplified created restriction sites and direct sequencing: a step in disease control. 31(1):49-62. Retrieved from http://www. ncbi. nlm.nih. gov/sites/entrez.

17. Krepia, N., Roupa, Z.,Gourni, M., Mastorakou, F., Efthimia Vojiatzi, Kouyioumtzi,A and Shell, S. (2006). A Qualitative Study on the Experiences of Mothers Caring for Their Children with Thalassemia in Athens, Greece. Journal of Pediatric Nursing. Volume 21, Issue 2, April, Pages 142-152.

18. Kugler, M. (2008). Thalassemia: Old Diseases, New Research. Retrieved from http://rarediseases.about.com/c/a.htm.

19. Mahmoud, M. (2009). Thalassemia around the world: Egypt. In Cooley's anemia Foundation. Retrieved from http://www. thalassemia. org/index. php? option=com_content &view=article&id = 222: thalassemia- around- the- world- egypt and catid =1: latest-news.

20. Ministry of Health. (2009). Blood Transfusion and the Role of the Nurse. Retrieved from http://www. Gnd moh. Com/vb/show thread. Php.

21. Mitra, J and Mashayekhi, S. (2004). Demographic and clinical aspects in thalassemic or hemophilic patients referred to pediatric hospital in Tabriz City, 2004, Iran. Research Journal of biological sciences, 2(5): 543 – 545.

22. Monson, K. (2007). Folic acid. Health information brought to life, eMedTV, Retrieved from http://www.emedtv.com/.

23. Navuluri, R. (2001). Documentation: What, Why, When, Where, Who, and How? Research for Nursing Practice.

24. Olivieri, N.F. (1999). The β-thalassemia. New England J. Med., 341:99-109.In Hashem, S. (2006). Thalassemic children and their mother's understanding: Effect on compliance to thalassemia management plan. Doctorate degree. Mansoura University.

25. Parks, MS. (2007). Thalassemia – Home Treatment. Retrieved from http://www. Health grades. com/kbase/topic/mini/hw 184660/overview. html.

26. Pignatti, B. C., Rugolotto, S and De Stefano, P. (2004). Survival and complications in patients with thalassemia major treated with transfusion and deferoxamine. Hematological; 89: 1187-1193.

27. Rosenthal, R. MS, (2007). Transfusion Basics. Retrieved from http://www.resourcenurse.com/career_center.html.

28. Sadati, A. (2004). The study of endocrinal complications of major thalassemic patients.TBZ. Med., 297:418-493.

29. Salem, M. (2007). Thalassemia Anemia. Moon Dragon's Obgyn Information. Retrieved from http://www. moon dragon. org/obgyn/anemia/anemia index.html.

30. Sazama, MD., Phillip J., DeChristopher., MD., Dodd, PhD., Chantal, R,. Harrison, MD., Ira, A. Shulman, MD., E. Cooper, MD., Richard J. Labotka, MD., Harold, A. Oberman, MD., Christopher, M. Zahn, MD, A., Greenburg, MD., Stehling, MD., Karla, J. Lauenstein, MT., Thomas, H. and Lee K. (1999). Practice Parameter for the Recognition, Management, and Prevention of Adverse Consequences of Blood Transfusion.

31. Truong, E and Ferguson, S. (2003) Welfare reform at the crossroads: Pediatric nurses bridging the gap between self-sufficiency and health. Journal of Pediatric Nursing 18 (2003, Feb), pp. 60–63 in Krepia, N., Roupa, Z., Gourni, M., Maotorakou, Γ., Efthimia VoJlatzi, Kouyıoumtzı, A and Shell, S. (2006). A Qualitative Study on the Experiences of Mothers Caring for Their Children with Thalassemia in Athens, Greece. Journal of Pediatric Nursing. Volume 21, Issue 2, April, Pages 142-152.

32. Tsiantis, Th., Dragonas, C., Richardso, D., Anastasopoulos, G., Masera and Spinett, J. (2004). Psychosocial problems and adjustment of children with β-thalassemia and their families. Journal of European Child and Adolescent Psychiatry. Retrieved from http://www. springerlink. com/content/w2036 wp747585267/full text. pdf?page=1.

33. Vahey, D., Swan. B., Lang, N., and Mitchall. P. (2004). Measuring and Improving Healthcare Quality: Nursling contribution to the state of science, Journal of Nursing Outlook. 52 (1).

34. Weatherall, D., Akinyanju, O., Fucharoen, S., Olivieri, N and Musgrove, P. (2006). Inherited Disorders of Hemoglobin. Chapter 34. Retrieved from http://www.dcp2. org/pubs/DCP.

33. Wong's Nursing Care of Infants and Children. (2007). (8th ed). Mosby Company. Canada. Chapter 35. Page 1529.

Chapter 4

Herbals in Promoting Nutrition among Children and Women

Aarati Saxena

Associate Professor in Botany
Sri Venkateswara College, University of Delhi South Campus
Presently Studying History of Medicine, Jamia Hamdard, New Delhi
E-mail: aaratisaxena@gmail.com

ABSTRACT

"Never before has the average man and woman been better fed and so poorly nourished," a one line statement that says all. One obvious reason is the distancing of man from nature. This has direct fallout on the family, society more so on young women and growing children. There are numerous ailments which can be cured safely by selecting natural foods which are endowed with an array of minerals, vitamins, trace elements and other magic substances. They have amazing curative properties and can provide 'comfort foods' rather than 'convenience foods'. Formerly rather sceptical of herbal food medicine, modern science now has taken a startling turn around and are re-reading old manuscripts to decipher magical drugs from natural laboratories of forests and fields. Use of simple herbs has many benefits. Besides their active principles they are also endowed with resin, gums, sugars, vitamins, inorganic salts. Herbal medicine and foods yield benefits as a consequence of synergistic effects of all the constituents some known and many unknown. Treatments in indigenous system of medicine always attempts with food as medicine first and then other formulations. The presentation would focus on simple interventions and remedies for problems faced by women during pregnancy, post natal care, new born and infant care as well as of adolescent girls taking inputs from folklore, heritage and authentication.

Keywords: *Herbals, Nutrition, Mother and child health, Medicines.*

Introduction

"Never before has the average human been better fed but poorly nourished", an urban reality on one hand and the rural poor battling hunger for survival or lack of food on the other hand. With the passage of time we seem to have lost the simplicity and serenity in food habits. Elements of serendipity are gift of discovery "which culminates in making pleasant, valuable and useful discoveries by accident", it has been the sole guiding phenomenon which has enriched our knowledge bank but is now a casualty. Or else how except for serendipity would we know that neem tree is like a village dispensary and parijat (Nyctanthes arbor tris tris) is a source of drug which keeps away from a sea of sorrow and is believed to be wish granting.

Plants including weeds are the treasure house of medicines ranging from ailments like headache to killer diseases like cancer. Over a billion years these plants develop countless chemicals combinations that help them ward of microbes and many provide protection to plants from insects and herbivores.

There is an alarming loss of biodiversity due to population pressure and aberrations in climate. In this context women being the home maker are inherently weak being daughters of anaemic mothers will find tough to raise healthy children.

The Indian system of medicine consists of two major components – folklore and codified or documented. Folk traditions are handed down orally from generation to generation and the codified have theoretical foundations like ayurveda, unani, sidha and others.

The above knowledge of herbs is relevant in that once again if we can bring it to mainstream foods, these herbs that are recognised since ancient times with proven healing power to alleviate pain and illness, can rescue us.

Heritage

Aristotle (384-324 BC) in his book "Golden Cabinet of Secrets" gave many formulae and prescriptions regarding certain herbs mentioned about tonic sedatives, aromatics, laxatives, purgatives.

Usage of medicinal plants is documented in the Rig Veda (4500 – 1600 BC). Text in Charak Sanhita on general medicine described the usage of about 350 plant species.

With the advent of Unani medicine in India between 10th and 11th century number of plant species grew manyfold for medicinal uses. Ibn Senna wrote 5 master piece books, Canon of Medicine (Al Qanun) mentions 700 simple drugs. The magic of herbs wove its spell over the people of the middle ages and the greatest body of knowledge ancients left is of herbs.

Seeds for Health

Primitives preferred consuming seeds instead of meat. It was easier to store, comforting in winter, had high protein content, saved them from hunting and much else. They used seeds of pumpkin, sesame, acorn, hemp, cucumber, sunflower, betel nut and fenugreek and others.

Aristotle said, "Nature does nothing without a purpose" it becomes clear as that more one delves into medical history the more one becomes convinced of the fact that it repeats itself. Man has learnt lessons from nature with sheer power of observation. Like the medicine tree papaya. Early explorers were impressed that Caribbean island natives could take exceptionally heavy meals of meat and fish followed by papaya desert. Ancient explorers also saw native's tenderized tough meat by wrapping green papaya leaves overnight. The raw papaya has protein digesting enzyme "papain" and the tablets of the same are now used for aiding digestion of proteins. Protein digesting enzymes in other botanical is bromelin of pineapple and even ripe fruit retains it.

Primitive medicine originated through prehistoric observations of animal behaviour like phlebotomy by rhino, emetics by canines, eating of sarpa ghandha (snake root plant) by mongoose before snake combat and licking of salt by cow. Their behaviour followed the inner compulsion which animals practiced for their own health, protection and survival.

Food as Medicine or Vice Versa

Use of simple herbs has many benefits besides having active principles other constituents like raisin, gum, sugar, vitamin and inorganic salts have synergistic effects of all the constituents present, some known and many unknown. A belief shared by people that an all wise providence has supplied man in the great natural labs of forests and fields.

Treatment with herbs always attempted first with food nutrition then medicine in this order. In Unani medicine there is practice of Ghizai: Dawai and Dawai: Ghizai.

Ghizai or diet is the one that is assimilated by the body and is part of the body after metabolism for example like cereals, pulses, vegetables etc. Whereas medicine or Dawai is one which enhances the metabolism like a catalyst but is not assimilated for example saffron or zafran which has proved anti oxidants properties and reverses age related macular degeneration and now it is dawned that how it has changed from a culinary luxury to a pill or turmeric in the kitchen is the staple has a range of medicinal properties it ought to have special space in grocery store and in the pharmacy too. There are many like aloes, olives, pepper and they are administered in prescribed doses like medicine. A special case is that of snake root (Rauwolffia serpentina) is a drug from ancient Indian Pharmocoepia. For thousands of years natives chewed the root for calming effects to alleviate nervous depression. It is believed that even Mahatma Gandhi used to dip the root in tea for calming effects. It is believed that not less than 1 million Indians regularly chewed the herb. In 1931 the west took note of it and in 1952 discovered the potent resource reserpene in roots which is a modern day tranquilizer. A drug company executive said "we finally figured that 1 million Indians could not be wrong" and now CCRUM central council on research in Unani medicine has developed a tea with saffron and almond which are both eye and brain tonic. They have also made Ashwagandha cookies which is a health tonic. In essence one needs to learn to create a wave of bio nutrients known for long and forgotten and to incorporate them in mainstream food.

The Confluence

The history of culture is inextricably bound with plants which usher in the state of well being. It is now felt than ever before the mystic of magical curative properties of herbs. Plurality of medicines in a multi cultural society with an innate historical consciousness is bound to happen.

Since time immemorial primitive man was not wrong in following his instinct and intuition, for in plants he found everything for daily needs.

A cursory look at the dietary ingredients based on the history of sure use indicates that plants listed in Ayurveda, Unani and even in Homeopathy share a common material medica. To an extent it is even safe to have datura – opium in the correct dose for the right result. In homeopathic bouquet Arnica Montana leaves chewed by guides while climbing realised they never have stiffness and were never tired, the same now is prescribed in homeopathy and Ayurveda as well. There are 573 herbs shared by Ayurveda, Unani, Sidha and Homeopathy. The following list of medicines is an indication

Bambusa (Bans Lochan) to improve assimilation in pregnant women.

Acorus calamus (Wacha) for indigestion.

Allium cepa for cold.

Daucus carota and *Ruta graveolens* for menstrual cycle problems

Cures for Problems during Pregnancy, Post Natal, New Born, Infant Care and Problem of Adolescent Girl

Concept of Contraception

To have healthy progeny, its proper care and upbringing is dream of every individual. History of fertility control can be traced back 4000 years on Egyption papyrus. It was a topic of discussion for ancient greek philosopher Aristotle and Plato. In ancient India emphasis was on healthy and wise progeny which created 'supraja' or healthy generation. Some references of female contraceptives are like application of seed powder of Palash with honey, fumigation with nimba kushtha, application of Datura root powder. Application of Pippali, Jagery, Latex of Euphorbia neerifolia, Glycyrrhiza all are on record in the traditional systems of medicine.

Health of uterus is vital as deficiency in vitamin, minerals and oxidants in daily diet are the main causes of weakening of uterus and loss of hormonal balance. Every third woman suffers from Leucorrhoea. The remedy is Kushta bazai murgh (Calcinated egg shell), Kushtae Marjan (coral) and mazu (Dyer's oak) with cows milk for one month. Urinary track infection: juice of Phyllanthes. Remedy for hormonal imbalance Musali black and white (Chlorophytum), fennel, satavari (Asparagus), Ashwagandha (Withania), Kalonji (Nigella), Amla (Embelica), rose petals, mochras (bombax) daily.

In Ayurveda there is a comprehensive explanation of woman and child health in Kaumara bhritya, which is an explanation of a child carrying, bearing, supporting, nourishing phase in a woman's life. According to WHO there is a 40 per cent loss in pregnancies and maternal death due to haemorrhages, infection, abortion and lack of healthcare in developing countries.

A diet regimen is advised in Ayurveda as follows:

1st Month

Yashtimadhu (Glycyrrhiza), Parushaka (Grewia), Madhukapushpa (Madhuca) with butter and honey.

2nd Month

Grapes, pomegranates and oranges

Shatavari (Asparagus), Ashwagandha (Withania), Yashtimadhu, kharjura (Phoenix) with milk.

3rd Month

Sariva (Hemidesmus), Madhukapushpa and Shatavari

Carrot, beetroot and leafy vegetables. Apple and grapes

4th Month

Sariva, Rasna(Pluchea), Yashtimadhu with milk

5th Month

Brihati (Solanum indicum), Kantakari (Solanum surattense), Gambhari (Gmelina), Nyagrodha (Ficus bengalensis), Udumbara (Ficus glomerata), Ashwattha (Ficus relegiosa) Dalchini (Cinnamomum) etc.

6th Month

Yashtimadhu, Ashwagandha, Shatavari, Sariva, Draksha (Vitis), Kharjura, Gokshura (Tribulus terrstris)

Khichri with 1 part rice, 1/4th part green gram, 6 parts water, ginger, turmeric, salt and powder of gokshura and sigru (Moringa)

7th Month

Follow 6th month also include Punarnava (Boerhavia), Eranda (Ricinus), Singhara (Trapa), Kamalakanda (Nelumbo) stem etc.

8th Month

Kapittha (Feronia), bilva (Aegle), Ikshu (Saccharum) etc.

9th Month

Ashwagandha/Shunthi, Devdaru (Cedrus), Yasthimadhu etc.

Generally diet should contain rice, rice flakes, wheat and green moong dal. Fruits like ripe banana, jackfruit, gooseberry and grapes are advisable.

Meat soup is recommended.

For morning sickness parched rice powder with honey, Zizyphus fruit pulp, pomegranate juice with honey etc.

For nausea plain ginger paste, cardamom with grapes

For anaemia sugar cane juice, shunthi churna with jaggery

Nutrition for lactating mother – lettuce seeds, purslane seeds, Asparagus roots, chilgoza pine seeds, almond, ashwagandha, pistachio,dates etc.

Massage for new borne – til oil with neem and nirgundi leaves

For children – ORS formulation 4:1 sugar and salt, saunf, soda bicarb and lemon.

Juice of Zyziphus as preventive and curative in swine flue.

Points to Ponder

With a population of a billion plus and a large number suffering from malnutrition India will pay for the disease prone population in the next decay. The state will spend millions of rupees to ensure medication.

Recommendations

Authentication of medicinal plants and a database is the need of the hour. This will promote their therapeutic validation and to minimize unfair trade practices.

Herbs with therapeutic value to be brought to the mainstream cuisine

An interface between different systems of medicine to be formulated where drugs in ayurvedic and unani systems are made available in homoeopathy. Further research is required to look into the possibility of same efficacy in treatment.

References

Ayurveda

1. Ashtang Hridaya
2. Ashtang Sangraha
3. Bhava Prakash
4. Charaka Samhita
5. Harita Samhita
6. Sushrut Samhita

Unani

7. Ibn Rushid : Kitab al Kulliyat, Urdu translation published by Central Council for Research in Unani Medicine 1987 page 212.
8. Ibn Sena : 'Al-Qanoon', Urdu translation by G.H. Qantoori, Aasif Javed Book Printers, Lahore 1992 page 131
9. Rabban Tabri : Firdaus Al Hikmat, Urdu translation by Sheikh Mohd. Basheer and sons, Lahore 1996 page 115-118
10. Proceedings : International Conference on Unani Medicine, organized by Central Council for Research in Unani Medicine, AYUSH, Vigyan Bhawan, New Delhi, February 2005.

General Books

11. Bakhru 1994: Foods that heal the natural way to good health, Orient Paperbacks
12. Richard Lucas Parker 1966: Nature's Medicine, the folklore, romance and value of herbal remedies, Publisher: Publishing Company Inc. West nyack N.Y.
13. Rustom Jal Vakil 1966: Our Glorious Heritage. The Times of India Press,Bombay

Chapter 5

Empowering Women in India through better Reproductive Healthcare

Devendra Kothari

Professor,
Population and Programme Management and Director,
Forum for Population Action, Suite 203, Pearl Mount View,
14-A Tilak Nagar, Jaipur – 302 004, India
E-mail: kothari42@dataone.in

ABSTRACT

The paper aims to provoke a discussion and mobilize support for reproductive health services. While India's population continues to grow by 16-17 million people annually, 25 million women, mostly in poor performing states, seek to postpone childbearing, space births, or stop having children, but are not using a modern method of contraception. Often, these women travel far from their communities to reach a health facility, only to return home "empty handed" due to shortages, stock outs, and/or non availability of doctors and paramedical staff. When women are thus turned away, they are unable to protect themselves from unwanted/unplanned pregnancies and sexually transmitted infections, including HIV/AIDSs and this type of incomplete control over the reproductive process leads to relatively high levels of unwanted childrearingt. It is argued that until the policy makers take a focused and long term interest in the advancement of women by ensuring reproductive rights backed by quality healthcare services, it will be rather difficult to achieve a breakthrough on the process of women empowerment. The paper also suggests that women centered reproductive healthcare may alter patriarchal constructs despite strong structural resistance. The paper uses the data provided by the National Family Health Surveys and the Reproductive Health Study conducted in the slums to present its argument.

Keywords: *Empowering women, Health, Poor performing states, Ferility and infertility.*

Introduction

The Government of India had ushered in the new millennium by declaring the year 2001 as "Women's Empowerment Year" to focus on a vision 'where women are equal partners like me'. The last few decades have witnessed some changes in the status and role of women in the country. However, on considering some of the basic parameters of progress and development, one finds the lack of education, poor health conditions and discrimination in opportunities for work and income, still haunt women in India in general and particularly in its poor performing and States. It appears most of women still wear the restrictive chains that drag them down. There is a need to re-think as how to expedite the process of women empowerment in a patriarchal and traditional society like India (Malhotra *et al.*, 1995).

The word 'empowerment' is often narrowly defined in terms of women's education and employment, both of which have a positive but limited impact on her life. Empowerment, however, covers a large canvas where a woman is enabled to negotiate better space for herself in the family, society and polity. In this paper we find it useful to rely on Naila Kabeer's definition (2001:3): "the expansion in people's (here women) ability to make strategic life choices in a context where this ability was previously denied to them." According to Kabeer, empowerment cannot be reduced to a single aspect of process or outcome. How women exercise choice and the actual outcomes will depend on the individual. Choices will vary across class, time and space

In this paper we seek to explore an alternative approach to empower women in India with a special reference to the poor performing States[1]. It is argued that by ensuring the "basic right to decide freely and responsibly the number and spacing of their children and to have the information, education and means to do so" (UNICPD 1994: Principle 8)[2] could be another but effective way to expedite the process of women empowerment in India. This calls for an efficient but pro-women reproductive healthcare system catering to the needs of women in general and the needy, unprivileged and economic backward sections of humanity in particular. Therefore, addressing inequalities in access to and use of reproductive health services including contraceptive services will be a powerful tool in empowering the women.

The paper uses the data provided by the National Family Health Surveys (NFHSs) and the Reproductive Health Study conducted in the Jawahar Nagar Kachi Basti (slums), Jaipur, Rajasthan in 2010 to suggest a framework for empowering women by

---

1. The poor performing States also known as BIMARU (Hindi for sick) States of Bihar, Madhya Pradesh, Rajasthan and Uttar Pradesh are having very poor reproductive health and gender indicators. These States, comprising around 40 per vent of India population, have high fertility, high maternal and infant mortality, low contraceptive prevalence, low female literacy and a poor sex ratio amid poor socio economic development. These States, along with nine other States, are officially called as the "Focus States" in the National Rural Health Mission (NRHM), which was constituted in the Ministry of Health and Family Welfare, Government of India in April 2005.
2. In 1994, at the International Conference on Population and Development (ICPD) held in Cairo, 179 countries accepted this principle. For details see UNICPD, 1994.

meeting their reproductive health needs. The use of reproductive health services by women particular poor women, measured in terms of antenatal care, immunization and contraceptive practices, shows a wide variation across the States of India. On the basis of this, the States of India could be divided into two categories: Poor Performing and Better Performing. The information collected from Rajasthan[3] - one of the poor performing States, and Andhra Pradesh[4] - one of the better performing States has been used to make the point. It is interesting to note that although these two States differ significantly as far as use of reproductive health services is concerned, there is no difference on the literacy front: 61 per cent versus 61 per cent, as revealed by the Census of India 2001.

The NFHS programme, initiated in the early nineties, has emerged as an important source of data on population, health, especially reproductive health and nutrition for India and its States. The NFHS-3 (2005-06) was preceded by NFHS-1 in 1992-93 and NFHS-2 in 1998-99. The NFHS-3 collected information from a nationally representative sample of 109, 041 households, 1,24,385 currently married women age 15-49 and 74,369 men age 15-54. The NFHS-3 sample covers 99 per cent of India's population living in 29 States. Field work for NFHS-3 was conducted from November 2005 to August 2006[5].

Additionally, a reproductive health study was conducted by the Forum for Population Action[6] in the largest slum area of Jaipur, the capital city of Rajasthan, India, to understand the poor women's perceptions about fertility control and their decision-making within the context of their family dynamics and complex realities. A total of 392 currently married women aged 15-49 were studied in the late 2009 to understand their fertility behavior. The study made use of individual interviews and focus-group discussions. During group discussions, women felt comfortable as the

---

3. The State of Rajasthan has an area of 3,42,239 sq. km. and a population of 56.51 million (2001). There are 33 districts, 237 blocks and 41353 villages. The State has population density of 165 per sq. km. (as against the national average of 312). The decadal growth rate of the State is 28.41% (against 21.54% for the country) and the population of the State continues to grow at a much faster rate than the national rate. For details, see: Kothari, Devendra. "Stalled Demographic Transition In Rajasthan: Implications for Sustainable Development, in Vijay Vyas et al. (eds), Rajasthan: the Quest for Sustainable Development. Academic Foundations, New Delhi, 2007. pp. 101-28.

4 The State of Andhra Pradesh has an area of 2.75,045 sq. km. and a population of 76.21 million (2001). There are 23 districts, 1128 blocks and 28,123 villages. The State has population density of 277 per sq. km. (as against the national average of 312). The decadal growth rate of the State is 14.59% and the population of the State is growing at a slower rate than the national rate. For details, see: Mahendra Dev S. Inclusive Growth in Andhra Pradesh: Challenges in Agriculture, Poverty, Social Sector and Regional Disparities. Working Paper No. 71. Centre for Economic and Social Studies, Hyderabad, 2007.

5. For details, see India: National Family Health Survey (NFHS-3) 2005-06. IIPS, Mumbai, 2007.

6. The Forum for Population Action (FPA), a registered society, came into existence in the year 2000. It works towards population stabilization in the broader concept of reproductive rights and informed choice by providing a platform for advocacy, development and promotion of alternative and innovative measures. The Management Board, which manages the Forum, includes public servants, representatives of Industry & Trade, NGOs, journalists, demographers, etc. as its members. For details, contact: the Director, Forum for Population Action at kothari42@dataone.in .

group setting was in their own locality and most of them came from similar cultural backgrounds. These discussions were informally structured with a checklist of open ended questions. The focus group discussions lasted around 2 to 3 hours each. In total 10 focused group discussions were planned involving 100 women, selected randomly from the list of women interviewed. The study followed the ethics of ensuring privacy and confidentiality of the women[7].

Women Empowerment: A Reality or Myth

Since the 1980's the Government of India has shown increasing concern for women's issues through a variety of legislations, promoting the education and political participation of women (Collier 1998). International organizations like the World Bank and United Nations have focused on women's issues especially the empowerment of poor women in rural areas. The non-governmental organizations have also taken on an increased role in the area of women's empowerment (Handya and Kassamb 2004). In spite of all these efforts, the gender gap in India runs deep, as revealed by the Global Gender Gap Report 2009 released by the World Economic Forum[8]. India ranks pathetically at 114 among the 134 countries considered. For the emerging markets group countries comprising of Brazil, Russia, India and China (BRIC), in terms of the overall Gender Gap Index, Russia (51) leads the way, followed by China (60), Brazil (81) and India (114). The Gender Gap Index rankings reveal the following order of performance within South Asia: Sri Lanka (16), Bangladesh (93), Maldives (100), Nepal (110), India (114) and Pakistan (132). That is a shameful reflection of the condition of the women in a country that is on a growth song.

The condition of women in India has undoubtedly improved since independence. However, the extent of this improvement is limited and mainly confined to the middle classes. According to Professor Beteille,[9], "the middle class family has become more supportive of the education of its daughters and their ambitions for professional development". It was perceived that the lower social class will follow the trend. The "trickle-down" mechanism, however, could not work in general. Even among the middle class families, Professor Beteille observes further that this change has been very slow and "it has benefited only a small proportion of women, mainly in the educated middle class and that too in metropolitan cities". Women from this class have achieved remarkable success and are piecing the glass ceiling, but they are still the exceptions.

---

7. For details, see; The Status of Reproductive Health in Jawahar Nagar Kacchi Basti (Slums), Jaipur, India. Forum for Population Action, Jaipur, 2010.
8. The Global Gender Gap Index, introduced by the World Economic Forum in 2006, is a framework for capturing the magnitude and scope of gender-based disparities and tracking their progress. The Index benchmarks national gender gaps on economic, political, education- and health based criteria, and provide country rankings that allow for effective comparisons across regions and income groups, and over time. For details, see: The Global Gender Gap Report 2009, World Economic Forum, Geneva, Switzerland, 2009.
9. Dr. Andre Beteille is professor emeritus of sociology, University of Delhi. For detail, see: "Look for Real Solutions", Times of India, Monday, March 29, 2010.

There are several reasons behind this situation. While formulating or implementing women programmes, we generally consider Indian women as a close-knit "homogeneous" group. However, one has to recognize that women do not constitute a homogenous group, and all women are not equal. Ours is not only a deeply caste-divided society, it is also a deeply class-divided one. Overall, women are more 'disadvantaged' due to the overall status of caste, economic status and religion within which they are placed. The quota within quota demand in the Women's Reservation Bill indicates that women do not constitute a homogenous group[10].

One of the background characteristics used throughout the NFHS-3 Report is an index of the economic status of households called the Wealth Index. The economic status index was constructed using 33 household asset data and housing characteristics[11]. The Table 5.1 provides some basic information about women by this index. The table reveals that differences by economic status are large for every selected variable. For example, only 11 per cent of women in the lowest economic strata have completed standard six and above of education, compared with 84 per cent of women in the highest economic class. The table also indicates that women belonging to lowest strata suffer most. Unless we focus on this segment, which constitutes around two-third of total female population, achieving women's empowerment within a reasonable time span will be a dream. Here the 'Bottom of the Pyramid' approach, coined by Prof. CK Prahlad (2006), could be of great help. In other words, we need not only area-specific but also class-specific measures to empower women in India.

Table 5.1: Distribution of Currently Married Women (15-49) by Selected Indicators according to Household Economic Status, 2005-06

Indicators	*Economic Status*			
	Lowest	*Middle*	*Highest*	*All*
Completed standard 6 and above (per cent)	11	37	84	45
Median age at first marriage (Years)	15	16	20	17
Institutional deliveries (per cent of total)	13	39	84	39
Birth order 4+ (per cent)	42	21	06	25
Number of children per woman (TFR)	3.9	2.6	1.8	2.7
Protected by modern contraceptives (per cent)	35	50	58	48

Source: National Family Health Survey- 3, 2005-06, IIPS, Mumbai 2007.

10. The Women's Reservation Bill has been a political raw nerve for more than a decade now. It has always triggered heated debates in Parliament and outside. Its advocates say it would lead to gender equality in Parliament, resulting in the empowerment of women as a whole. Opponents argue that reservation would only help women of elitist groups gain political power, aggravating the plight of the poor and deprived sections. The proposed legislation aims to reserve 33 % seats in Parliament and State legislatures for women. The Bill was introduced in the Lok Sabha on September 12, 1996. Though it has been introduced in Parliament several times since then, the Bill could not be passed because of lack of political consensus.
11. For details, see India: National Family Health Surrey (NFHS-3), 2005-06, IIPS, Mumbai, 2007.

How to Forge Ahead?

The India Gender Gap Review 2009, a supplement of The Global Gender Gap Report 2009 indicates that between 2006 and 2009, Indian women and girls have narrowed the gap with men and boys on education, economic and political participation; relative to men, however, "they are slipping further on health" (WEFa 2009:11). It is because they have unequal access to basic health resources especially reproductive healthcare services and lack adequate counseling as well as follow-up and management of side effects. The result is an increasing risk of unintended or unwanted, early pregnancies, HIV infection and other sexually transmitted diseases. Further, as per NFHS-3, around a third of married women are below 18 year, the legal age for them to get married. This in turn, leads to a disturbing result – over 54 per cent of pregnant women are anemic, locking the child they are carrying into a health deficit in the womb itself. Just 23 per cent of women get required iron and folic acid supplements, and only about half of them get the required three or more antenatal check-ups from the health workers (NFHS-3 2007).

Furthermore, available studies indicate that women in poor performing States by and large, no matter how poor or subjugated they may be, have a strong desire to control their fertility. However, as per the latest National Family Health Survey (NFHS-3 2007), every fifth birth has been classified as unplanned or unintended (that is mistimed or unwanted at the time the women became pregnant). It is estimated that more than 26 million children are born in India every year and out of this about 5.5 million births have been classified as unplanned. Approximately two-thirds of the unintended pregnancies resulted from non-use of contraceptives; clearly indicating the need for revamping the Family Welfare Programme. In addition, around one-third of unintended pregnancies resulted from the ineffective use of contraceptives, which suggests the need for improved counseling and follow-up of couples that adopt the method (Kothari and Tewari 2009).

The level of unwanted fertility can also be measured by comparing the total wanted fertility rate with the total or actual fertility rate. The total wanted fertility rate represents the level of fertility that theoretically would result if all unwanted births were prevented. The proportion of births that were unwanted was the highest for births to women from the "bottom of pyramid". Table 5.2 reveals that in India, the total wanted fertility rate of 2.4 children per woman, belonging to the lowest economic strata is lower by 1.5 children (that is by 38 per cent) than the actual or total fertility of 3.9 children per woman. This means the women belonging to low economic strata have more children than they actually want and this can be seen throughout the country (NFHS-3 2007). The table also indicates that the level of unwanted fertility decreases sharply among women from the lowest economic strata to the women in the wealthiest strata from 1.5 children per woman to 0.3 children per woman. One can argue that total fertility rate would drop substantially among women from the lower strata if their unwanted fertility could be eliminated.

Table 5.2: Level of Unwanted Births per Woman by Economic Status, Selected States, 2005-06

Economic Status	*Rajasthan*		*Andhra Pradesh*		*India*	
	Actual Number of Children/ Woman	*Number of Unwanted Children/ Woman*	*Actual Number of Children/ Woman*	*Number of Unwanted Children/ Woman*	*Actual Number of Children/ Woman*	*Number of Unwanted Children/ Woman*
Lowest	4.5	1.6	2.4	0.5	3.9	1.5
Middle	3.1	0.9	1.8	0.3	2.6	0.8
Highest	2.1	0.4	1.5	0.2	1.8	0.3
All	3.2	1.0	1.8	0.3	2.7	0.8

Source: National Family Health Survey-3, 2005-06, IIPS, Mumbai, 2007.

Unmet need for family planning[12] is an important indicator of assessing the potential demand for family planning services. In spite of poverty and illiteracy, the prevailing unmet need for family planning services is surprising, especially in the lower economic strata. Table 5.3 indicates that unmet need for family planning decreases with an increase in economic status of households. The table also indicates that poor performing States like Rajasthan have much more unmet need for family planning services as compared to better performing States like Andhra Pradesh: 15 per cent versus 5 per cent. In other poor performing States like Bihar and Uttar Pradesh, more than 22 per cent of married women have unmet need for family planning services, and overwhelming proportion of them belong to lower economic strata (NFHS-3 2007).

Table 5.3: Level of Unmet Need for Contraception by Economic Status, Selected States 2005-06

Economic Status	*Level of Unmet Need for Family Planning Services (per cent)*		
	Rajasthan	*Andhra Pradesh*	*India*
Lowest	18.6	06.5	18.2
Middle	15.1	04.0	12.8
Highest	09.1	02.1	08.1
All	14.6	04.7	12.8

Source: National Family Health Survey-3, 2005-06, IIPS, Mumbai, 2007.

12. The standard definition of unmet need depends upon the apparent inconsistency between a woman's contraceptive behavior and her Stated reproductive preferences. The concept of unmet need was highlighted first time in India in a study conducted by the author in Rajasthan in 1988 on behalf of Ministry of Health and Family Welfare, Government of India. Based on the field data, the study revealed that there was sizable number of eligible couples that were not using contraceptive methods but did not want another child. According to the study, 15 % of currently married couple in Rajasthan had unmet need for family planning services in 1988-89. For details, see Devendra Kothari, Family Planning Programme in Rajasthan: Beyond the Existing Approach, Indian Institute of Health Management Research, Jaipur, 1989.

It appears that in the changed situation most of the women, belonging to the lower economic strata, do not want more children. But, they still have them, primarily due to their 'subordinate' position in the family as well as due to in complete control over the reproductive process because of lack of client centered reproductive healthcare. During the focused group discussions in the Kacchi Basti, it was observed that most of the women with large number of children are dependent on their husbands and other family members. Usually in such a situation, the social identity and status of women is tied to that of their husband. Because of this dependence (or powerlessness) women find little space to express their opinions, or make decisions, whether for their own life or the family. The reflection of her subordinate position or low status is particularly more glaring when it comes to matters of sexuality and reproduction, since these directly threaten to challenge the power equations. If such a challenge is posed, it is ruthlessly dealt with. It is thus not coincidence that wife beating or domestic violence has been found to be most common form of violence in India. The findings of NFHS-3 corroborate this observation. Table 5.4 clearly shows that prevalence of emotional, physical or sexual violence does vary by economic status. It declines sharply from a high of 52 per cent for women in the lowest strata to a low of 21 per cent for women in the highest strata. Despite differentials by economic strata, these data suggest high rates of all forms of violence in even the wealthiest households in the poor performing States like Rajasthan.

Table 5.4: Percentage of Married Women in Reproductive Ages who have Experienced Emotional, Physical, or Sexual Violence Committed by their Husbands by Economic Status, some Selected States, 2005-06

Economic Status	*Percentage of Women Experienced Domestic Violence*		
	Rajasthan	*Andhra Pradesh*	*India*
Lowest	52	45	52
Middle	50	41	42
Highest	39	18	21
All	50	37	40

Source: National Family Health Survey-3, 2005-06, IIPS, Mumbai, 2007.

It is interesting to note that the prevalence of domestic violence increases with the number of children. Table 5.5 shows that one in two women with five or more children report have experienced some form of domestic violence. Why this violence against women? Experts believe that as tradition-bound practices and belief systems crack up under pressure from socio-economic changes and women try to become less submissive and pliant, the entrenched ideology of domination will desperately fight against what is seen as a threat. And, the primary weapon for that is physical, emotion or sexual violence (Varma 2010).

During the focus group discussions, it was observed that most of the women in the Kacchi Basti are keen to control fertility, as shown by the prevailing unmet need for family planning services. But, they are not in position to do so since the existing family planning programme is not in a position to serve the women. It appears that the existing reproductive healthcare is a source of frustration for women in general and poor in particular. Women in the study area in a resounding manner reported dissatisfaction with their hospitals and health centers as well as doctors and health workers. Seventy per cent of married women aged 20-29 were dissatisfied with the reproductive healthcare services provided by the public health institutions located in the area. More specially, they were irritated by the amount of time they spent waiting for doctors and nursing staff. Making matters worse, women generally pay for reproductive services provided by the private hospitals and/clinics. Further, there is rampant inability of the current reproductive healthcare delivery infrastructure to meet the basic requirements for proper screening, counseling, administration, follow up and managements of side effects of contraceptives.

Table 5.5: Percentage of Married Women Age 15-49 who have Experienced Domestic Violence Committed by their Husbands by Number of Living Children, Selected States, 2005-06

Number of Living Children	*Rajasthan*	*Andhra Pradesh*	*India*
0	38	31	31
1-2	45	34	35
3-4	54	42	44
5+	61	42	52
All	50	37	40

Source: National Family Health Survey-3, 2005-06, IIPS, Mumbai, 2007

Smaller families are slowly becoming the norm in India. Fertility has continued to decline since NFHS-2, dropping to an average of 2.7 children per woman in NFHS-3 from 2.9 children per woman, though the rate of decline was slow. For the first time ever around, half of the currently married women in reproductive ages in India are using modern contraception. However, its use increased slowly from 43 per cent to 49 per cent between NFHS-2 and NFHS-3. Economic status has a positive effect on contraceptive use, with use increasing from 35 per cent among married women in households in the lowest economic strata to 58 per cent among those in the highest strata. The use of any three modern spacing methods (The Pills, IUCD, and Condom are the part of government family planning programme) increased sharply from 4 per cent among women in the lowest strata to 22 per cent among in the highest one (Table 5.6). The use of condoms increased sharply from 1 per cent among men in the lowest economic strata to 3 per cent among men in the middle strata to 13 per cent among the men in the highest strata. This indicates that the use of existing spacing methods is not very popular among women and men belonging to lower economic strata mainly due to lack of choice and follow up, as well as management of the ensuing side effects. Such a situation leaves couples with no choice except sterilization. This choice is not widely preferred by couples in the light of prevailing of high infant and child mortality[13].

Table 5.6: Percentage Distribution of Married Women in Reproductive Ages using Modern Contraception by Economic Status, Selected Status, 2005-06

Economic Status	*Rajasthan*		*Andhra Pradesh*		*India*	
	Modern Methods	*Spacing Methods*	*Modern Methods*	*Spacing Methods*	*Modern Methods*	*Spacing*
Lowest	28	3	60	(0.1)	35	4
Middle	42	6	66	(0.3)	50	7
Highest	63	24	74	5	58	22
All	44	9	67	1	49	10

Source: National Family Health Survey-3, 2005-06, IIPS, Mumbai, 2007.

The Family Welfare Programme of India offers limited contraceptive choices like IUCD, oral pills, male condom, tubal ligation and vasectomy. There is a substantial unmet need of 13 per cent for contraception; of which about 50 per cent is for spacing methods (NFHS-3, 2007). There is an urgent need to give a 'wider choice' of contraceptives including injectables to young women in order to enable them to decide when a pregnancy would be most convenient for them. In other words, the wider choice of contraceptives will give every woman total control over her own body, thus freeing her from many patriarchal constraints.

The findings of the group discussions indicate that women in the Kacchi Basti want wider choice of methods like injectable contraceptives to be part of the official Family Welfare Programme to improve 'choice' and 'convenience'[14]. Although injectable contraceptives have been kept out of the programme for even now, they are available in the private health sector. In our study area a large number of women knew about injectable contraceptives and some of them were using Depo-Provera, an injectable contraceptive (once in three months), though they found it expensive. However they considered it more convenient in comparison with taking pills every day, or inserting an IUCD or telling their husbands to use condom. The women of the

---

13. Households in the highest economic strata experienced only one-third of the under-five mortality rate of household in the lowest strata (NFHS-3, 2007). This is mainly due to the poor coverage of immunization, especially in poor performing States. Overall, there was only a small improvement in full vaccination coverage, with 44 % of children ages 12-23 months receiving all recommended vaccinations in 2005-06, up from 42 % seven year ago.

14. It may be noted that the injectable contraceptive Depo-Provera was approved for marketing by Government of India in 1993. However, women's groups launched an intensive campaign against the introduction of injectables and succeeded in filing a petition in the Supreme Court, seeking a ban on such contraceptives. After much lobbying and pressure from women's groups, in early January 2002, The Ministry of Health and Family Welfare, Government of India finally dropped its plan to introduce injectables in the Family Welfare Programme. Although injectables like Depo-Provera are not included in the Family Welfare Programme of India, the doctors are prescribing them.

study area were convinced that an injectable is actually a more convenient means of contraception than the existing ones. One of the women told in the group discussion:

> *"I was not keen on the third child since I was already having two children - a boy and a girl. I had a lot of arguments with my husband because of this. I tried to convince him, but in vain. I came to know about injection from my friend and took it from the local clinic Aadhar (a clinic run by the Parivar Seva in the Basti). I had some health problems like bleeding, back pain, nausea, joint pain and headache. Despite these problems, for me the injection was a blessing, as I was relieved from conceiving again and again".*

Although injectable contraceptives are not included in the Family Welfare Programme of India, it is surprising that more than half of the currently married women are aware of this spacing method. And in some poor performing States like Uttar Pradesh, the awareness was more than 80 per cent among women. Further, the proportion of women who know about injectable contraceptives increased significantly from 19 per cent in NFHS-1 to 52 per cent in NFHS-3. And the level of awareness is relatively high among women belonging to lower strata. Although the use of injectable contraceptives is extremely low in India, it is relatively more popular among the women belonging to lowest strata (NFHS-3, 2007).

The foregoing analysis indicates that incomplete control over the reproductive process leads to relatively high levels of unwanted childrearing. There is little doubt that women are in dire need of contraceptives that are both convenient and safe. India's Family Welfare Programme has largely failed to encourage the use of effective reversible methods, particularly among young women who are in the most fertile years of their reproductive period, and are most prone to unplanned pregnancies. As such, there is an urgent need to make the management of reproductive health service delivery more responsive to the women, and this will a "powerful tool in the battle to reduce the adverse outcomes of unintended and unwanted pregnancy" (Ortayli and Malarcher 2010: 107). In other words, "sexual and reproductive health and rights can be mere words unless they are backed by functional policies and servicers that include a full range of safe and effective family planning methods and the contraceptives and abortion information and services to fulfill individuals' choices" (Sen 2010:143). And for this, one must focus attention on the lacunae in reproductive healthcare, as argued by the well known community health physician- Dr. Saroj Pachauri[15].

Discussion and Conclusion

The consequences of unintended pregnancy are serious, imposing significant burden on women and families, and in turn slowing down the process of women's empowerment. Unintended pregnancy breeds powerlessness and powerlessness breeds subordination (quality of obedient submissiveness) and subordination breeds unintended pregnancy and women find themselves in a vicious circle, as shown below;

---

15. For details, see: Saroj Pachauri , "Investing in Women", Times of India, August 4, 2010, p.12

Unwanted Pregnancies and Women Empowerment

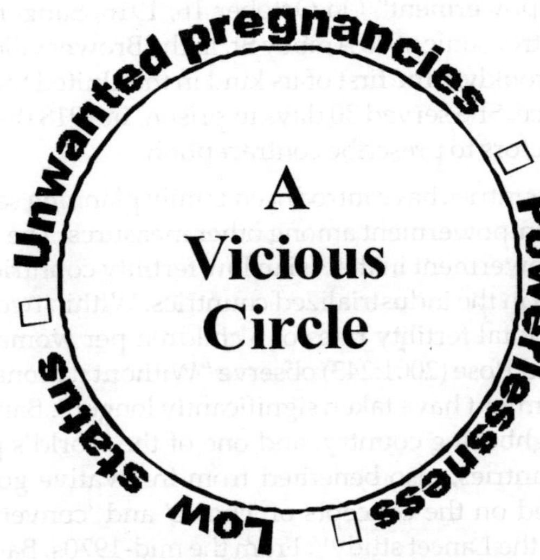

There is only one cure for women to come out from the vicious circle, and that is to stop breeding powerlessness. In a patriarchal society, where power relations make women passive and subordinate, reproductive technology can help them to break this vicious circle. It appears that the reproductive healthcare is an important pre-requisite to create an environment where people especially women can take decisions regarding the number, timing and spacing of their children. For example, in the early twentieth century women in the developed countries including USA raised the movement to have pro-women family planning services to have children by choice. They held very rightly that women could never be free if they are not given the right to protect their body. Margaret Sanger[16], who did a lot to establish the birth control movement in the United States to empower women, said: "A woman must have her freedom, the fundamental freedom of choosing whether or not she will be a mother and how many children she will have. Regardless of what man's attitude may be,

16. Margaret Higgins Sanger Slee (September 14, 1879 – September 6, 1966) was an American birth control activist, and the founder of the American Birth Control League. As Sanger worked in New York's Lower East Side slums with poor women who were repeatedly suffering due to frequent childbirth and self induced abortions, she began to speak out for the need of women to become knowledgeable about birth control. Sanger felt that in order for women to have more "equal footing" in society and to have physically and mentally healthy lives, they needed to be able to decide when a pregnancy would be most convenient for themselves. For details, see: Sangar, Margaret. The New Motherhood. London: Jonathan Cape, 1922. Also see: Sanger, Margaret, An Autobiography. New York: Cooper Square Press, 1938.

that problem is here - and before it can be his, it is hers alone. She goes through the vale of death alone, each time a baby is born. As it is neither the right of the man nor of the State to coerce her into this ordeal, so it is her right to decide whether she will endure it". She observes further: "Birth control is the means by which women attain basic freedom and empowerment" On October 16, 1916, Sanger opened a family planning and birth control clinic at 46 Amboy St. in the Brownsville neighborhood (a slum community) of Brooklyn, the first of its kind in the United States. It was raided 9 days later by the police. She served 30 days in prison. In 1918 the New York Court of Appeals allowed doctors to prescribe contraception.

Since then many countries have introduced family planning services to expedite the process of women empowerment among other measures. The fertility transition as well as women empowerment in the Asian low fertility countries has occurred at a much faster pace than in the industrialized countries. Within two to three decades, fertility declined from total fertility rates of 6 children per woman to replacement fertility of 2.1. Frejka and Rose (2001:243) observe "Without national family planning programs, this decline might have taken significantly longer". Bangladesh, which is India's immediate neighboring country, and one of the world's poorest and most densely populated countries, also benefited from innovative government family planning policies, based on the concepts of 'choice' and 'convenience', says John Cleland, lead author of the Lancet study[17]. From the mid-1970s, Bangladesh adopted a community-based approach, recruiting married, literate village women trained in basic medicine and family planning to go door-to-door dispensing contraceptives and referring women for clinical contraception. The approach was successful. Fertility rates in Bangladesh halved from about six children per women in the early 1970s to three children per women now. And it has had a positive impact on the status of women.

In 1952, the Indian Government was one of the first in the world to formulate a National Family Planning Programme which was later expanded to encompass maternal and child health, and nutrition. The family planning programme, officially known as "Family Welfare Programme", is a centrally sponsored programme. The States receive 100 per cent assistant from the Government of India for the purpose as per approved plans. The policy principles are laid by the Centre. The administration and implementation of the programme is organized through an integrated structure of health and family welfare services at the States. Within the general policy guidelines framed by the Centre, the States have a measure of flexibility to adopt the programme according to local conditions and requirements. They can make changes in the framework within which they have to operate. Here the political and administrative will of a State government can play an important role in the success of the programme. Andhra Pradesh is one such example. During the early nineties, the State government decided to revamp its reproductive healthcare delivery system looking to the needs of

17. John Cleland. 2008. Defusing The Population Bomb: *Bangladesh* Vs. Pakistan , *the Lancet study.*

women[18]. It was a political decision and this increased the use of reproductive health services significantly. As per the NFHS-3, two-thirds of married women in Andhra Pradesh used modern contraception in 2005-06, one of the highest rates in India. It had dramatic impact on fertility by reducing unwanted pregnancies. Andhra Pradesh, along with Tamil Nadu, exhibits the lowest fertility among major States of India[19] – 1.8 children per woman. It is interesting to note that women with no education or less than 5 years of education are more likely to use contraception than women with more education, since reproductive health services are easily available looking to the needs of clients. As a result, only 5 per cent of currently married women have an unmet need for family planning, down from 8 per cent in NFHS-2 and 10 per cent in NFHS-1. Currently, 94 per cent of the demand for family planning is being satisfied, up from 82 per cent in NFHS-1. The impact of client centered reproductive healthcare could be seen from a comparison of the birth order distribution in NFHS-1, NFHS-2, and NFHS-3 for married women. The proportions of births of order four or higher decreased from 22 per cent in NFHS-1 to 15 per cent in NFHS-2 and 10 per cent in NFHS-3. All these had an impact on the level of unwanted fertility. Andhra Pradesh recorded one of the lowest unwanted children per woman in India as per NFHS-3 (0.3 children per woman), as shown in Table 5.7. Not only in family planning but in other areas of reproductive healthcare, Andhra Pradesh has done equally well. In the State, 85 per cent of women had at least three antenatal care visits for their last birth. About two-thirds of children in Andhra Pradesh who were born in the past five years were delivered in a health facility.

By managing the reproductive healthcare looking to the needs of 'the bottom of pyramid', Andhra Pradesh was able to bring significant changes in basic reproductive health variables in nineties, and this in turn has improved the status of women measured in the terms of participation in decision making[20] and the level of domestic violence (Table 5.7). In the NFHS-3, married women were asked who made decisions

---

18. Among many initiatives of the Government of Andhra Pradesh, the establishment of "Round the Clock Women Health Centres" wan an important one. 470 PHCs (Primary Health Centres) in the backward areas have been designed as Round the Clock Women Health Centres in the nineties. Normal delivery services are being provided round the clock in these centres by nursing staff of PHC. 450 ANMs (as well as doctors) have been taken on contract in these PHCs. Specialist clinics by Gynecologist and Pediatrician are being provided in these institutions on a fixed day once in a week. Additional facilities like telephone and vehicle for transportation are also provided to improve communication and referral system for emergency cases. For detail, see document: Brief of the Family Welfare Department, Office of Commissioner of Family Welfare, Government of Andhra Pradesh, Hyderabad, 20.06.2003.

19. The major States are those having total population of 25 million or more. There were 14 such States in India, as per the Census of India 2001.

20. The ability of women to make decisions that affect the circumstances of their own lives is an essential aspect of empowerment. In order to assess women's decision- making autonomy, NFHS-3 collected information from married women (15-49) on their participation in four different types of decisions: their own healthcare, making large household purchases, making purchases for daily household needs, and visiting their family or relatives. Women were asked who usually makes each decision. Available data indicate that in our society women does not play important role in decision-making, though there was a significant difference between States.

about their own healthcare, major household purchases, purchases for daily household needs, and visiting their own family or relatives. More than half of currently married women in Andhra Pradesh (53-66 per cent) reported participating in making each of these decisions. And around 40 per cent participated in making all four decisions. The level of domestic violence could be another indicator of women's empowerment. In all, 34 per cent of women age 15-49 in Andhra Pradesh have experienced physical, emotional or sexual violence. Although it appears to be high, it was significantly lower as compared to Rajasthan.

Table 5.7: Reproductive Health Variables and Status of Women, Selected States of India, 2005-06

Indicators	*Rajasthan*	*Andhra Pradesh*
A. Variables indicating reproductive health status		
☆ Number of children per woman	3.2	1.8
☆ Number of unwanted children per woman	1.0	03
☆ Women with birth order 4+ (per cent)	35	08
☆ Couples using modern contraceptives (per cent)	44	67
☆ Pregnant women received 3 + antenatal care visits	41	64
☆ Children 12-23 months old fully immunized (per cent)	26	59 (NFHS-2)
B. Variables indicating status of women empowerment		
☆ Women alone or jointly with their husbands made all four decisions* (per cent)	23	41
☆ Women experienced emotional, physical, or sexual violence	46	34
C. Source of female sterilization		
☆ Public hospitals/clinics	94	78
☆ Private hospitals/clinics	06	22

Source: National Family Health Survey-3, 2005-06, IIPS, Mumbai, 2007.

Note: * Four types of decisions: 1.Own healthcare, 2. Making large household purchases, 3. Making purchases for daily household needs, and 4. Visiting their family or relatives.

Andhra Pradesh Family Welfare Programme has made remarkable progress over the last ten to fifteen years due to continuous political and administrative commitment, innovative programme approach, government and non-government collaboration, strong IEC programme, and commitment of the field-level functionaries. The programme has also taken into account women's isolation and dependence.

On the other hand, fertility in Rajasthan is the third highest among the major States of India. The largest differentials in fertility are by economic status and education. At current fertility rates, women with no education will have twice as many children as women with 10 or more years of schooling (3.7 children per woman compared with 1.8). Among the major States of India, total unwanted fertility is the third highest in Rajasthan (one child per woman). Despite a 15 per cent age point increase in current contraceptive use among currently married women since NFHS-1, less than 45 per cent of women in Rajasthan are currently using any modern contraceptive method. Around 15 per cent of married women in Rajasthan have an unmet need for family planning, down from 18 per cent in NFHS-2. Currently, 76 per cent of the demand for family planning is being met, up from 70 per cent in NFHS-2 and 62 per cent in NFHS-1. The distribution of births by order is yet another way to view fertility and performance of reproductive healthcare service delivery system. Around one third of total births in Rajasthan in 2005-06 were of order four or higher, which was the third highest among the major States of India. Further, no significant decline was seen in the higher order births between NFHS-2 and NFHS-3: 34 per cent versus 32 per cent. Despite substantial improvement in the coverage of antenatal care for mothers, only 4 in 10 women in Rajasthan received at least three antenatal care visits for their last birth in the past five years. The per cent age of births in Rajasthan delivered in a health facility is much lower than the national average. Full immunization coverage is lower in Rajasthan than in any other State except Uttar Pradesh. A little more than one-quarter (27 per cent) of children age 12-23 months are fully vaccinated against six major childhood illnesses: tuberculosis, diphtheria, pertussis, tetanus, polio, and measles.

The poor reproductive health status had an adverse impact in the process of women empowerment in Rajasthan. Only 23 per cent women participate in making all four decisions as compared with 41 per cent in Andhra Pradesh. Further, the percentage of ever-married women who have experienced domestic violence is higher in Rajasthan than in any other State except Bihar- another poor performing State.

The above discussion indicates that meeting women's demand for reproductive healthcare, as in case of Andhra Pradesh, increases the health and stability of their families, and results in women's empowerment over time. On the other hand, as it stands, the public reproductive healthcare in Rajasthan does not reach everyone, and even where it does it is stretched to the limit. The system is also plagued by lack of trained healthcare providers, which impedes delivery of services. Further, the private sector has not been encouraged to come in. It appears that the poor performing States are reluctant to encourage the private sector involvement.

While population of India continues to grow by 16-17 million people annually, 25 million women, mostly in poor performing States, seek to postpone childbearing, space births, or stop having children, but are not using a modern method of contraception Often, these women travel far from their communities to reach a health facility, only to return home "empty handed"[21] due to shortages and stock outs[22],

21. Population Action International (PAI) is an international non governmental organization that utilizes research and advocacy to improve global access to family planning and reproductive healthcare. Empty Handed, a documentary produced by PAI, tells the story of women's lack of access to reproductive health supplies in sub-Saharan Africa, and its impact on their lives. The film documents the challenges at each level of the supply chain and identifies key areas for improvement.

22. At the time of writing of this paper (July 2010), the Jawahar Nagar Kacchi Basti, the study area, has been suffering from the acute shortage of spacing methods like condoms and pills as well as iron folic acid tablets for last six months , as reported by the Public Health Workers working in this area.

and/or non availability of doctors and paramedical staff[23]. To make matters worse, most doctors hardly turn up to these centres. When women seeking family planning services are turned away, they are unable to protect themselves from unwanted/ unplanned pregnancies and sexually transmitted infections, including HIV/AIDs. This type of situation leads to relatively high levels of unwanted childrearing. Around 26 million children are born in India every year and out of this about 5.5 million births have been classified as unplanned.

We have to agree that the poor performing States of India have neglected the reproductive health programme. Had the poor performing States been meticulous enough to provide client centered reproductive health services and to frame appropriate policies to manage the programme, India could have, by now, improved the status of women and reduced the gender gap significantly, as observed in many developing countries (WEF 2009). The paper argues that ongoing challenges in obtaining reproductive healthcare can have devastating consequences on our way to empower women and to break the vicious circle. Expedition of the process of women's empowerment by ensuring reproductive rights, backed by quality reproductive healthcare, as has been seen in the Andhra Pradesh, is a proven, effective way to improve the prospects of women's empowerment, and by that coin, society at large.

In conclusion, the paper aims to provoke discussion and mobilize support for reproductive health services to expedite the process of women empowerment in order to reduce the gender gap. In the changed situation, most women in India do not want more children, but that they have them is mainly due to non-availability and inaccessibility of quality reproductive healthcare services. They have been trapped in a vicious circle. The women need help to have children by choice and not by chance. This requires steady political as well as administrative will, which sadly has, so far, been inconsistent. The need of the hour, thus, is to create confidence among policy makers and programme managers that a breakthrough is possible by adopting a feminist agenda for women's empowerment. There is no need to implement coercive measures or to provide incentives and disincentives. The real need is to provide services in un-served and underserved areas by realigning the capacity of health system to deliver quality care to suit the needs of clients, especially those belonging to the "bottom of pyramid". Therefore, reproductive healthcare is an essential plank in empowering the women. We need creative policies to strengthen this foundation.

The observation of the theatre personality and social activist, Shabana Azmi, appropriately sums this up: "I believe men and women are different not better, nor worse. And the difference needs to be celebrated. For far too long, solutions of all problems have sought to be resolved from male point of view. One has to take women's perspective into account, since women think differently". One has to recognize that

---

23. Throwing light on the abysmal situation of basic healthcare, the latest rural health statistics reveal massive vacancies in primary and community health centres across the country in general and poor performing States in particular. Primary Health Centres, for example, alone have vacant slots for 5,224 doctors, 7,243 healthcare workers and 1701 health assistants. For details, see: Bulletin of Rural Health Statistics- 2009, Ministry of Health and Family Welfare, Government of India, 2010.

women don't need patronage. They need opportunities "to decide freely and responsibly the number and spacing of their children and to have the information, education and means to do so". The paper suggests that the women centered reproductive healthcare may alter patriarchal constructs despite structural resistance, and this alteration is worth the initiative required, both for elevating women's status and for reducing the gender gap. And this feminist agenda will contribute significantly towards women's empowerment.

References

1. Collier, Paul. 1998. Women in Development: Defining the Issues, *Policy, Planning and Research Working Paper 129*, Washington D.C: Population and Human Resources Department, World Bank.
2. Dev, S. Mahendra. 2007. Inclusive Growth in Andhra Pradesh: Challenges in Agriculture, Poverty, Social Sector and Regional Disparities. Working Paper No. 71. Centre for Economic and Social Studies, Hyderabad.
3. Frejka, Thomas and John Ross. 2001. "Path to sub-replacement Fertility: The Empirical Evidence", Population and Development Review, A Supplement to Vol. 27, New York: Population Council, 213-254.
4. Handya, Femida and Meenaz Kassamb. 2004. Women's empowerment in rural India, Paper presented as the ISTR conference, Toronto Canada, July 2004
5. Kabeer, Naila. 2001. "Reflections on the Measurement of Women's Empowerment." In Discussing Women's *Empowerment-Theory and Practice*, Ida Studies No. 3. Novum Grafiska AB: Stockholm.
6. Kothari, Devendra. 2007. "Stalled Demographic Transition in Rajasthan: Implications for Sustainable Development", In Vijay Vyas *et al.* (eds.): Rajasthan: the Quest for Sustainable Development. New Delhi: Academic Foundation, 101-28.
7. Kothari, Devendra and S. Krishnaswamy. 2003. "Poverty, Family Planning and Fertility vis-a vis Management of Family Planning Services in India: A Case Study". In Maria Eugenia COSIO-ZAVALA (Ed.). Poverty, Fertility and Family Planning, Paris: CICRED, 335-58.
8. Kothari, Devendra and Sudha Tewari. 2009. Slowing Population Growth in India: Challenges, Opportunities and the Way Forward. MIPD Policy Brief No. 2, Management Institute of Population and Development, (Parivar Seva Sanstha, New Delhi).
9. Malhotra Anju, Reeve Vanneman, and Sunita Kishor. 1995. Fertility, patriarchy and development in India. Population and Development Review, Vol. 21(20, 281-306.
10. NFHS-1. 1995. India: National Family Health Survey, 1992-93. International Institute for Population Sciences, Mumbai.
11. NFHS-2. 2000. India: National Family Health Survey, 1998-99. International Institute for Population Sciences, Mumbai.

12. NFHS-3. 2007. India: National Family Health Survey, 2005-06. International Institute for Population Sciences, Mumbai.
13. Ortayli, Nuriye and Shawn Malarcher. 2010. "Equity Analysis: Identifying Who Benefits from Family Planning Programs." Studies in Family Planning 41 (2):101-108.
14. PAI. 2010. "Empty Handed", Documentary film produced by Population Action International, Washington D.C.
15. Prahlad, C. K. 2006. The Fortune at the Bottom of Pyramid: Eradicating Poverty through Profit. Pearson Education, Inc.
16. Sen Gita. 2010. "Integrating Family Planning with Sexual and Reproductive Health and Rights: The Past as Prologue", Studies in Family Planning 41 (2):143-146.
17. UNICPD. 1994. Programme of Action, International Conference on Population and Development. 5-13 September, New York: United Nations.
18. WEF. 2009. The Global Gender Gap Report 2009, World Economic Forum, Geneva, Switzerland.
19. WEF. 2009a. The India Gender Gap Review 2009, World Economic Forum, Geneva, Switzerland.

Chapter 6

The Role of Awareness, Comprehension and Attitude Constructs in Behaviour Adoption towards Alleviation of Nutritional Anaemia: A Before-and-After Study of Adolescent School Girls

Sanjana R. Bhat[1] *and Nirupama Prakash*[2]

[1]*Gynaecologist, Medical Centre BITS–Pilani*
Assistant Professor, Pharmacy Group,
Birla Institute of Technology and Science, Pilani, Rajasthan, India
[2]*Group Leader Humanistic Studies,*
Chief, Centre for Women Studies and Societal Development Unit
Co-ordinator, Hospital and Health Systems Management
Birla Institute of Technology and Science, Pilani, Rajasthan, India

ABSTRACT

Objectives

1. To measure the level of awareness, comprehension and attitude (behaviour intention component) of adolescent girls (in residential and in a non-residential school) towards Nutritional anaemia.
2. To measure the level of awareness, comprehension and attitude (behaviour intention component) towards Nutritional anaemia after Direct (nutritional

counselling of students) and Indirect promotional methods (nutritional counselling of teacher's) of Intervention. To compare the relative effectiveness of the direct and indirect methods of promotional interventions.

3. To measure the relative effectiveness of Indirect promotional intervention in the residential and the non-residential school setting.

Material and Methods

A before-and-after study on awareness, comprehension and attitude in behaviour adoption towards nutritional anaemia was undertaken in adolescents studying in a residential and a day school in Pilani. The students of the residential school were divided into two Groups (1 and 2) and subjected to the direct and indirect methods of intervention respectively while those in day school (Group 3) were subjected to indirect intervention only. A pre-tested questionnaire was used to collect the information both before and after the intervention. Results were analysed using paired t-test of difference between means.

Results and Conclusions

Direct method of intervention in a residential school setting leads to a statistically significant increase in awareness about anaemia. In the case of indirect intervention, in a residential setting there is an increase in awareness about anaemia but not about the inhibitors and enhancers of iron absorption, calories provided per gram of different foods or the food types–areas that require expert knowledge. The indirect method of intervention in a day school setting led to a statistically significant increase in awareness about the optimal level of haemoglobin and the effect of menstruation on iron requirement, rich sources of iron, iron-fortified locally available foods–areas that involve transfer of simple information.

Neither the direct nor the indirect method of intervention in either setting(residential or day school) showed any statistically significant increase in comprehension or in behaviour intention to change–as these seem more complex and difficult to change and require perhaps an attitudinal change through other methods.

Keywords: Anaemia, Iron deficiency, Nutritional counselling, Adolescents, Haemoglobin, Awareness.

Introduction

The focus on adolescent health issues gained importance with the declaration of 1985 as the International Year of Youth and when discussions were focussed on the health of the youth in the World health assembly in 1989 (Kurz *et al.*, 1994)

Among adolescents, girls constitute a vulnerable group. India has the dubious distinction of being one of the countries with the highest prevalence of anaemia due to various factors, such as poverty, inadequate diet, and poor availability of iron, chronic blood loss due to hook worm infestation and malaria and lack of access to quality healthcare services. The incidence of iron deficiency among adolescents is on a rise (Maeda M *et al.*, 1999). A multi-center study carried out by Indian Council of Medical Research (ICMR) in 16 districts from 11 states in India showed an overall prevalence of anaemia of 90.1 per cent (Toteja *et al.*, 2003). Even in a developed nation like Britain, a study on 1700 young people showed that 44 per cent of adolescent girls aged 11-19 years had low iron intake (Thane *et al.*, 2003).

The health consequences of anaemia in children and adolescents are well documented. In children anaemia affects their physical growth and mental development. As children mature, anaemia leads to reduced levels of energy and productivity, dip in memory and concentration leading to a fall in academic performance and an impaired immune system making them prone to recurrent infections (Agarwal *et al.*, 1987). Persistent iron deficiency during childhood may have long term consequences in adulthood such as abnormal behaviour (Lazoff B *et al.*, 2001).

The poor nutrition and health status of adolescent girls is often compounded by the socialization factors including discriminatory care practices, early marriage, early and frequent pregnancies. Anaemia during pregnancy leads to high maternal morbidity and mortality and a greater risk of delivering low birth weight babies. Anaemia has inter-generational consequences also (anaemic mothers giving birth to low birth weight infants with low I.Q and stunted growth).

In India, the prevalence of anaemia is almost universal. Data from the district household survey 2004 revealed that 98 per cent of adolescent girls suffer from some form of anaemia. The latest data from National Family Health Survey 3 (NFHS) 2005-06 shows an increasing trend of anaemia in children and women of reproductive age which is a cause of concern as adolescents comprise 22 per cent of India's population. Adolescent girls are our potential mothers. An uncared anaemic adolescent results in an anemic pregnant mother. As pregnancy further increases iron demand, an iron deficit occurs resulting in negative reproductive consequences like premature births and low birth weight babies leading to an increase in perinatal and neonatal mortality. In India anaemia is directly responsible for 20 per cent of maternal deaths while in another 40 per cent it is a contributory factor. 50 per cent of the currently married girls are less than 18 years, 1.5 million girls are married below 15 years, out of which 20 per cent are already mothers.

Despite having so many National programmes for control of anaemia, we have not been able to achieve the desired results. One of the possibilities is a complete *lack of awareness* about anaemia, the importance of having an optimal haemoglobin level or the importance of iron in the diet (Kanani S.1995) Erratic feeding habits, unhealthy lifestyle combined with high nutritional requirements further aggravates the problem among adolescents. Rarely is haemoglobin checked during adolescence. But adolescence is a critical period for addressing anemia in girls in order to improve their quality of life.

As *prevention starts with awareness*, Haemoglobin awareness in every child should be such that he/she must be inquisitive about knowing his/her haemoglobin and if less than 12g/dl,should be curious to know why is it less and how to make it 12g/dl.

There is little research in India however about the effectiveness of promotional interventions *viz. direct* (one-to- many interaction of the health worker that will improve awareness, comprehension and positive health seeking behaviour among adolescents) and *indirect* (one-to-one interaction of the health worker with opinion leader *e.g.* the teacher in a school setting who is also a role model and remains in touch with the students for a longer period of time) in creating awareness, comprehension and attitudinal changes in adolescents.

The present research study seeks to address this research gap in school going adolescent girls both in the context of a residential as well as in a non-residential school.

Material and Methods

A quasi- experimental before- and- after study was done from December 2008-February 2009 enrolling adolescent girl students of class 10th from a Residential and a Day school in Pilani-Rajasthan (India) after seeking permission from the concerned authorities. The Residential school has a pan India representation with students being drawn from all parts of the country while those in the day school belong to middle class families in Pilani. The girl students of class 10th were chosen as they represent the median age group in adolescents (10-19years).

A total of 114 students participated in the study—83 from School 1 (the Residential school) and 31 from School 2 (the Day school). Figure 6.1 below showing plan of the study.

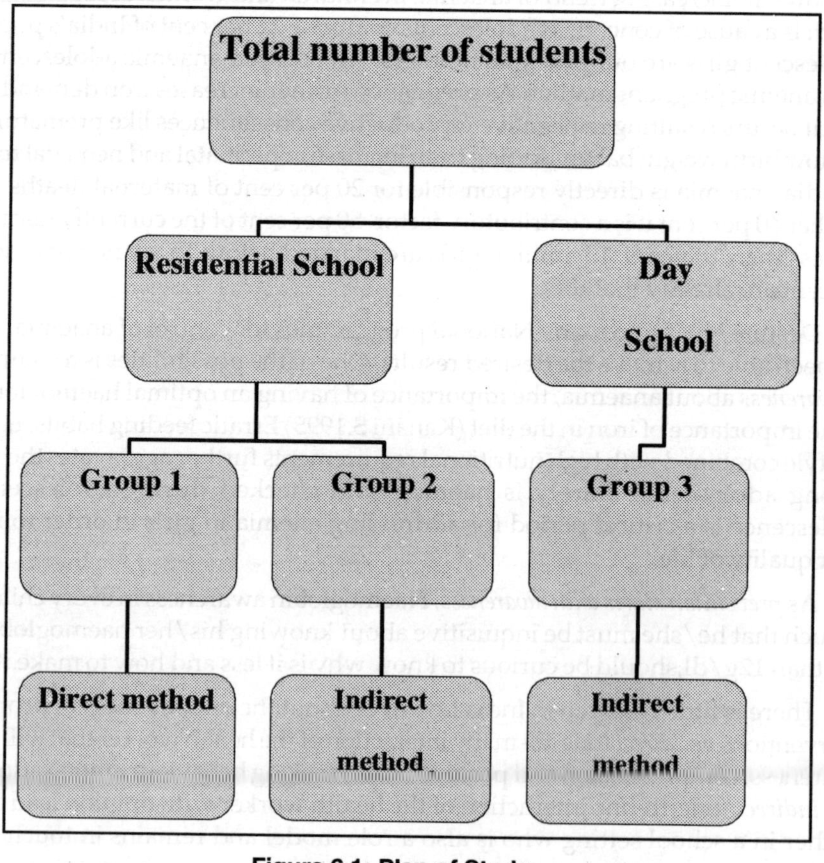

Figure 6.1: Plan of Study

The students of School 1 were randomly assigned into two groups (1& 2) while those from the day school comprised Group 3

- *Group 1*: Residential Group/Direct Intervention
- *Group 2*: Residential Group/Indirect Intervention
- *Group 3*: Day school/Indirect Intervention

Two different methods were adopted for creation of awareness in these three groups.

1. *Direct Method* (Nutritional counselling with students)
2. *Indirect Method* (Nutritional counselling with teachers)

In the *Direct method* interactive sessions spread over a period of one week were held directly with the students in Group 1. All the aspects related to Nutritional anaemia-its definition, causes, ill-effects on the present and future health and educational performance of adolescents were discussed in detail. Visual aids like charts and posters were used and presentation highlighting all aspects of iron deficiency anaemia made.

Educational material related to combating anaemia; rich dietary sources of iron, folic acid and vit.B12; a chart depicting calorific value of commonly used food preparations was given to the participants to make them aware of the necessity of having a well balanced diet, dietary modifications to be made to enhance absorption of iron in our diet–a simple measure being addition of vitamin C rich foods like lemon, amla, guava etc. Stress was laid on the need to avoid erratic intake of meals and junk-foods and avoiding skipping meals.

In the *Indirect method*, one-to-one interactive session was held with the teachers wherein all the aspects of Nutritional anaemia were discussed in detail.

Phase I

After explaining the reason for conducting the study and obtaining oral consent from the participants, all the participants in Group 1, Group 2 and the Group 3 were asked to fill a structured questionnaire that tested their awareness, comprehension and their attitude towards Nutritional anaemia.

Group 1 was then subjected to the direct methods of creating awareness about Nutritional anaemia.

In Group 2 and Group 3, the indirect methods of creating awareness about nutritional anaemia were used.

Phase II

(After a gap of 3weeks)The participants were again asked to fill a questionnaire to test their awareness, comprehension and attitude towards Nutritional anaemia.

After data collection, each questionnaire was assessed for its completion.The questionnaires of the respondents, who had not filled more than 50 per cent of the questions in each of the 3 section of the questionnaire pertaining to awareness, comprehension and attitude towards nutritional anaemia were rejected. This left 32 paired questionnaires in Group 1, 21 pairs in Group 2 and 13 paired questionnaires for the final analysis. One mark each was given to a correct response, thereby converting the qualitative data into the quantitative one. The scores obtained by the respondents were added and divided by the total possible score thereby getting the average score for each question in all the groups, both before and after the intervention. The results were statistically analysed using paired t-test for difference between means at 95 per cent confidence level with $\alpha = 0.05$.

Results

The mean age of the respondents was 14.5 years and ranged from 13–15 years.

Table 6.1 shows the effect of the direct and indirect methods of intervention on mean awareness scores in Groups 1,2 and 3 and the results of the statistical test also (S*representing significant difference while N.S* representing not–significant difference in mean score post intervention).

Awareness regarding the nutritional deficiency disorders before the interventions in Group 1, 2 and 3 was 61.25 per cent, 79.04 per cent and 35.38 per cent which increased across all the groups to 87.5 per cent, 86.66 per cent and 43.07 per cent respectively. Awareness regarding rich sources of Iron and other nutrients before the interventions in Group 1, 2 and 3 was 67.91, 70.15 per cent and 56.92 per cent which increased across Groups 1 and 2 to 81.2 per cent &79.36 per cent respectively and increased to 68.28 per cent for Group 3. Awareness regarding nutrients required for the formation of haemoglobin in Group 1, 2 and 3 was 31.25 per cent, 25.39 per cent and 28.20 per cent which increased across all the Groups to 62.5 per cent,46.03 per cent and 30.76 per cent respectively. Awareness regarding the symptoms due to anaemia in Group 1, 2 and 3 was 37.5 per cent, 9.52 per cent and 28.20 per cent which increased across all the Groups to 62.5 per cent, 19.04 per cent and 41.02 per cent respectively. Awareness regarding the iron-fortified foods available easily in the local market in Group 1, 2 and 3 was 14.58 per cent, 30.15 per cent and 12.82 per cent which increased across all the Groups to 47.91 per cent, 65.07 per cent and 25.64 per cent respectively. Awareness regarding the normal haemoglobin level in adolescent girls in Group 1, 2 and 3 was 579.3 per cent, 52.38 per cent and 69.23 per cent which increased across all the Groups to 87.5 per cent, 76.19 per cent and 92.30 per cent respectively. Awareness regarding the symptoms due to anaemia in Group 1, 2 and 3 was 579.3 per cent, 52.38 per cent and 69.23 per cent which increased across all the Groups to 87.5 per cent, 76.19 per cent and 92.30 per cent respectively. Awareness regarding the calories provided by one gram each of carbohydrates, proteins and fats in Group 1, 2 was very poor at 0.10 per cent, 9.52 per cent which slightly increased to 39.58 per cent and 19.04 per cent respectively. There was however no correct answer to this question from those in Group 3 both before and after indirect intervention. Awareness regarding the effect of menstruation on iron requirement in Group 1, 2 and 3 was 56.25 per cent, 57.14 per cent and 30 per cent which increased across all the Groups to 84.37 per cent, 80.95 per cent &53.84 per cent respectively. Awareness regarding the inhibitors and enhancers of iron absorption before the interventions in Group 1, 2 and 3 was 42.96 per cent, 52.9 per cent and 40.38 per cent which increased

Table 6.1: The Effect of the Direct and ndirect Methods of Intervention on Mean Awareness Scores in Groups 1, 2 and 3 and the Results of the Statistical Test (S*representing significant difference while N.S* representing not-significant difference in mean score post intervention)

Sl.No.	Question	Awareness								
		Group 1			Group 2			Group 3		
	Awareness about....... Per cent Correct/ Mean Score	Before	After	S. Test#	Before	After	S. Test#	Before	After	S. Test#
1.	Nutritional disorders	61.25/3.062	87.5/4.375	S*	79.04/3.952	86.66/4.33	S	35.38/1.769	43.07/2.158	N.S**
2.	Rich sources of iron and nutrients	67.91/10.187	81.2/12.187	S	70.15/10.52	79.36/11.90	S	56.92/7.69	51.28/8.53	S
3.	Nutrients for Hb synthesis	31.25/0.93	62.5/1.87	S	25.39/0.761	46.03/1.38	S	28.20/0.846	30.76/0.923	N.S
4.	Symptoms of anaemia	37.5/1.125	62.5/1.875	S	9.52/0.285	19.04/0.571	S	28.20/0.846	41.02/1.230	N.S
5.	Locally available iron fortified foods	14.58/0.437	47.91/1.4375	S	30.15/0.90	65.07/1.952	S	12.82/0.384	25.64/0.76	S
6.	Normal Hb Level	59.3/0.593	87.5/0.875	S	52.58/0.523	76.19/0.761	S	69.23/0.692	92.30/1.0	S
7.	Caloric requirement/ day	15.62/0.156	53.12/0.531	S	23.80/0.238	52.38/0.523	S	7.69/0.076	15.38/0.153	N.S
8.	Calories/gram of different foods	0.10/0.031	39.58/1.187	S	9.52/0.285	19.04/0.571	N.S	–	–	–
9.	Effect of menstruation on iron need	56.25/0.562	84.37/0.843	S	57.14/0.571	80.95/0.809	S	30/0.307	53.84/0.538	S
10.	Inhibitors and Enhancers of iron absorption	42.96/3.43	69.53/5.56	S	52.9/4.23	56.52/4.52	N.S	40.38/3.23	57.69/4.61	S
11.	Types of foods	48.75/2.43	65.62/3.28	S	40.95/2.04	44.76/2.23	N.S	35.38/1.76	40/2.0	N.S

* S: Statistically Significant; N.S.: Statistically not-significant.

across all the groups to 69.53 per cent,56.52 per cent and 57.69 7 per cent respectively. Awareness regarding the role of various foods in the body as energy giving, body building and protective foods in Group 1, 2 and 3 was 48.75 per cent, 40.95 per cent and 35.38 per cent which increased across all the groups to 65.62, 44.76 per cent,&40 per cent respectively.

Table 6.2 shows the effect of the direct and the indirect method of nutritional counseling on the comprehension scores in group 1, 2 and 3 respectively. Although there was an increase in the scores post–intervention, but the difference was not statistically significant except in Group 1 regarding calorific values of different foods.

Table 6.2: The Effect of the Direct and the Indirect Method of Nutritional Counseling on the Comprehension Scores in Groups 1, 2 and 3 Respectively

Sl.No.	Question	Comprehension								
		Group 1			Group 2			Group 3		
	Comprehension About.... ($\bar{\rho}$ Score)	Before	After	S. Test#	Before	After	S. Test#	Before	After	S. Test#
1.	Vit. C Content of different foods	0.3	0.65	N.S	0.136	0.20	N.S	0.115	0.215	N.S
2.	Iron content of different foods	–0.125	0.33	N.S	–0.03	–0.1	N.S	–0.31	–0.35	N.S
3.	Calorific value of different foods	0.082	0.524	S*	–0.044	0.224	N.S	–0.084	–0.27	N.S

* S: Statistically Significant; N.S.: Statistically not-significant.

Table 6.3 shows the effect of the direct and the indirect method of nutritional counseling on behavioral intention to act in Group 1, 2 and 3 respectively. Neither the direct method of intervention nor the indirect method of intervention in either of the settings (residential or day school) show any significant increase in behavioral intention to act except in the case of not sharing their health related problems with either teacher or the doctor in the groups where indirect method of intervention was used. In general it indicates that adolescents don't intend to share their health related problems with others.

Discussion

As the prevalence of nutritional anaemia in adolescents is very high especially in the developing countries like India, this issue has to be tackled on a war footing as the quality of our future generations, too, is dependent on how healthy our adolescent girls are.

The direct method of intervention (*i.e.* counseling of students) in residential setting leads to a significant increase in awareness about all aspects of nutritional anaemia. In the case of the indirect method of intervention (*i.e.* counseling of teachers) in a residential setting, the results show a significant increase in awareness about nutritional anaemia except in the case of awareness about calories provided per gram of different foods, inhibitors and enhancers of iron absorption and food type–

areas that may require in-depth knowledge of the subject. The results also show that the indirect method of intervention (*i.e.* counseling of teachers) in a day school setting did lead to a significant increase in awareness about nutritional anaemia in, areas which involve transfer of simple information. These findings are consistent with those of Shojaeizadeh *et al.* (2001), who found poor knowledge, unfavorable attitude in 57.3 and 54.1 per cent of secondary school girls respectively, in Iran regarding Iron deficiency anaemia. Kaur *et al.* (2001) and Sachdeva *et al.* (2008) found an increase in awareness and positive attitude towards anaemia in the intervention group given health education/nutritional counseling, compared to control group in a study on young women and in elderly males in rural and urban areas respectively.

Table 6.3: The Effect of the Direct and the Indirect Method of Nutritional Counseling on Behavioral Intention to Act in Group 1, 2 and 3 Respectively

Sl.No.	*Question*	*Group 1*			*Group 2*			*Group 3*		
	Beh. Intention about....(X Mean Scores)	*Before*	*After*	*S. Test#*	*Before*	*After*	*S. Test#*	*Before*	*After*	*S. Test#*
1.	Sharing health related problems with									
	a) Peers	5.91	7.91	N.S	7.21	8.14	S	7.63	8.09	N.S
	b) Parents	5.24	8.72	N.S	8.75	9.45	S	9.25	9.41	N.S
	c) Teachers	6.42	6.28	N.S	5.46	6.07	N.S	6.45	6.72	N.S
	d) Doctor	8.07	8.03	N.S	6.07	7.78	N.S	7.66	6.91	N.S
	e) None of above	4.28	5.0	N.S	3.0	4.5	N.S	5.4	5.2	N.S
2.	Consult a doctor when symptomatic	2.84	3.43	N.S	2.66	3.0	N.S	3.38	3.92	N.S
3.	Preference for diagnostic method									
	a) Vinger prick	8.52	8.34	N.S	7.0	7.61	N.S	7.83	8.58	N.S
	b) Venous sample	8.68	7.89	N.S	7.0	7.88	N.S	7.58	8.58	N.S
	c) Physical examin.	8.27	8.04	N.S	5.8	7.53	N.S	6.90	6.63	N.S
4.	Intention towards compliance per cent	46.8	62.5	N.S	64.7	82.3	N.S	64.7	82.3	N.S

* S: Statistically Significant; N.S.: Statistically not-significant.

The above results indicate that neither the direct method of intervention (*i.e.* counseling of students) nor the indirect method of intervention (*i.e.* counseling of teachers) in either of the settings (residential or day school) show any significant increase in comprehension about nutritional anaemia. This may be probably due to the fact that although nutritional education can create awareness but comprehension requires knowledge that includes relating information to different contexts.

These results indicate that neither the direct method of intervention (*i.e.* counseling of students) nor the indirect method of intervention (*i.e.* counseling of teachers) in either of the settings (residential or day school) show any significant increase in behavioral intention to act about nutritional anaemia except in the case of not sharing their health related problems with either teacher or the doctor in the groups where indirect method of intervention was used. In general it indicates that adolescents don't intend to share their health related problems with others.

Finally although nutritional education through counseling of students and teachers in both residential and day school can lead to a significant increase in the level of awareness but comprehension and behavioral intention change is perhaps much more complex and difficult to create and would require an attitudinal change through methods else than counseling. What these effective methods could be is a matter of future research.

Conclusions/Recommendations

Based on our research findings, it can be safely recommended that for creation of awareness among students regarding nutritional anaemia on most of the factors, the methods of counseling of students and counseling of teachers by experts (Doctors) should be resorted to by the schools.

While the objective of creating awareness can be attained by the above recommended method, as per our research findings the same cannot be said to be the case with most of the factors in terms of comprehension and behavioral intention.Our recommendation on this aspect will be to explore more involved means of knowledge transfer in which students understand the mechanisms and processes involving cause-effect relationship. It is recommended such an input be incorporated in their curriculum and interesting pedagogy to impart the same in a fun way could be the solution.

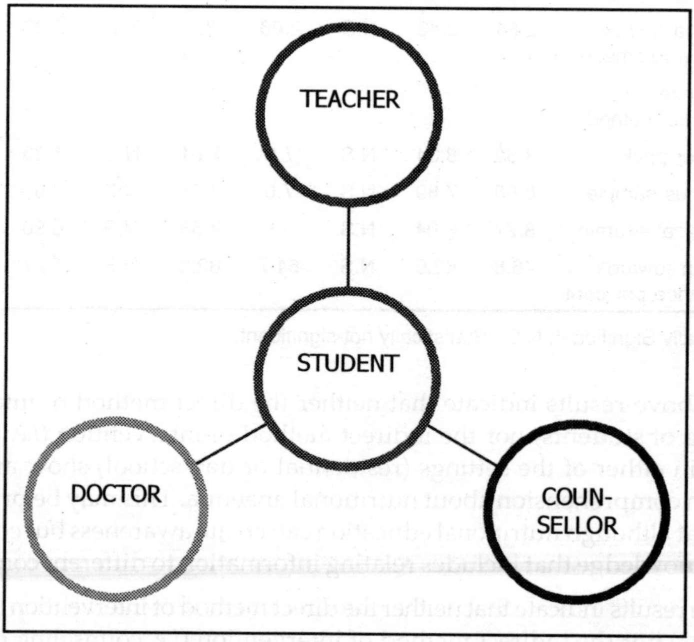

Figure 6.2: Recommended Model for Anaemia Alleviation for a Residential School

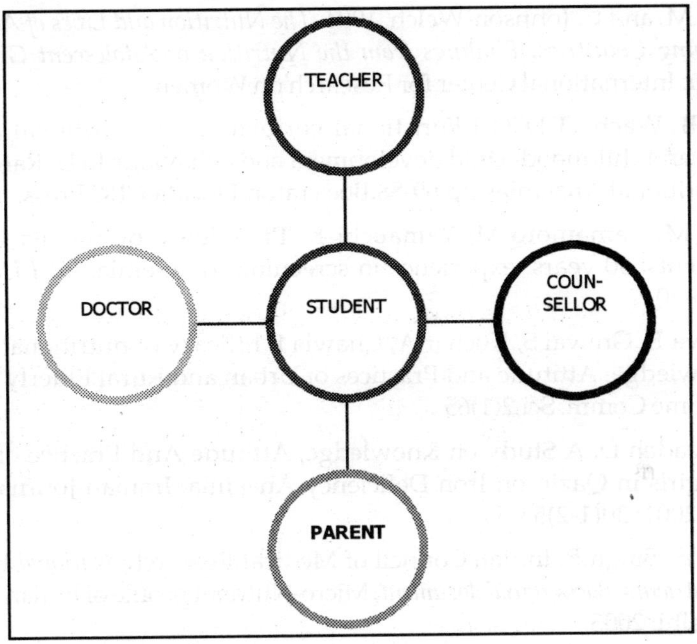

Figure 6.3: Recommended Model for Anaemia Alleviation for Non-Residential School

Our research indicates a general reluctance on behalf of the students at their critical life-cycle stage of adolescence to share their health related problems. It is hence suggested that regular counseling sessions by an expert counselor be institutionalised to effect an attitudinal change which will moderate the relationship between awareness levels to action. It should be though ensured that the counselors have professional competence who respect confidentiality so that student's find them both trustworthy and easy to approach. Additionally, during interaction with management of day school, it was felt that parents who have a strong influence on the attitude formation of their children should also be counseled regarding all aspects of nutritional anaemia. The recommended models for anaemia alleviation are, therefore, given in Figure 6.2 and 6.3 for the residential and the day school respectively.

References

1. Agarwal DK, Upadhyay SK, Tripathy AM, Agarwal KN. Nutritional Status, Physical Work Capacity and Mental Function in School Children. Nutrition Foundation of India, New Delhi, *Scientific Report No. 6*, pp1987; 16-23.

2. Kanani S. Strategies for combating anemia in adolescent girls. *Ind J Pediatrics* 1995,2; 375-77.

3. Kaur M, Singh K. Effect of Health Education on Knowledge,attitude and Practices About Anaemia among Rural women in Chandigarh. Indian Journal Of Community Medicine 26;(3) 2001-07-2001-08.

4. Kurz K.M, and C. Johnson-Welch. 1994. *The Nutrition and Lives of Adolescents in Developing Countries: Findings from the Nutrition of Adolescent Girls Research Program.* International Center for Research on Women.

5. Lazoff,B, Wachs T.D2001.Functional correlation of nutritional anaemia in infancy and childhood- child development and behaviour.In U. Ramakrishnan, ed, Nutritional Anaemias,pp.69-88.Boca raton,Florida,CRC Press.

6. Maeda M; Yamamoto M; Yamauchi K. Prevalence of anemia in Japanese adolescents: 30 years' experience in screening for anemia. *Int J Hematol* 1999 69(2):75-80.

7. Sachdeva R, Grewal S, Kochar A, Chawla P.Efficacy of nutritional counseling on Knowledge, Attitude and Practices of Urban and Rural Elderly Males.2008 Stud.Home Comm. Sci,2(1)65

8. Shojaeizadeh D.`A Study on Knowledge, Attitude And Practice of secondary school girls in Qazin on Iron Deficiency Anaemia. Iranian Journal Of Public Health 2001; 30(1-2)53-56

9. Toteja GS, Singh P, Indian Council of Medical Research, *National Workshop on Micronutrients, Background document*, Micro-Nutrient profile of Indian Population, New Delhi, 2003.

10. Thane CW, Bates CJ, Prentice A. Risk factors for low iron intake and poor iron status in a national sample of British young people aged 4-18years. *Public Health Nutr. 2003;* 6: 485-496.

Chapter 7

Health and Nutrition Concerns of Women in Reproductive and Post-Reproductive Years in Developing Countries

Sheel Sharma

Professor,
Department of Food Science and Nutrition,
Banasthali University, Rajasthan – 304 022, India
E-mail: sheelsh56@yahoo.com, sheelsh@rediffmail.com

ABSTRACT

In the year 2000, United Nations general assembly expressed grave concern over the unacceptably high rates of maternal mortality and morbidity in most of the countries all over the world. Since for every woman who dies, approximately 30 more suffer injuries, infection and disabilities during pregnancy or parturition. The problem needs to be viewed as an unmitigated disaster affecting no less than 15 million women in a year out of which more than 0.5 million actually die. In fact, 80 per cent of maternal deaths occur due to direct causes like hemorrhage, infection, complications related to unsafe abortion and hypertensive disorders for want of skilled obstetric care at critical moments during pregnancy and childbirth. But the same does not become available to the women even because of reasons, such as: failure to recognize the signs of life-threatening complications; postponing the decision to seek care despite being aware of owing to delay in reaching the appropriate care delivery centre; and getting a raw deal at the care delivery centre itself, either due to lack of facilities or non cooperation on the part of care providers at the delivery centre's. As for ageing in the context of women, they ought to be treated as an especially vulnerable group because of two realities. One, the women have a longer life expectancy than men though they have higher morbidity rates, thereby implying that they live more to suffer more sickness for obvious reasons, and Second, the problems of elderly women are compounded because of their postmenopausal status. In fact, this post reproductive period of life is a juncture of readjustments as it brings in its wake characteristic physiological and psychological problems needing nutritional, medical, social and often psychological- psychiatric care. Making motherhood a safer time in women's reproductive years and caring for them at the stage of life of lengthening shadows require commitment at all levels: in the home, in the community, in the hospital, in the country and across the globe. This calls for a long term investment in terms of imparting awareness and providing attention and intervention to the women in need The society owes this to their prime progenitors; the women. Otherwise, our avowed resolve of achieving millennium development goal of reducing the maternal motility ratio by three quarters between 1990 and 2015 and of adding lively years to the lives of elderly women would only remain a pipe dream.

Keywords: *Healthcare, Nutrition, Reproductive and post-reproductive, Developing countries.*

Introduction

Coming face to face with ground realities that prevail in the developing world, the most important issue that is linked to women health is physiological and nutritional stress of being expectant mothers taking up the perilous journey to child birth. By considering the nutritional intake and healthcare of a young girl, a nutritionist or health practitioner can ensure safer physiological events in the later reproductive phase. However, in the low income rural setting of developing countries like India, many undernourished girls remain stunted during their growth periods leading to their pelvic bones remaining small. Later on, in the reproductive, child bearing age, this causes difficult and risky child birth or parturition that, more often than not, results in death (Holloway, 1994).

It is a sheer irony that people celebrate the birth of a new baby, societies expect women to bear children and own them for their role as mothers, yet in most of the world, pregnancy and childbirth continues to be a perilous journey. In less developed countries, more than half a million mothers die from causes related to this life-giving event each year. For many women, motherhood spans decades. The period when mothers are most at risk of death, however, is during pregnancy, delivery, and the 42-day period following childbirth.

A pathetic portrayal of the situation comes in the words of Fred Sai (2000), a former President of International Planned Parenthood Foundation: *"No country sends its soldiers to war to protect their country without seeing to it that they will return safely, and yet mankind for centuries has been sending women to battle to renew the human resource without protecting them"*. Evidence shows that motherhood can be safer for all women if the indifference in creating the maternal health and obstetric care and in equities in its availability is removed. Over the past decade, experts have largely come to agree on a set of lifesaving strategies that can work even in low-resource settings. Governments around the globe have signed international inventions that advocate significant reductions in maternal mortality. In 2000, however, the United Nations General Assembly acknowledged that "despite progress in some countries, rates of maternal mortality and morbidity remain unacceptably high in most countries".

According to the estimates developed by WHO, UNICEF and UNFPA (Geneva, WH: 2001) 515,000 women die annually from maternal causes. 99 per cent of these deaths occur in the less developed world, making maternal mortality the health indicator that reveals the largest disparity between developing and developed countries. The situation is most dire for women in sib-Saharan Africa, where one of every 13 women dies of pregnancy-related causes during her lifetime, compared with only one in 4085 women in industrialized countries. These deaths are only a part of landscape which has bigger dimensions. For every woman who dies, approximately 30 more women suffer injuries, infection, and disabilities during pregnancy or childbirth – at least 15 million women a year. The cumulative total of those affected has been estimated at 300 million, or more than a quarter of adult women in the developing world. These pregnancy-related health problems include severe anemia, infertility and damage to the uterus and reproductive tract sustained during childbirth. Many women are too ashamed to speak about these and other conditions or to seek treatment for them. This "culture of silence" is exacerbated in setting where women are not empowered to make choices and act freely to take care of their health (WHO, 1999).

The majority of maternal deaths occur after childbirth, mostly within 24 hours. About a quarter take place during pregnancy, and about 15 percent happen at the time of delivery. The most common medical cause is hemorrhage; a swift and severe loss of blood before, during, or after delivery (Loudan, 1992).

Hemorrhage is considered a "direct" cause of death, because it is directly associated with pregnancy and childbirth. Four-fifths of maternal deaths are due to direct causes; hemorrhage, infection, complications related to unsafe abortion and hypertensive disorders. Figure 7.1 shows how much each of these direct causes contributes to maternal mortality. The remaining 20 percent of maternal deaths have indirect causes, conditions that are aggravated by pregnancy, such as malaria, diabetes, viral hepatitis, rheumatic heart disease and anemia, all conditions aggravated by pregnancy. Other indirect causes include ectopic pregnancy, embolism and anesthesia-related deaths. Most of the deaths from the direct causes could be prevented if women received skilled are at critical moments during pregnancy and childbirth. Unfortunately, many women deliver without the assistance of a skilled attendant – a health professional such as a doctor, nurse or a midwife who can manage normal deliveries and treat the life-threatening complications of pregnancy and childbirth or stabilize and refer women for appropriate care. Experts estimate that about 15 per cent of delivers have complications that require skilled medical intervention. Yet only about half of deliveries in less developed countries currently take place with a skilled attendant present Figure 7.2 depicts a region wise account of skilled care at delivery juxtaposed with maternal deaths as per the estimates developed by WHO, UNICEF and UNFPA (Geneva: WHO, 2001)

Maternal mortality is influenced by the social, economic and political context of the healthcare system and the cultural and biological realities of women seeking care. This complex interaction means that even when skilled care is available, women may not seek it out or receive it. At several stages of the journey through pregnancy and childbirth, women face delays in receiving skilled care. These delays pose barriers

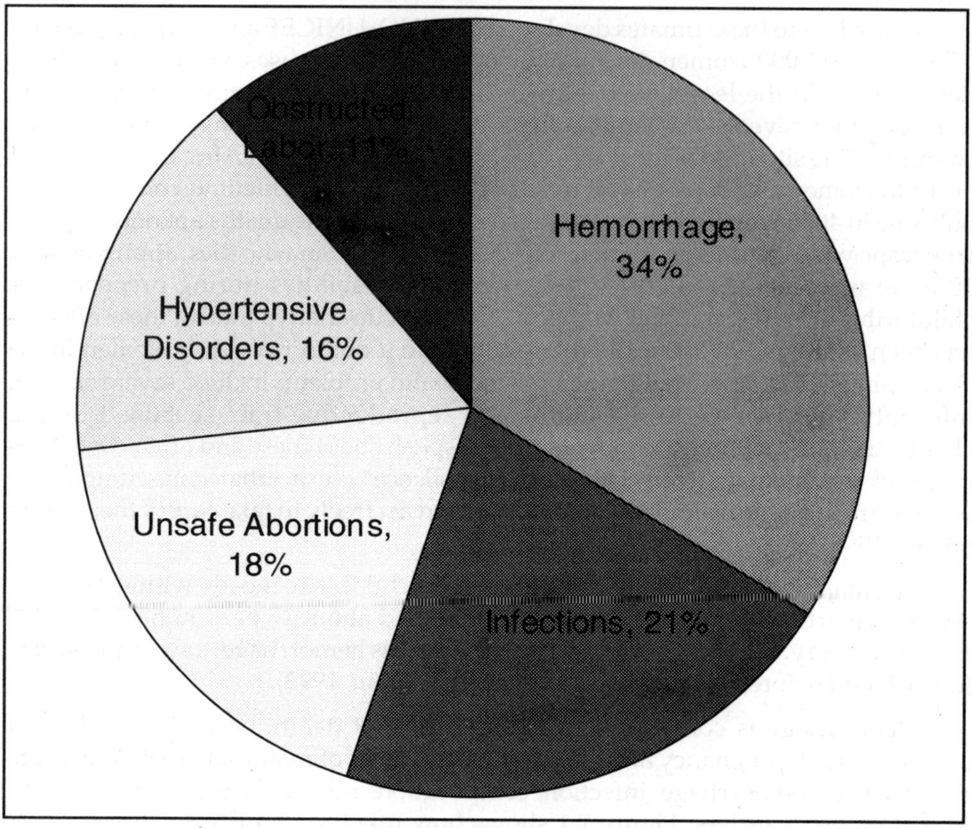

Figure 7.1: Direct Causes of Maternal Deaths (WHO, UNICEF and UNFPA (Geneva: WHO, 2001)

to safe motherhood. Women and their families or caregivers may not recognize the warning signs of life-threatening complications. Women may have difficulty reaching a decision to seek medical care; they also may fear opposition from husbands and elderly ladies in the house, high fees or substandard care at health facilities. Women may also face delays in reaching health facilities in time. Even deliveries in health facilities may be needlessly risky because of poor quality obstetric care and the lack of medical supplies or blood. These delays are interrelated and reflect a country's level of socioeconomic development (Hind and Khattab, 1992; Adamson, 1996).

Maternal morbidity and death is fraught with dangerous consequences, for a vast majority of women who die from or are seriously injured by maternity-related causes are in the prime of life, their illnesses and deaths have dire social and economic outcomes for both families and communities. Families forgo a woman's crucial role in household management and care for children and other family members. Consequently, families that lose mothers are likely to suffer declining nutritional status. Surviving children may have lower rates of school enrollment. Maternal disabilities related to pregnancy and childbirth, such as anemia and malnutrition,

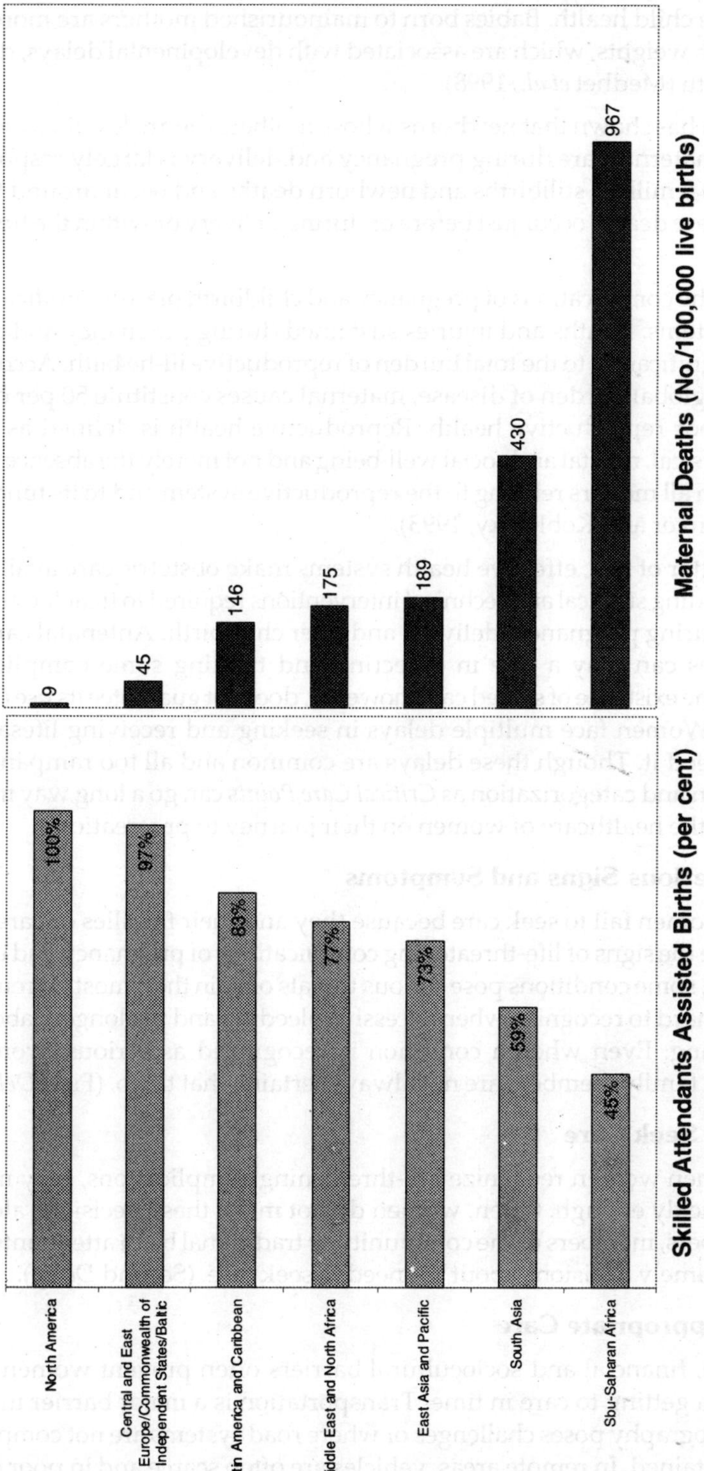

Figure 7.2: Skilled Care at Delivery and Maternal Deaths, Regional Comparisons [WHO, UNICEF and UNFPA (Geneva: WHO, 2001)]

also influence child health. Babies born to malnourished mothers are more likely to have low birth weights, which are associated with developmental delays, disabilities and even death (Medhet *et al.*, 1998).

Research has shown that newborns whose mothers die are less likely to survive. Insufficient maternal care during pregnancy and delivery is largely responsible for the estimated 8 million stillbirths and newborn deaths and occur around the world each year. These deaths occur just before or during delivery or within the first week of life.

Finally, the complications of pregnancy and childbirth place a significant burden on health systems. Deaths and injuries sustained during pregnancy and childbirth contribute significantly to the total burden of reproductive ill-he4alth. According to a study on the global burden of disease, maternal causes constitute 50 per cent of the burden of poor reproductive health. Reproductive health is defined as a state of complete physical, mental and social well-being and not merely the absence of disease or infirmity in all matters relating to the reproductive system and to its functions and processes (Tinker and Koblinsky, 1993).

As a matter of fact, effective health systems make obstetric care available to all women, including surgical and technical interventions required to treat life-threatening conditions during pregnancy, delivery and after childbirth. Antenatal care, among other services can play a role in detecting and treating some complications of pregnancy. The existence of skilled care, however, does not guarantee its use (Koblinsky *et al.*, 2000). Women face multiple delays in seeking and receiving lifesaving care when they need it. Though these delays are common and all too rampant yet their crystallization and categorization as *Critical Care Points* can go a long way in bridging the hiatus in the healthcare of women on their journey to procreation.

Realizing Serious Signs and Symptoms

Many women fail to seek care because they and their families or caregivers do not recognize the signs of life-threatening complications of pregnancy and childbirth. Furthermore, some conditions pose serious threats only in their most extreme form. It is especially hard to recognize when excessive bleeding and prolonged labor become life-threatening. Even when a condition is recognized as serious, women, their spouses, and family members are not always certain what to do. (First *Delay*).

Deciding to Seek Care

Even when women recognize life-threatening complications, they may fail to seek care quickly enough. Often, women do not make these decisions alone; other family members, members of the community or traditional birth attendants may also fail to make timely decisions about the need to seek care. (Second *Delay*).

Reaching Appropriate Care

Physical, financial and sociocultural barriers often prevent women and their families from getting to care in time. Transportation is a major barrier in countries where the geography poses challenges or where road systems are not comprehensive or well-maintained. In remote areas, vehicles are often scarce and in poor condition.

The costs of arranging emergency transportation can be heavy and beyond the paying capacity of the family. (Third *Delay*).

Availing Care at Health Facilities

Even when women with complications arrive at a healthcare facility, they may not receive the care they need quickly enough to save their lives. Sometimes the healthcare facility does not have an efficient system to make sure that emergency cases are seen promptly. This is often due to the inability of facility staff to recognize obstetric emergencies. Shortages of skilled attendants at healthcare facilities mean that women receive substandard care at the moment when they most need high-quality care. (Fourth *Delay*).

Thus not recognizing the signs of life-threatening complications; or postponing the decision to seek care despite knowing them; or getting delayed in reaching the appropriate care delivery centre, due to one reason or other; or getting a raw deal at the care delivery centre itself. One or more of these delays put the life of the mother in jeopardy and become no mean contributors to the heavy toll of maternal mortality

Women will stop dying in childbirth when they are able to plan their pregnancies, give birth under the supervision of a skilled attendant and have access to high-quality treatment if pregnancy complications occur. These improvements are feasible even in low-income settings, but require con continuous and focused improvement of health systems.

Many events occurring in daily life bring challenges that impinge upon our body, mind and emotions and the body's reaction perceiving them as threats constitute *stress* for us. Way back at the turn of 20th century, Walter Cannon, an American physiologist, coined the term 'homeostasis' which meant the capacity to maintain the consistency of our internal environment. An organism is said to be in 'homeostasis' when its internal environment; level of nutrients and other metabolites, such as electrolytes, water, blood sugar; other factors like body temperature, remain within normal limits. However, a disturbance in homeostasis with respect to one or more of such aspects can cause stress which snowballs into a disease of one or the other kind if consistency limits are not restored in due course. The events that cause upheavals in the homeostasis are termed stressors. The stressors may be exogenous (coming from outside); such as heat, cold, infection, lack of oxygen, or else endogenous (surfacing from within the body) such as pain, anxiety, unpleasant thoughts, variations in body temperature or blood sugar. In fact, the events remain the same but their perception by the body and mind make them stressors of different intensity.

Consider for instance a long distance walk thrust upon an individual not used to walking marathon distance-the exercise a patent stress for him. But the same event causes little discomfiture, much less a stress, in a habitual jogger or sprinter. Consider another case, a person running a kilometer on a routine exercise schedule, experiences negligible stress. However, the same person, running the same distance chased menacingly by a dog would experience an intense stress. Stress perception, therefore varies from individual to individual and circumstances to circumstances and accordingly varies the body's response to it.

If one perceives ones ability to cope with the threatening events as weak, the level of stress one experiencing will be high. Conversely, on self perception of one's coping capacity being high, the intensity of stress experienced will be comparatively low.

While perceiving threat to our dignity, health, value system, self respect and ego; we react with fear, anger, anxiety and frustration. While doing so the response of our body is reflected through nervous and endocrine systems. This includes a wide range of bodily changes termed by Hans Selye, a reknowned authority on stress, as *General Adaptation Syndrome*. The premier endocrine ensemble – the hypothalamus pituitary axis, sends messages to the various tissues/organs, more or like distress signals, to prepare them for the coping action. The three phases of body response 'alarm reaction, *resistance reaction* and exhaustion' have been widely deliberated upon. Where as alarm reaction is an instant 'fight or flee' response, resistance reaction is longer and steady affair at providing sustained energy supply and other important substances for the functioning and maintenance of nervous system and other traumatized tissues. Exhaustion is a rarely reached yet dismal situation of being down and out. Situations like, post menopausal state, are long term, taking on toll both body and mind. Observational studies also point out that ovarian changes associated with menopause might be a cause of depression anxiety and irritability. As we all know that human brain is an amazingly complex and versatile organ as its different parts regulate body and mental functions. Limbic system; the part of the brain that punctuates our mood, anxiety and irritability, has also its intercellular communication through chemical messengers or neurotransmitters; most important of which are serotonin and norepinephrine. Their circulating levels become determinants for the quality of mood and level of happiness. However, stressors make neurotransmitter levels plummet precipitating, mood swings, and irritability, anxiety and depression tendencies. Further, there could also be a causal relationship between the menopausal transition and difficulty in thinking, forgetfulness or other cognitive disturbances. Like wise, menopause accompanies the prevalence of somatic symptoms including back pain, tiredness, stiff and painful joints and other symptoms associated with osteoporosis.

Menopause related symptoms seem to occur due to ovarian aging and a consequent drop or cessation of their ability to produce female reproductive hormones.

The vasomotor symptoms of hot flashes- sudden sensation of intense heat with sweating and flushing typically lasting 5 to 10 minutes and night sweats have been reported in high frequency in postmenopausal women. As a mater of fact vasometer symptoms are severe and create a burden on daily life. Though sleep disturbances tend to increase with age irrespective of gender yet evidence from longitudinal cohort and cross sectional observational studies indicate that such disturbances get accelerated in the case of postmenopausal women. Various components of sexual dysfunction during menopausal transition have also been identified. They include decrease in libido arousal and other aspects of sexuality.

As for ageing in the context of women, they ought to be treated as an especially vulnerable group because of two realities. For one, the women have a longer life expectancy than men though they have higher morbidity rates, thereby implying that they live more to suffer more sickness. Further, the problems of elderly women are compounded because of their postmenopausal status. In fact, this post reproductive period of life is a juncture of readjustments as it brings in its wake characteristics physiological and psychological problems needing medical, nutritional, and often psychological-psychiatric attention. Some of the problems accompanying postmenopausal status can be summed up as under:

Physiological

- ☆ Hot flashes in the chest and face
- ☆ Sweating of palms and forehead
- ☆ Headaches and dizziness
- ☆ Wrinkling/dryness of skin
- ☆ Loss of muscle strength and tone
- ☆ Brittle bones and increased risks for osteoporosis
- ☆ Risk of heart attacks and malignancy
- ☆ Sexual dysfunction

Psychological

- ☆ Irritability
- ☆ Mood swings
- ☆ Anxiety/tension
- ☆ Fatigue
- ☆ Low self esteem
- ☆ Depression
- ☆ Forgetfulness
- ☆ Sleep disturbances

Most of these problems are attributed to hormonal changes, especially the reduced level of estrogen and a consequent rise in pituitary hormone (Sen *et al.*, 1994).It has been pointed out that unfavorable lipid profile, mostly with respect to TG and LDL cholesterol, occurs in postmenopausal women, possibly owing to a slackening of homeostatic control of metabolism by the neuroendocrinal mechanisms as a consequence of menopause (Imahori, 1992; Rosenbrg, 1997).

Whereas some women seek to supplement their declining estrogen level through medical intervention with Hormone Replacement Therapy (HRT), others choose to be benefited from natural plant estrogens known as phytoestrogens. Estrogen (conjugated estrogen) alone, or often in combination with progestin (medroxy progesterone acetate), has been studied in randomized clinical trial (RCTs) for management of postmenopausal complication. Reassuringly, estrogen, either by itself or with progestin, has proved most consistently effective therapy for hot flashes, night sweats, mood and sleep disturbances, sexual dysfunction and quality of life symptoms. However, incessant use of HRT for 3-4 years or were has been found to increase the risk for stroke, coronary and thrombolitic events, pulmonary embolism and breast cancer. Incidentally, interest in the physiological role of a number of bioactive compounds present in plants has increased dramatically over the last decade, of which *phytoestrogens* remain of utmost interest. (Cassidy, 2003) Though, weaker than human estrogen; when supplemented in diet through food stuffs, rich in them, the phytoestrogens seem to increase body estrogen activity considerably (Whipple, 2000). In fact substantial number of studies of phytoestrogens and isoflavones have been conducted, motivated by epidemiological data showing differences in levels of menopausal symptoms in countries with different levels of these nutrients in their diets.

Duncan *et al.* (2003) stated that phytoestrogens are estrogenic compounds found in plants, consisting of isoflavones, lignans and coumestans. Epidemiological studies provide evidence for a protective role of isoflavones, and to a lesser extent lignans, and other members against the development of numerous chronic diseases, including coronary vascular disease (CVD), osteoporosis and certain cançers. As a matter of fact, structural similarity of phytoestrogens to the endogenous estrogen has given credence to the hypothesis that phytoestrogens exert hormonal effects and their wide availability and appropriateness put them on a pedestal as a prudent dietary alternative to *none too side effect free* HRT therapy. *Phytoestrogens'* is an area of active and advancing research with high potential to affect human health favourably.

Also known as plant chemicals or phytochemicals, isoflavones a type of phytoestrogens are primarily found in soybeans and foods made from them. In particular, the significant therapeutic properties of soybeans have been generally attributed to soy isoflavones. Soy isoflavones play an important role in reducing plasma cholesterol levels and cancer prevention, particularly, of tumours under endocrine control (breast and others) as well as in prevention/treatment of post menopausal symptoms of osteoporosis (Sirtori, 2001).

It has been estimated that a daily feeding of 75 mg of soy isoflavone to the postmenopausal women for 1-2 years can cause a decrease in menopausal symptoms along with a positive health promoting effect on lipoprotein metabolism causing decrease in LDL-cholesterol and triglycerides levels with an attendant raise in the HDL- cholesterol. Further, a meta analysis of 38 clinical trials at Milan (Italy) aimed at examining the relationship between soy protein intake and serum lipids, reported that the consumption of soy in women is associated with a significant decrease in serum total and LDL cholesterol and triglyceride levels. The association was all the stronger for subjects with higher initial levels of cholesterol (Kang *et al.*, 2002).

In the same vein, red clover leaf (Trifolium pretense) contains phytoestrogens compounds and is believed to work as weak estrogen mitigating postmenopausal symptoms. Another sought after herbal remedy; ginseng root (Panax ginseng or Panax guinguefolius) could also help as it has been found effective against well being and mood and sleep disturbances symptoms.

In Asian cultures, plant based prudent diets rich in phytoestrogens, high in mutually supplemented protein and omega-3 fatty acids, as well as low in saturated fats, have been consumed. Available evidence suggests that *plant based diets* is a contributing factor to the low rate of menopausal symptoms, breast cancer, heart disease and osteoporosis among Asian women. Complimentary and alternative approaches such as acupuncture, mind- body approaches including yoga, homeopathy and Ayurveda can also often remedial hope but to date there is a pancihj of well designed studies. Similarly, behavioral interventions could also be an area one can look forward to, the advantage being the absence of side effects (Singh and Kaushik, 2000). Health education and awareness is a must to improve knowledge about menopause related symptom and the availability and efficacy of the remedies and therapies with risk benefit information to promote self care behaviour and decision making for opting HRT or complementary and alternative approaches to impart and ensure quality in the lengthening shadows of life.

The doctrine " *Let food be thy medicine*" espoused by Hippocrates nearly 2500 yrs ago, ought to be given a renewed emphasis if the ill nourished and marginalized common folks in general and the vulnerable groups of the women in particular have to become a part of the mainstream healthy and well nourished society.

Healthy women in reproductive and graying years, add value to the society. Their survival and well being are not only important but also central to solving much broader economic, social and developmental challenges. When women die untimely deaths or live sickly lives; their families, communities and nations suffer as well. Improving their survival and well being would not only consolidate the health of societies; but also go a long way in alleviating inequity and poverty.

Making motherhood a safer time in women's reproductive years and caring for them at the stage of life of lengthening shadows require commitment at all levels: in the home, in the community, in the hospital, in the country and across the globe. This calls for a long term investment in terms of imparting awareness and providing attention and intervention to the women in need The society owes this to their prime progenitors; the women. Otherwise, our avowed resolve of achieving millennium development goal of reducing the maternal mortality ratio by three quarters between 1990 and 2015 and of adding quality years to the lives of elderly women would only remain a pipe dream.

References

1. Cassidy, A. (2003). Potential risks and benefits of phytoestrogen rich diets. *Int J Vitam Nutr. Res.*, *73*(2), 120-6.
2. Duncan, A.M., Phipps, W.R., Kurzer, M.S. (2003.) Phytoestrogens. *Best Pract Res Clin Endocrinol Metab*,*17*(2), 253-71.
3. Hind and Khattab (1992) The Silent Endurance: Social Conditions of Women's Reproductive Health in Rural Egypt (Amman, Jordan: UNICEF Regional Office of the Middle East and North Africa; and Cairo: Population Council Regional Office of the Middle East and North Africa).
4. Holloway, M. (1994). Trends in women's health: A global view. *Sci. Ame*, Aug, 67-73.

5. Sai, F. (2000). Saving lives: skilled attendance at childbirth. Tunisia, Nov. 13-15.
6. Imahori, K. (1992). How students understand ageing.
7. *Nutr Rev, 50*(12), 315-322.
8. Kang, H.J., Absbacher, R., Hammoud, M.M. (2002). Use of alternative and complementary medicine in menopause. *In J. gynecol Obstet., 79*,195-207.
9. Koblinsky, M., Conroy, C., Kureshy, N., Stanton, M.E., Jessop, S. (2000). Issue in Programming for Safe Motherhood. Arlinton, VA: Mother Care/Johm Snow, Inc
10. Loudon, I. (1992). The transformation of maternal mortality. *British Medical Journal, 305*,1557-60.
11. Medhet, F., Becker, S., Berendes, W.H. (1998). Contextual determinants of maternal mortality in rural Pakistan. *Social Science and Medicine, 46* (12),1587-98.
12. Rosenberg, I.H. (1997). Nutrition and Senescence. *Nutr Rev, 55* (1), 569-577.
13. Sen,G.,Germain,A.,Chen,L.C.(Eds.).(1994). Population Policies Reconsidered: Health Empowerment and Rights.USA: Harvard School of Public Health Publication.
14. Singh, M. and Kaushik,S.S. (2000). A comparison of relaxation, meditation and cognitive therapy for enhancing stress-coping skills of middle aged women at risk of depression. Indian Journal of Clinical Psychology, 27(1):89-96.
15. Sirtori,C.R. (2001)Risks and benefits of soy phytoesterogen in cardio vascular disease, cancer climacteric symptoms and osteoporosis.*Drug Saf,24*(9),665-82
16. Tinker,A.,Koblinsky,M.with contributions from Daly P (1993).Making Motherhood Sage.*World Bank Discussion Paper* 202, Washington, DC: World Bank.
17. Unfer,V.,Casini, M.L.,Costabile, L. (2004). Endometrial effects of long term treatment with phytoestrogen:a randomized double blind, placebo control study. *Fertil Steril,82*,145-148
18. WHO/UNICEF (1989).Ten seps to sccessful beast feding. potecting, pomoting spporting beast feding: The secial rle of halth srvices. *A Joint WHO/UNICEF* statement, World Health Organization, Geneva.
19. WHO (1999).Reduction of Maternal Mortality. *A Joint WHO/UNFPA/UNICEF/* World Bank Statement.
20. World Health Organisation (WHO), United Nations Children's Fund (UNICEF),United Nations Population Fund (UNFPA).(2001). Maternal Mortality in 1995.

Chapter 8

Assessment of the Prevalence of Under-nutrition and Anaemia in Adolescents Residing in Villages around Pilani Area of Rajasthan State in India

Nirupma Prakash[1], *Suman Kapur*[2], *Devinder Kumar*, *Urvashi Kaushik*[3], *R.P. Pareek*[4] *and Taniya Mozumder*

Birla Institute of Technology and Science, Pilani, Rajasthan, India

***E-mail:** [1]nirupama.prakash@gmail.com, [2]mssuman@gmail.com, [3]urvashi.dr@gmail.com, [4]pareekrp@gmail.com,*

ABSTRACT

The objective of the study was to address anaemia in adolescents and emphasize on its prevention and control. Adolescence is the building phase of life and as the child grows rapidly the iron requirement also increases rapidly during this phase. At least 60-70 per cent of adolescent girls in India are anaemic. 20 per cent of all maternal deaths are attributed to anaemia during pregnancy. Measures to overcome anaemia of nutritional origin at an early stage of life, can substantially impact the high maternal mortality rate and high incidence of low birth babies in India. This can only be achieved by way of more education, parasite control, nutritional supplementation and regular assessment and follow-ups. The present study has been conducted in schools located in villages adjoining Pilani with an aim to assess prevalence of anaemia in adolescents (age group 11 to 19 yrs) and control/prevent anaemia by education, de-worming and iron supplementation. Total of 304 students (175 boys and 129 girls) were studied for their nutritional status, anthropometry and haemoglobin levels.

The nutritional status of all students was found to be less than the Indian Council Medical Research (ICMR) prescribed standards and both wasting and stunting was observed in a significant percentage of students. All 312 adolescents were screened for haemoglobin levels and 77 per cent subjects were found to be anaemic with very few children having a level of 12gm per cent. More concerted efforts and steps need to be taken by to address the widespread public health issue of under-nutrition and anaemia.

Keywords: *Under nutrition, Anaemia in adolescents, Assess prevalence, Villages around Pilani area of Rajasthan.*

Introduction

Anaemia is characterized by low level of haemoglobin (Hb) in the blood. Haemoglobin is necessary for transporting oxygen from the lungs to other tissues and organs of the body. Anaemia mostly results from a nutritional deficiency of iron (iron-deficient anaemia), folate, vitamin B12, or other nutrients such as Vitamin C. Iron deficiency is the most widespread form of malnutrition in the world, affecting more than two billion people (1). Anaemia is an important and uncontrolled public health problem in India and affects an estimated 50 percent of the population in India (2). Recognizing the fact that nutritional anaemia is a preventable and controllable condition, several national programmes have been instituted (1). The main purpose of these programmes was to control and prevent anaemia in women of reproductive age group and pre-school children with the help of Fe-Folic acid supplementation. However, even after several efforts by the union and state governments the problem is still prominent in society leading to decreased productivity by individuals and thus the nation as a whole.

Anaemia has detrimental effects on the health of women and children, and is the major under-lying cause of maternal and perinatal mortality. Anaemia during pregnancy is an important public health problem not only in India but also in most of the south East Asian countries. About 4-16 per cent of maternal deaths are due to anaemia. Anaemia also results in an increased risk of premature delivery and low birth weight (2). Early detection of anaemia can help prevent complications related to pregnancy and delivery as well as address child development related problems. The National Family Health Survey of India (NFHS)-3 highlighted the high prevalence of anaemia in both women and children in comparison to previous surveys. Prevalence of anaemia in Rajasthan has been reported to be 53.1 per cent among women (Hb <12.0g/dl) and 23.6 per cent among men (Hb <13.0g/dl) between the age group 15-49 years. Among the 15-19 years olds an estimated 55.8 per cent girls and 30.2 per cent boys are anaemic. National statistics also reveal that the rural and poor are more vulnerable to anaemia.

Anaemia in adolescent group has been overlooked and this group has been neglected even now. NFHS-2 &3 did not address the problem in this age group as it considered only females of reproductive age group (15-49 years) and males were not considered at all. In view of this present scenario it is very important to tackle the problem of anaemia and hit the right target at the right time. Adolescence is the age when the human body prepares itself for future, the physical and cognitive development is at peak and several health impacting habits are being formed. Adolescents with worm infestations, regular blood loss (in case of girls), under-nutrition, high growth rate and physical over activity are more prone to iron deficiency anaemia. The minimum daily requirement of dietary iron during adolescence is 10-15 mg/day and is almost equivalent in both the sexes, however, young women and girls may require more, due to regular loss of blood during menstruation resulting in a higher incidence of anaemia in this group. Through this paper we are trying to address the problem of anaemia in this age group as it offers an opportunity to impact both, nutrition and health status, by adopting school-based targeted intervention programs to minimize and/or eradicate anaemia.

Materials and Methods

Subjects, Study Area and Investigations

A total of 304 students (175 boys and 129 girls) were studied in the government and private schools in villages of Chapra and Chirawa in district Jhunjunu. Ethical permission and consent from all concerned (Principal, parents and adult subjects) were obtained prior to the study and the study was approved by the Institutional Ethics Committee (IHEC) of BITS, Pilani. A simple stratified technique was used to recruit students between the ages of 11-19 years. A 24-hour food recall method was used to know the nutritional status and daily calorie and protein intake of the subjects. Each subject was subjected to anthropometric measurements (height and weight) and Body Mass Index (BMI) was calculated using Quetlet's index. Criteria of underweight normoweight/overweight were used as per ICMR guidelines. Waslow's weight for height and height for age were used in order to see stunting and wasting respectively. Simple prick method was used to draw a drop of blood from the ring finger and haemoglobin percentage was estimated using Sahli's haemoglobinometer.

Intervention Tools Used

1. *Education*: Students were provided with basic knowledge of food composition and dietary principles. Important food items which can prevent anaemia of nutritional origin, such as green vegetables and local seasonal fruits, were brought to their notice. Knowledge about practices for personal hygiene and clean/healthy habits to prevent infections and parasite infestations was also imparted through interactive classroom sessions. Concept of anaemia and its consequences were also made clear to them.
2. *De-worming*: Participants found to be anaemic (Hb per cent < 12.0g/dl) were administered with a suitable de-worming agent.
3. *Iron supplementation*: After one week of de-worming all the participants with anaemia were put on weekly Iron supplementation for 4 months.

Data Analysis

Data was digitized and analysed on SPSS 10.0 statistical software.

Results and Discussion

Anthropometric Measurements

The nutritional and health status of all participants in the study were found to be below WHO standards for both weight for height and weight for age. The BMI shows variable trends in different age groups (Table 8.1). The observed mean BMI also revealed under nutrition in both the sexes (Table 8.2) of the cohort studied.

Table 8.1: Mean Height, Weight and Body Mass Index in Different Age Groups

Per cent Tiles of Age	*Height (cm) Mean ± SD*	*Weight (kg) Mean ± SD*	*Body Mass Index (kg/m^2) Mean ± SD*
11-12, N=127	143.40 ± 10.15	33.88 ± 7.89	16.395 ± 3.121
13-14, N=106	151.01 ± 13.28	40.34 ± 8.54	17.551 ± 2.393
15-16, N=64	161.05± 9.63	49.48 ± 7.50	19.052 ± 2.062
17-18, N=7	168.14 ± 8.84	54.71 ± 5.31	19.386 ± 1.871
Total, N=304	150.34 ± 13.29	39.90 ± 10.15	17.426 ± 2.847

Table 8.2: Height, Weight and Body Mass Index with Respect to Sex of Subject

Sex of Subject	*Height (cm) Mean ± SD*	*Weight (kg) Mean ± SD*	*Body Mass Index (kg/m^2) Mean ± SD*
Male, N=175	151.86 ± 15.11	40.63 ± 11.74	17.294 ± 2.739
Female, N=129	148.27 ± 10.03	38.90 ± 7.95	17.605 ± 2.988
Total, N=304	150.34 ± 13.29	39.90 ± 10.15	17.426 ± 2.847

Further analyses revealed that only 54.6 per cent students were within the 90 per cent tile of ICMR prescribed weight for their height and only 70 per cent met the national standard for the prescribed height for their age. A bigger concern was that even with an operational midday meal program for school children, run under the aegis of Integrated Child Development Scheme of the Government of India, >24 per cent adolescents showed sever wasting while nearly 29.3 per cent depicted severe stunting (Figures 8.1a and b). As expected there was a positive correlation between age of the subject and BMI (Figure 8.2).

Haemoglobin Percentage

As shown in Table 8.3 the mean Hb per cent in all groups was below the standard norm of 12 g/dl, and the trend was similar in both boys and girls. An extremely small minority, merely 16 boys (9.14 per cent) and 10 girls (7.75 per cent) in the cohort met the norm of 12gm per cent for girls and 13gm per cent for boys. Thus, only 8.5 per cent adolescent children were not anaemic in this cohort of school going adolescents. Age stratification further revealed that children with ideal Hb levels ranged from 0 to 22.6 per cent only (Table 8.4) leaving a wide gap between the desired and the observed situation from public health perspective. Mean Hb level for the cohort was only 10.36gm per cent even with all the Government of India programs in schools.

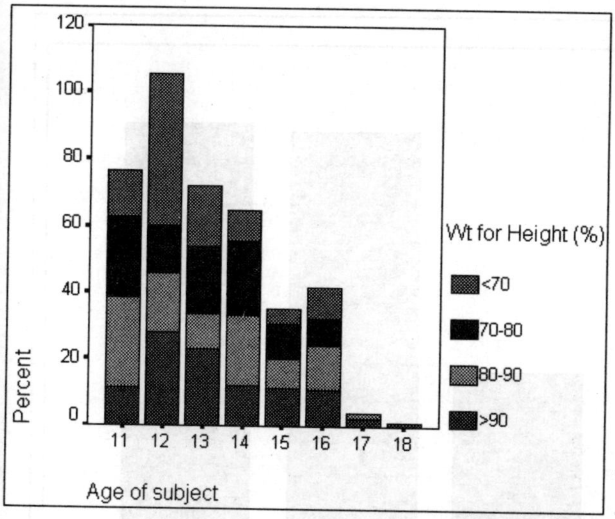

	Frequency	*Percent*
>90	166	54.6
80-90	67	22
70-80	49	16.1
<70	22	7.2
Total	304	100

Figure 8.1a: Weight for Height

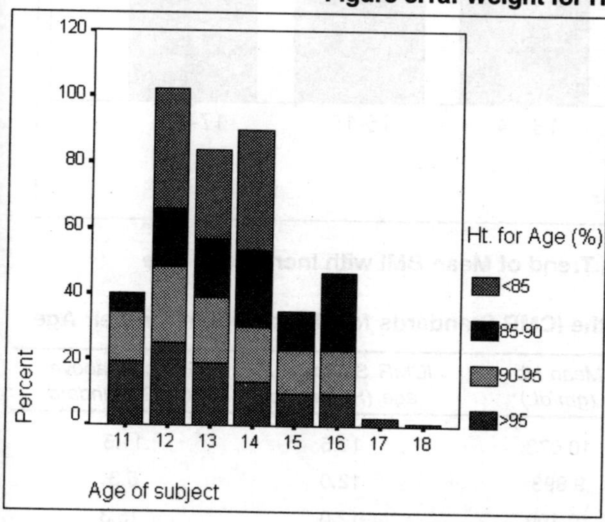

	Frequency	*Percent*
>95	215	70.7
90-95	61	20.1
85-90	17	5.6
<85	11	3.6
Total	304	100

Figure 8.1b: Height for Age

Table 8.3: Haemoglobin Levels in Different Age Groups

Per cent Tiles of Age	*Haemoglobin (gm per cent) Mean ± SD*
11-12, N=127	9.97 ± 1.08
13-14, N=106	10.06 ± 1.06
15-16, N=64	11.51 ± 1.58
17-18, N=7	12.63 ± 1.02
Total, N=304	10.39 ± 1.48
Males, N=175	10.67 ± 1.56
Females, N=129	9.99 ± 1.28

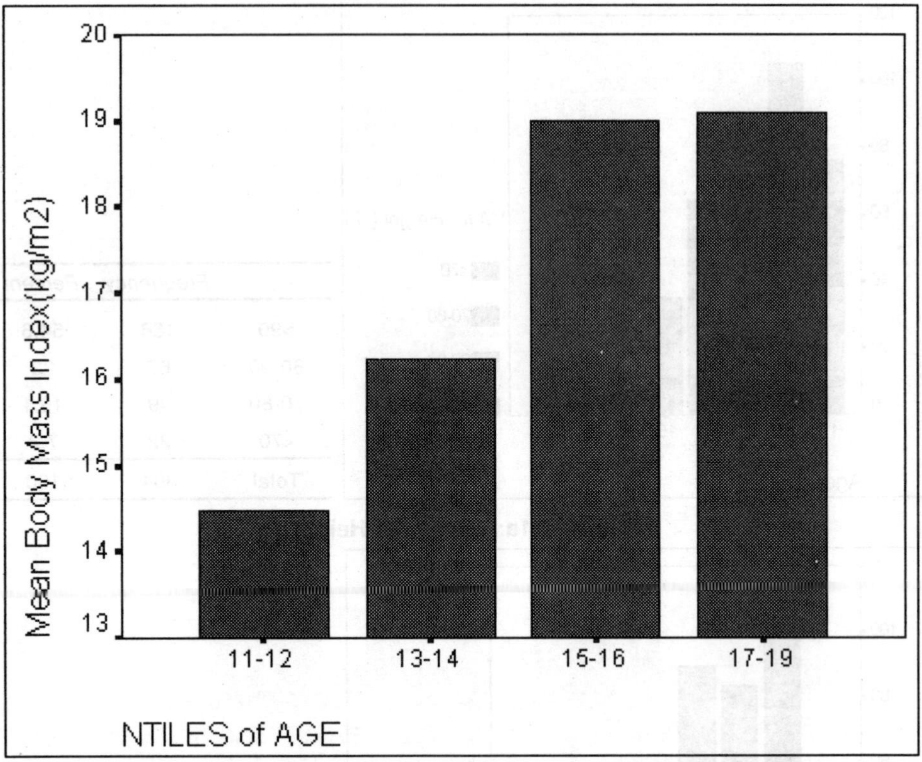

Figure 8.2: Increasing Trend of Mean BMI with Increase in Age

Table 8.4: Adolescent Meeting the ICMR Standards for Haemoglobin for their Age

Age (in years)	*N*	*Mean Hb (gm/dL)*	*ICMR Standard for age (Hb gm/dL)*	*Per cent above ICMR Standard*
11	52	10.073	11.5	11.5
12	75	9.893	12.0	5.3
13	59	10.100	12.0	15.3
14	47	10.013	>12.0	8.5
15	31	11.061	12.5	22.6
16	33	11.927	13.0	21.2
17	5	12.200	13.5	0
18	2	13.700	14.0	50

Nutritional Intake

The nutritional intake was calculated on the basis of 24 hour recall method. The calorie and protein intakes of participants of both the schools were found to be below the Recommended Daily allowances (RDA).

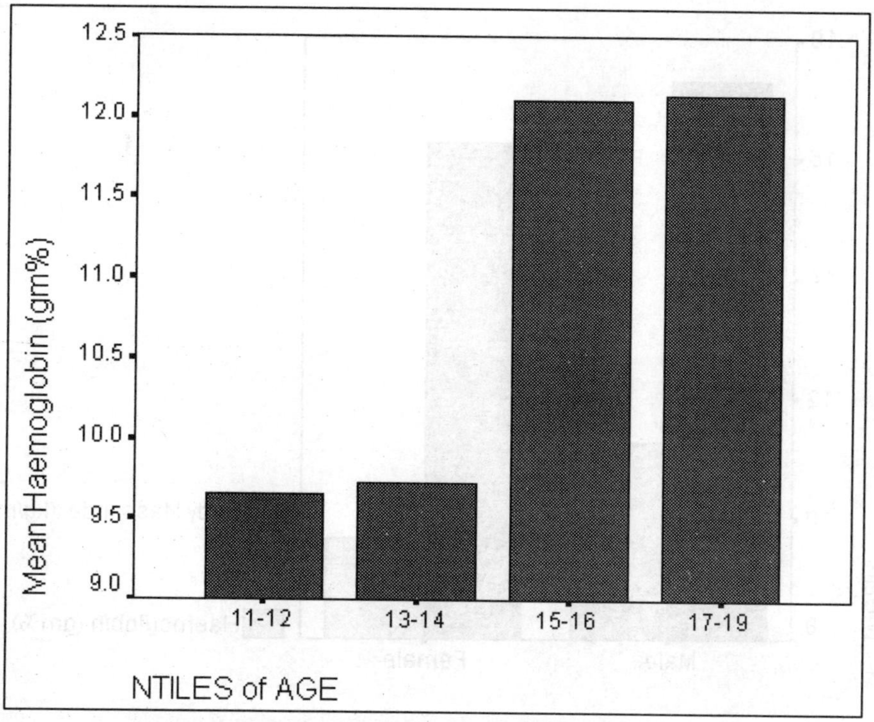

Figure 8.2a: Mean Hb Per cent in Different Age Groups

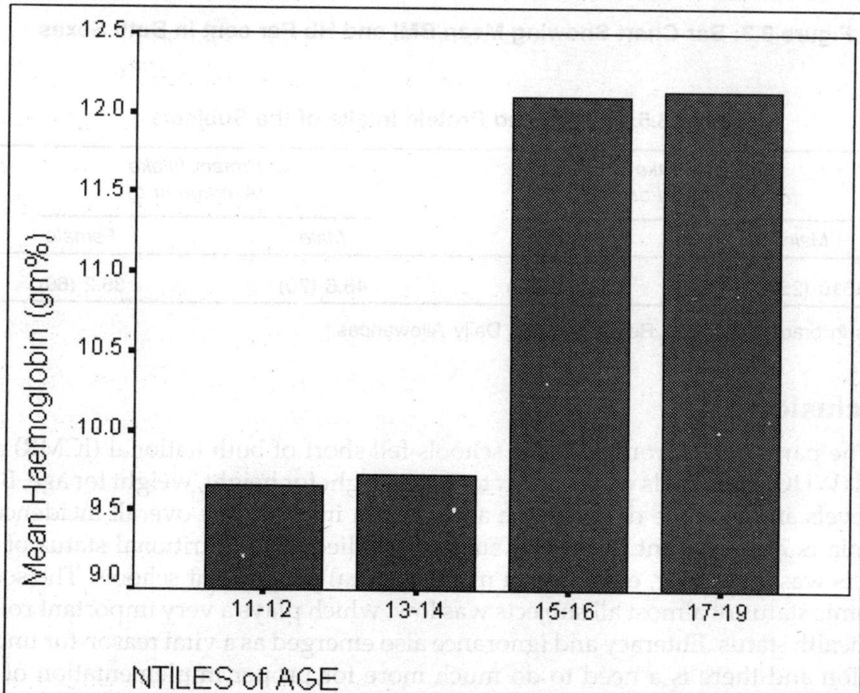

Figure 8.2b: Mean BMI in Different Age Groups

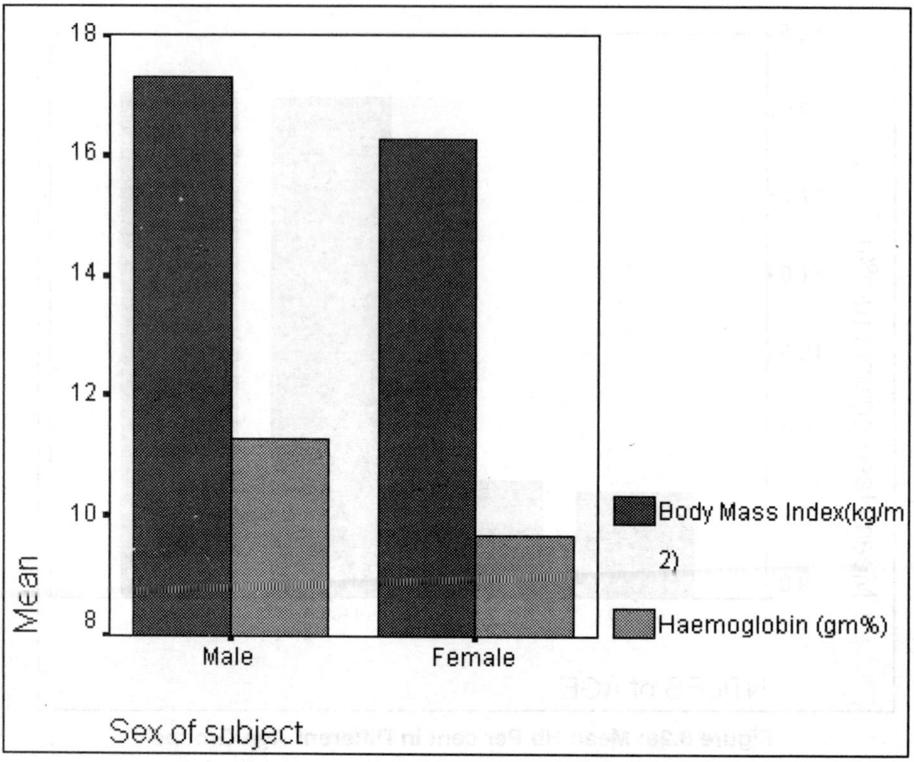

Figure 8.3: Bar Chart Showing Mean BMI and Hb Per cent in Both Sexes

Table 8.5: Energy and Protein Intake of the Subjects

Energy Intake (Average Kcal/day)		*Protein Intake (Average in g)*	
Male	*Female*	*Male*	*Female*
1510 (2500)	1380 (2000)	48.6 (70)	36.2 (60)

Figures in brackets are the Recommended Daily Allowances.

Conclusions

The participants from both the schools fell short of both national (ICMR) and global (WHO) standards with respect to their weight for height, weight for age, BMI, Hb Levels and average daily calorie and protein intakes. The overall incidence of anaemia is 77.4 per cent in the 304 subjects studied. The nutritional status of the subjects was very poor, even with a mid-day meal program at schools. The socio-economic status of almost all subjects was low, which plays a very important role in their health status. Illiteracy and ignorance also emerged as a vital reason for under-nutrition and there is a need to do much more for proper implementation of the present schemes, introduction of contextually effective micronutrient supplementation programs and regular periodic follow-ups to effectively overcome the problem of iron-deficient anaemia and malnutrition.

References

1. Park, K (2007), *The Textbook of Preventive and Social Medicine*, 19th edition, 10:492-493; 504-506.

2. http://www.12 by 12 initiative.com, *12 by 12 initiative (haemoglobin 12 gm per cent by 12 years of age.*

3. http://www.nfhsindia.org/nfhs3.html, *NFHS-3 national fact sheet.*

Chapter 9

The Impact of Decentralization Health Authority on Safe Motherhood Program in Indonesia

Sri Setiawati

Assistant Deputy to the Minister for Ethics and Harmonization of Science and Technology, Indonesia
E-mail: asdep42@yahoo.com

ABSTRACT

Indonesia is a stable democratic nation facing challenges of the 21st century. One of those challenges is the health of its 225 million citizens, and half of populations are women. Indonesia is engaged in a major governmental transition from centralized planning into the decentralization of administrative responsibilities to the level of the Kabupaten (District) and Kotamadya (City) administration which consist of 33 provinces and 497 Districts/city. In Indonesia, democratization and subsequent reform including public sector decentralization may suffering safe motherhood program, since political and financial power became decentralized to regional governments. As a result, the capacity of the central government including the Health Ministry to command the district governments to prioritize maternal healthcare program weakened dramatically. Decentralization of health authority from central to provincial and regional governments has worsened the women and children health conditions. The prevalence of disparities in Indonesia before and at the starting of the decentralization process was very extensive. According to Health Ministry data, the country's maternal mortality rate (MMR) remains high at 228 maternal deaths per 100,000 live births in 2007 just decrease 20 point from 2006 result. In comparison, the maternal mortality rate reached only 39 per 100,000 in Malaysia and 6 per 100,000 in Singapore. Reducing the MMR has become the first priority in the Indonesian healthcare system. The high level of MMR also influence by women empowerment status that is due to structural and socio cultural constraints. Meanwhile, achievement of Infant Mortality Rate more better in 2009 has been 34 per 100.000 and targeted to be 24 per 100.000 in 2014. Indonesia is in a danger of failing to achieve the Millennium Development Goals (MDGs) if it fails to reduce its MMR, however an achieving IMR still on the track. Indonesia is likely to face difficulties in reducing MMR to be 118 by the end of 2014. Therefore, government in every level hand in hand with Parliament and other parties should have strategies and an increasing their commitment to speed up on providing better health for women and their family in the region. Begin 2010, holistic approach on seven pilot government agencies including health sector have new budget policy on the implementation of gender responsive budget for programmes.

Keywords: *Decentralization, Autonomy, Women empowerment, Safe motherhood.*

Introduction

Indonesia is an archipelago country that stretched from Sabang at the top of Sumatra Island to Merauke at the bottom of Papua across the equator for more than 5,000 kilometers from east to west and more than 2,000 kilometers from north to south, or from 6′ north to 11′ south latitude, and from 95′ to 141′ east longitude. It lies on a crossroads between two oceans, the Pacific and the Indian, and bridges two continents, Asia and Australia. It is an appropriate description of the archipelago as there are estimated to be a total of 17,504 islands, of which only about 6,000 are inhabited. There are five main islands and about 30 smaller islands. The five main islands are: Sumatra (446,687 square kilometer); Java/Madura (129,306 square

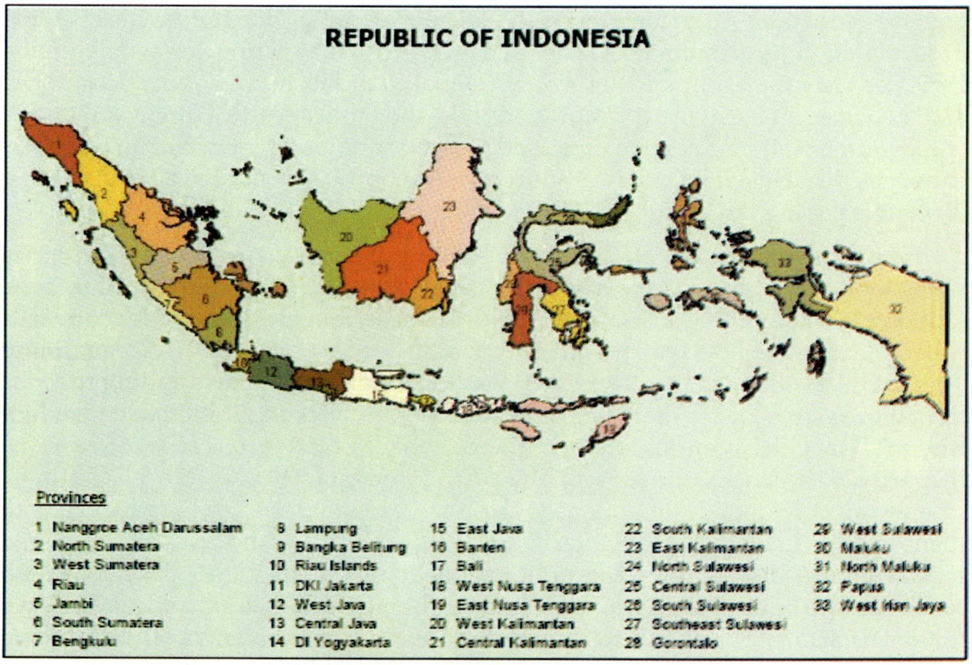

Figure 9.1: Republic of Indonesia

kilometer); Kalimantan, which comprises two thirds of the island of Borneo (507,412 square kilometer); Sulawesi (193,847 square kilometer); and Papua (424,501 square kilometer), which is part of the world's second largest island, New Guinea. Indonesia's Administrative regions in 2010 consist of 33 provinces, and 497 district/city. Based on BPS Statistic Indonesia, population number in 2006 was 225,642,124 that almost a half women population. Population density level was still dominated by provinces in Java that is population distribution was unequal as 58.70 per cent of total population lived in Java Island (the area with only 6.95 per cent of Indonesia), 21.03 per cent in Sumatra, 7.21 per cent in Sulawesi, 5.53 per cent in Kalimantan, 5.40 per cent in Nusa Tenggara and Bali, and 2.13 per cent in Maluku and Papua. In average, number of people lived in rural 56.88 per cent and 43.12 per cent in urban area.

The government of Indonesia has showed in many instances their special attention on women newborn and child health. There are several inter sector collaboration lead by the MOH, working on different scopes on maternal and child health in the country. The improvement of health services in general and for maternal and child care in particular is best achieved also through tight collaboration between healthcare and social welfare services. This collaboration will strive towards achieving the MDG 4 and 5 for reducing maternal, and child mortality and morbidity. To reduce maternal and child mortality, ensuring continuum of care for MNCH is important which spans from pregnancy, childbirth, postpartum, newborn and child care; as well as continuum care at individual, family, community, primary care and first referral levels. Through continuum of care approaches will beneficial for children to become a healthier next generation. These approaches are also an investment to high quality human resources, support economics development and an important role in poverty reduction. According to WHO (2006) stated that integrative intervention program such as economic, politic, and educational to empower women have indicated the greatest impact on women's quality of life, autonomy and authority and on policy changes, and on improved child and family health. Patient and family empowerment strategies have increased patients' abilities to manage their disease, adopt healthier behavior, and use health services more effectively, as well as increasing care-giver coping skills and efficacy.

The main issue of decentralization in health was intended to bring health service closer to the society and make it better particularly to inhabitants in the rural areas. However, a long 10 years of reform process, criticism of the government's decentralization policy centered on the lack of an adequate architecture to support it. The central government in effect functioned as an equalizer, redistributing revenue from the resource- rich to the resource-poor provinces. Decentralization would reduce the imbalance between Jakarta and the regions, but, paradoxically increase the disparity between the richer and the poorer regions. Second, the institutional framework at the local level to manage these resources and the functions that go with them may be inadequate to the task. Health decentralization has been hampered technically because of the weak political policy in provinces. Meanwhile, health sector tends to be more technical. For example, the mutation of health officers between regions is also very difficult to do. Further, budgeting problems and health data which are still not managed well between Central and Provincial regions have made health service less good. The budget allocated to poor and rural regions should be more than the wealthier ones. This also happens to public health insurance (Jamkesmas). In order to achieve the goal of health development, it is necessary to have awareness; willingness and ability of all components, if it is realize the healthy people as a source of strong resilience of nations.

The International Conference on Population and Development (ICPD) in Cairo 1994 and Millennium Development Goals (MDGs) recognized the importance of reproductive health and rights, as well as women's empowerment and gender equality, as the cornerstones of population and development programs. To reiterate the commitment to reduce maternal and neonatal mortality in Indonesia, in 2010 the Government of Indonesia launched the Making Pregnancy Safer strategic plan which focuses on strengthening the capacity of the health systems to secure the provision and utilization of interventions that target the major causes of maternal and neonatal mortality and morbidity through women empowerment in every aspect such economy, socio-cultural and political.

Current Health Status

Decentralization can be positive or negative benefit for the health status. It could improve the status of devolution of public health but also can weaken the public health status. In general, this is influenced by the priorities are made by local government and political commitment due to parliaments very powerful to vote budget allocation. Therefore, disparity among region in implementing public program such as health and education has been indicated as national problem to be solved an achieving welfare of the state.

Human Development Index (HDI) is one measure to describe the level of achievement of the result of development in a country, including of a health indicators. Meanwhile, the common health status has been indicated through the performance of Infant Mortality Rate (IMR), Maternal Mortality Rate (MMR) and Under Five Mortality Rate (UMR). Based on BPS (2007) indicated the trends of several indicator from 2003 until 2007 had been improved slowly as can be shown in Table 9.1 below. To increase HDI, The National Programme for Indonesian Children made the issue

Table 9.1: Performance Indicator on Health Status in Indonesia, 1994-2007

Parameter	*1994*	*1997*	*2003*	*2007*
TFR	2.9	2.8	2.6	2.6
IMR	66	52	43	39
USMR	81	58	46	44
MMR	390	334	307	228
Eo	67.7	64.3	65.8	69.6
CDR	-	7.6	8.0	6.9
HDI	0.66	0.67	0.72	0.73

Sources: 1. IDHS, 1994, 1997, 2003, 2007; 2. BPS, Bapenas, UNDP.

of the death of babies and young children as one of the most important parts. The program is part of the Indonesian Children's Vision 2015, a movement that involves all segments of society, from government, the private sector to academia and civil society. Together, these groups try to improve the quality of health and welfare of babies and children under 5. In addition to promoting healthy living for children and improving the quality of access to comprehensive health services, part of the Goal, is to increase the proportion of births assisted by trained personnel, so to expect changes in the behavior of the community to more actively seek health services, especially for young children and children under five. The risk of maternal death because of the birth process in Indonesia is 1 death in every 65 births. Each year 20,000 deaths estimated to occur because of maternal complications during childbirth and during pregnancy. The main causes of maternal death in Indonesia are haemorrhage, eclampsia, which causes high blood pressure during pregnancy, abortion's complications, infection and complications during the birth. Although Indonesia does not yet have good data collection system to obtain information on Maternal Mortality in Indonesia, experts estimate that the Maternal Mortality in Indonesia in 1992 is 425 and decrease to 228 in 2007.

Concerning to the poor community's health status is also influenced by the complex and interlinked gender issues disfavoring, mostly women, but also ignoring the importance of men involvement for example, in reproductive health issues. The Ministry of health, having fostered the enactment of the Presidential Instruction no 9 of 2000 on Gender Mainstreaming in all development sectors has implemented gender mainstreaming activity under the leadership of RH sub-directorate. Gender analysis and development of the work plans was conducted, initially in 6 priorities programs namely TB, malaria, maternal health, environmental health, Nutrition and STI/HIV/AIDS, and then expanded to other health programs.

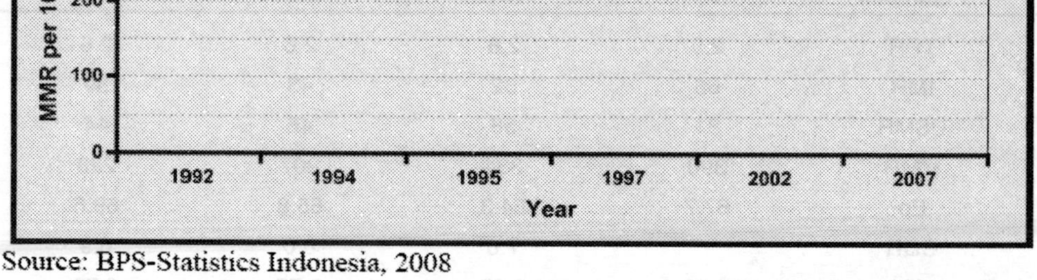

Source: BPS-Statistics Indonesia, 2008

Figure 9.2: Maternal Mortality Rate PER 100.000 Live Births, 1994-2007

Moreover, the threats to health especially in poor cities or districts are even higher due to the lack of understanding and awareness of new leadership of local governments, on the benefits of and funding for public health services. To ensure that local governments undertake certain public health measures, the Ministry of Health issued a decree pertaining to 26 types of minimum/essential public health services that the local governments must perform, including 54 indicators to be achieved. Of the 26 services, 18 are related to public health such as maternal and child health, promotion and prevention of prevalent diseases, school health and disease surveillance. For instant, Study was conduct by Zohra Andi Baso (YLK South Sulawesi) on the decentralization of health services in Makassar, showed that is by changes in local structures. As a result local expenditure swelling that local governments trying to increase local revenue (PAD) without structurally involve community participation. For example, in the Makassar budget allocation of health sector is only 6.5 per cent and 52.12 per cent of the budget used for administrative costs, salaries and expenses for business trips. Beside budget allocations more top-down, an initiative of the government and does not involve and accommodate community input.

The performance of district on managing public services such as health depend on the ability and innovation of the leader as head of region that do not merely of budget problem. For instance, Jembrana Distric in Bali Province that is famous as successful district on preparing public services to community mainly in health and education sector. With limited budget from central government and local revenue (PAD), the authority has policy to manage the budget allocation for hospital through Health Insurance managed by other institution.

The infant mortality rate in Indonesia is the highest among the other ASEAN countries. Nevertheless, Indonesia has actually reached the fourth goal of MDGs. Our job now is to ensure that Indonesia's children get their constitutional rights. Article No. 23 on Child Protection states that every child has the right to obtain health services and social security according to their physical, psychological and social needs. One third of the infant deaths in Indonesia occur within the first month after birth, 80 per cent of them occur during the first week of life. The main causes of death are acute respiratory infections, diarrhea and birth complications. Besides the main causes, some infectious diseases such as meningitis, typhus and encephalitis are also quite often the causes of infant mortality.

On health budget, Indonesia government spending has raise from about US$1 billion in 2001 to over US$4 billion in 2007, which for the first time reached 1 per cent of GDP 8 while 24 out of a total of 33 provinces allocate less than 10 per cent of their budgets for health (MOH, 2008). National health priorities include maternal and child health, services for the poor, improved capacity of health personnel, emergency responses to communicable diseases, malnutrition and health crisis caused by disasters and service delivery for remote, underdeveloped and border areas and outer islands. Water and sanitation are not considered high priorities at national level or below.

Devolving authority and obligation of health functions to the local governments poses threats to public health. Since the local government, including the local

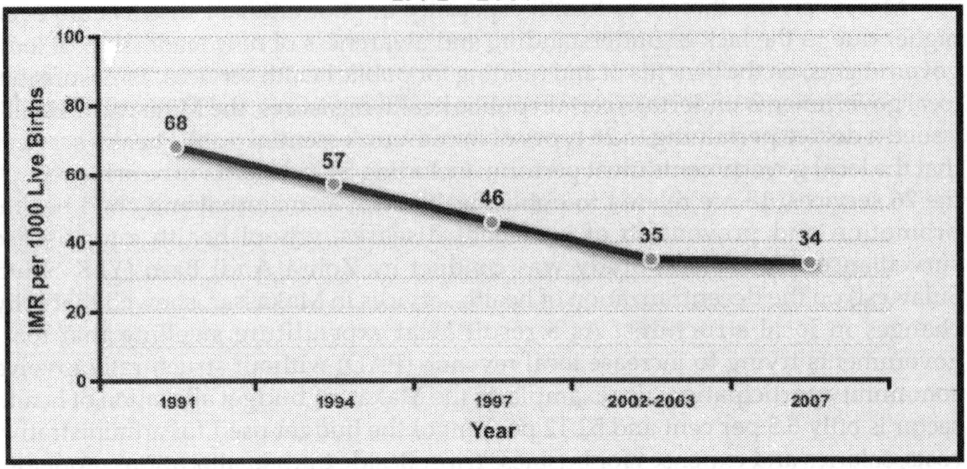

Source: Result of Indonesia Demography and Health Survey, BPS-Statistics Indonesia

Figure 9.3: Estimation of Infant Mortality Rate (IMR) PER 1.000 Live Births 1991-2007

parliament, is an elected body, the chances of elected officials not having an understanding nor commitment to public health are greater than in the previous 'less democratic' government. Not only the health sector, but also other sectors responsible for basic services such as education may also be at risk of lack of local government funding, jeopardizing the future development of the local areas. In order to ensure that public programs implemented under decentralized governments are equitable, accessible and affordable, the central government has set standards for guiding the local administration with minimum obligatory functions.

The new law on regional autonomy (the Act 32/2004) has rectified some problems which existed under the previous law. To date, it is very difficult to draw a map of the capacity of local governments. One general observation is the lack of fiscal capacity generated by the regions and the low priority given to public health. More than three quarters of local governments in Indonesia are fiscally dependent on the general allocation budget (*Dana Alokasi Umum*), allocated by the central government. As a residual effect of centralized government of the past, when good people in the municipalities and provinces were shifted to serve in the central offices, the capacity of human resources at the local governments is very limited and human resources mobility in the region become difficult due to local regulation. In such a situation, even if the central government might channel quite a large sum of funds, there is little chance that these funds will be given to the health sector. Even if the health sector receives an adequate budget, it is very likely that the funds will be used for capital items such as purchasing fancy medical equipment, constructing new or extending the existing facilities, rather than improving the human resource capacity.

Women Empowerment

Based on Law 22/1999 on local government and decentralization, local governments in have greater power and autonomy in deciding and conducting the development process at their regions. This new law which is based on principle of democracy and equity is intended to increase the capacity of civil society and community participation by strengthening the position of the people's representation in asking for accountability of the executive. However, local governments in face structural and cultural obstacles in realizing gender equity. The revival of local patriarchal values along with institutional constraints poses great challenges to women. Although the Article 27 of 1945 Constitution guarantees human rights equality for all people of Indonesia - both men and women, many found practices that discriminate and thus trigger the occurrence of gaps, especially at the local level. This includes the implementation of local regulations that contain elements of duality that is not in accordance with the 1945 Constitution.

According to a recent gender gap study conducted by the World Economic Forum, Indonesia ranking have been fluctuated from 2006 until 2009. The data show in 2006, Indonesia ranked 61 (117 countries), 2007 ranked 66 (128 countries), 2008 ranked 93(134) and 2009 ranked 93rd out of 134 countries. Indonesia ranked higher than Malaysia, which placed 101st on the gender gap list, and Cambodia (104th), but compare to other neighbors such as the Philippines (9th), Thailand (59th), Vietnam (71st) and Singapore (85th). The survey assessed gender equality in a number of areas that included education, economy, politics and health. Indonesia does not gain any positions in the overall rankings, The discrimination against women was even worse among the poor, as their chances of gaining access to quality education and health services dropped considerably. The Indonesia Government is currently doing a lot of strategies to support the achievement of the third goal of MDGs. In addition to the gender program in education sector, efforts are also made to increase opportunities for women to work in non-agricultural sector and equity rewards. The women empowerment sector is an important step for achieving the MDGs third goal and also an impact to achieve four and five goal of MDGs. including increased representation of women in the political aspects. Many regulation has been implemented to increase women empowerment and gender equality as follow:

- National Constitution (Articles 27, 28)
- Law No. 7/1984 on Ratification of CEDAW
- Law No. 39/1999 on Human Rights
- Law No. 32/2004 on Local Government
- Presidential Instruction No. 9 Year 2000 on Gender Mainstreaming in National Development to all actors of government at the national and sub-national leves;
- Law No. 7 Year 2005 on Mid-Term National Development (2004 – 2009), continued in 2010-2014 and already integrated in the Law No 7/2007 on Long Term National Development
- Finance Ministerial Decree No. 119 Year 2009 on the implementation of gender responsive budget in seven pilot government agencies programmes and budget starting 2010
- Home Affairs Ministerial Decree No. 15 Year 2008 on Manual for the Implementation of Gender Mainstreaming in the Region

However, some constraints still in place to implement such policy mainly in the structural and socio cultural. In the structural constraints such as some laws and regulations/policies are still discriminative and gender biased; lack of Commitment from decision makers, lack of gender expertise, lack of disaggregated data (gender profile) provide. In the socio-cultural constraints such as the patriarchal structures of the community contribute to the disproportionate share of responsibilities in care and housework related activities, communal and traditional obligation that women in have to carry. Thus, women have limited or no time to involve in community meeting or other public activities which are influential to local decision making.

Although, Indonesia Gender Gap still higher compared to other countries and need to be challenge that still has achieved much progress in addressing the issue of inequality between men and women. The 9-year compulsory education program has brought positive impacts in the reduction of inequalities in education. The ratio between the participation of students, men and women, both net and gross participation have almost reached 100 per cent at all levels of education. However, the success of this program still needs to be improved, particularly for the older age groups. There are still quite a gap and a false impression in the context of gender and role in society. This incorrect perception happens in almost all aspects of life, from the career (of equal opportunity and benefits) to representation in politics.

Further, decentralization allows the revitalization of local patriarchal values which strengthen the patriarchal structure of the community, thus threatening women's empowerment program at the local level. Local governments need to play active role in reconstructing more gender equal community by disseminating information and persistently campaigning on women's reproductive health aim at both men and women and that both men and women are responsible for women's reproductive health. - By emphasizing more on gender sensitivity of programs and service delivery such as women's reproductive health centers, credit scheme for women, sanitation, and other welfare related programs aims to equalize gender relation, local governments have strategic role in deconstructing this inequalities.

Policy Concern

Based on government experience and evaluation of previous five years program (2004-2009) especially in public sector, government make new policy that is construct development program whereas gender mainstreaming is the one of success indicator on implementing the programs for all sectors.

Dealing with the Indonesian target on development program, the classical problem of lack of efficient coordination between the central and local governments need to be concern, to cut off constraints that caused to the disparity of health status among regency/municipality. Indonesian government consistently relied on MPS strategy in accomplishing MDG 2015 which is similar in goal with difference in time of achievement toward Medium-term Health Indonesia that is to achieve "Healthy Indonesia 2010".

Therefore, the government needs to be more proactive in making sure its programs were carried out properly. Methods to monitor these programs and evaluate them have to be put in place, especially if the country hopes to achieve the Millennium Development Goals by 2015. The New Cabinet 2010-2014 have been establishing Midterm Planning 2010-2014 in which to meet the target of MDG's on 2015. In order to achieve the goal of national development, it is necessary to have awareness, willingness and ability of all component of the nation to realize that healthy people as source of countries Therefore, every ministry has been develop Strategic Planning 2010-2014 that should be an integrated program to dealing with the national vision and target.

Table 9.2: Target 4 and 5–Reducing MMR and IMR by 2015

Sl.No.	Indicator	1990	2007	Target
1.	Mother Mortality Rate	390	307	118
2.	Birth helped by trained Nurse	40.7 per cent	72,4 per cent	Indicator
3.	Under Five Mortality Rate	81	40	32
4.	Infant Mortality Rate (IMR)	57	32	19

Source: MOH, 2004, 2007 Indonesia Health Profile.

MOH, 2010, Strategic Planning 2010-2014.

Based on Finance Ministerial No 119/2009 there are 7 Government agencies namely Department of National Education, Health, Public Work, Agriculture, Finance, Ministry of National Development Planning/National Development Planning Board and Ministry of Women Empowerment to implement Gender Responsive Budget (GRB) in 2010. There are asked to prepare Gender Budget Statement in four parts: (a) Outcomes and outputs of the largest-sub- programmes and their implications for gender equality; (b) outcomes and outputs which specifically target women and girls; (c) outcomes and outputs which will benefit both men and women and promote gender equality (d) outcomes and outputs which will strengthen gender mainstreaming institutions (gender focal points, working groups etc) in their respective Work plan. Based on the national policies determined in the Middle-term National Development Plan 2010-2014 of Ministry of Health stated that Health Development Programs need to be emphasizing on increasing gender equity on giving opportunity for access, participation, benefit and control between women and men in health services. Therefore, Ministry of Health and Ministry of Women Empowerment make target and program to reduce IMR and MMR on 2010 that has been focused on;

1. The Attainment of Public Health, focus on Increase Maternal Health Service and Increase Child Health Service.
2. The Attainment of Personal Health, focus on Increase Reference Health Service
3. Protection and Elimination of Disease focus on Prevent and Recovery of Risk Disease and Finding/Recovering the Victim.

Further to Strengthening Mother and Child Health Program such program has been implemented mainly on community and family support for mothers and children as follow;

Birth Preparedness and Complication Readiness (BPCR/P4K)

BPCR/P4K using Sticker is one breakthrough to accelerate decreasing of maternal mortality which is the Sticker put it in each pregnant mother house. BPCR/P4K is also as one component of Alert Village/Desa Siaga Program. Through the BPCR/P4K every pregnant mother can monitor intensively by her husband, her family, community and midwife as well, early detection and prompt treatment when complication arise, safe and secure delivery assisted by skilled health provider and avoid maternal death. Through P4K with sticker also encourage and empower husband, family and community to be alert of pregnant mother through preparation and provision of saving, transportation, blood donors when pregnant mother needed. To improve knowledge of pregnant mothers for making birth plan, MCH Handbook is given to them during the first visit with health provider.

Mother Friendly Movement (Gerakan Sayang Ibu)

Ministry of Women Empowerment and Ministry of Health initiate Mother Friendly Movement/Gerakan Sayang Ibu (GSI) which are a movement among government and community to improve women quality of life especially to increase acceleration of MMR and IMR. GSI has programs for providing Birth Preparedness, ensuring good nutrition for pregnant mother and save deliveries.

Conditional Cash Transfer (CCT)/Program Keluarga Harapan

Ministry of Social Affair initiates Conditional Cash Transfer/Program Keluarga Harapan which are a movement among government and community to improve women quality of life particularly for poor pregnant or lactating mother and children between 0-15 years old to get the quality health services through cash supported to very poor household. The reason underlying CCT is basically to improve the quality of human resources of children as healthy next generation through compulsory basic education, health and social welfare services in line with the MDG's target. CCT program is crucial program since it is not merely social assistance but also to educate the poor people in spending money for basic and specific purpose in relation with health and social welfare and education needs.

Desa Siaga Program (Alert Village)

Desa Siaga (alert village) is a village which is prepared with trained resources and capability to prevent and respond health problems. In Alert Village facilities, consist of primary healthcare (village health post, sub health center), facilitated with community-based health unit (integrated health center). Also community-based preparedness and response for emergency situation, and operation on community-based budget.

Family and Women Empowerment Models

Through women organization or women groups conduct the program to improve women empowerment, to improve women knowledge and skilled, to support increasing income generating, giving the same opportunity in the community forums. The main activities of Community based Programs in supporting mother and child health that stated above are:

- Inform danger sign of mother, neonatal and under 5 children
- Encourage using of MCH Handbook
- Empowering health cadres
- Provide blood donors
- Provide transportation if needed to refer mother
- Provide saving for emergency situation

Regarding to availability of data, the government also needs to improve the monitoring system to achieve MDG 5. Improved data collection system, particularly the management aspects and the flow of information, especially basic health infrastructure data, and coordination between related institutions with the donor community also needs to be improved to avoid overlap and unnecessary activities, so the increase in maternal health can be achieved more effectively and efficiently. Dealing with problem of data, the Ministry of Health has been developing National Health Information System.

Conclusions

Indonesia is encountering massive changes in public functions, including the health sector, from centralized to decentralized systems. Since perception and understanding on the nature and the benefits of decentralized health systems, especially personal and public health, policies and program, vary widely across regions, competition to get a bigger pie of the government budget has left the health sector relatively under-funded in most regions. This lack of priority has increased the risk of poorer health status of the already chronically under-funded health sector in Indonesia.

The Ministry of Health has anticipated such a danger of neglected public health services, undertaking regulation measures such as issuing minimum healthcare/ service functions to be delivered by local governments. In practice, most local governments have difficulties in fulfilling the minimum functions due to lack of financial and human resources.

High disparity in fiscal capacity across regions and a severe shortage of good health personnel, who have moved to the central government offices, have made the risks of worsening health status within region.

In the mean time, the severe shortage and huge gaps between the present and estimated supply of human resources (as measured by conservative population ratios) have been coupled with the sprouting of multiple education institutions throughout the country.

Therefore, to achieve MDG's target on Women Empowerment, MMR and IMR on 2015, Indonesian government should have strong policy and commitment in improving the health status of the people of Indonesia. To address the urgent public health problems, the Ministry of Health together with Ministry of Women Empowerment, Coordinating Ministry of Welfare, Local Government, Parliament either in central and local and other community as whole should take a holistic approach and comprehensive action dealing with the problem to achieve MDG's in 2015.

References

1. BPS, 2007 Indonesian Demography and Health Survey.
2. BPS, 2006 Intercensus Survey
3. BPS-Statistic Indonesia, Bappenas, and UNDP. 2004. *National Human Development Report*
4. *2004, The Economics of Democracy, Financing Human Development in Indonesia.* BPS, Jakarta
5. Ministry of Health of Indonesia, ADB and EPOS (2006) The effect of Decentralization on the Health Status and Healthcare Utilization Pattern in Indonesia.
6. Ministry of Health of Indonesia, 2004 Indonesia Health Profile
7. Ministry of Health of Indonesia, 2007 Indonesia Health Profile
8. Ministry of Health of Indonesia, 2010. Strategic Planning Of Health 2010-2014
9. WHO (2006), What is the evidence on effectiveness of empowerment to improve health.
10. World Economic Forum, 2009 Women's Empowerment: Measuring the Global Gender Gap.

From Web

11. Target MDG's- Indonesia- The Effort to achieve the MDGs in Indonesia.

Chapter 10

The Role of Employment on Women's Mental Health

Akram Ghadimi[1] and Ghazaleh Nazifkar[2]*

[1]Member of Faculty in National Research Institute for Science Policy, Tehran, Iran

[2]Iranian Crescent Society

**E-mail: akram72000@yahoo.com*

ABSTRACT

Women who have jobs often oppose them to the careers which they see their families to be, and feel defensive when their priorities are perceived in any other light. Women who do not work in paid employment feel they have to counter the charge of not doing anything, or making anything of their lives (Apter 1993, p.54).

Mental Health has become a very important issue in Twenty First Century, yet it faces serious challenges. Goldstein defined mental health as existence of harmony between people and environment toward self-realization. Chaussans describes mental health as maximum effectiveness and contentedness resulting from social and individual interaction as well as having positive emotions toward self and others. Although mental health of people in general affects each country's drive for development, mental health of women-because of various roles they play in family and society-has a bigger impact. Among various factors affecting mental health of both men and women, employment plays a more crucial role. Development of each given society depends on providing employment to its citizens, hence contributing to the mental health of society at large. The impact of employment on the mental health of men has been investigated by Andre Michael? Who argues: "Employment and income earning of a husband or a father plays a crucial role in providing him with series of responsibilities which are necessary for the family system. That is why men are entitled head of the household".With transformation of the role of women in society and family in contemporary society, more often than, women have started playing the same role as providers and head of the household. Three views have emerged in regard to women's mental health emanating from their employment. These views might be categorized as positive, negative and conditional. In this paper, we shall try to analyze employment as a determining factor on women's mental health in both rural and urban areas, as well as investigating validity of the above mentioned contrasting views.

Keywords: *Employment, Mental health, Empowerment, Women.*

Introduction

Women and issues concerning them have reached the same prominence as shared values of human beings including freedom, equality, health and eradication of poverty and hunger.

Many organizations and institutions have made gender equality in various areas as a part of their agenda. Women constitute half of the population of all human societies, yet they are deprived of their rights in many parts of the world. Women's deprivation is not a result of their inability to perform their social duties but because of the prejudices which exist toward achievement of their rights.

One of the major challenges toward sexual equality is women employment. Swanson and Johnston believe that despite the increased participation of women in work force of many industrialized countries, the issue of women's employment remains controversial. They discuss controversies which exist in regard to the employment of women with children and refer to them as "Mother Wars".[1]

In regard to the consequences of women's employment, different views have emerged which we will allude to some of them in this paper. Psychological and emotional aspect of women's employment might be considered the most crucial aspect of their social life. Despite the fact that women mainly join the job market for economic reasons such as earning a living, employment has played a very important role in their psychological health.

The aim of this paper is to discuss the impact of employment on mental health of women by utilizing indicators such as sexual equality, definition of mental health, review of pros and cons of positive impact of employment on women's mental health.

Gender Equality

In the Fourth Conference on Women held in Peking in 1995, providing conditions for women participation in work force and women equality were considered a major factor in sustainable development. Cairo Conference, called for empowering women through providing more opportunities in areas such as access to education, technology and employment as a new strategy in this process.

Indicators for a functional definition of sexual equality vary for different groups and organizations. For Example Social Watch Organization which provides annual report on gender equality analyzes gender equality based on social indicators of education, economic participation, and political participation.[2]

---

1. Johnston & Swanson , Moms hating Moms: The Internalization of Mother war rhetoric , Sex Roles Journal , Springer Netherlands , 2004, p.497
2. Social Watch Report 2009.

Global Economic Forum analyzes gender cleavage by taking indicators such as access of each gender to political, economic, educational and health into consideration.

Although gender inequality is more prominent in developing societies, these cleavages exist to a lesser extent even in advanced societies.

As the then UN Under Secretary General and Associate administrator of UNDP on Millennium Development, Ad Melkert has indicated,[3] the main cause of all crises is the entrapment of women and young girls by poverty. He refers to the above phenomenon as silent crisis. Some of experts believe that societies have eventually come to grip with the reality of changing gender roles. He further indicates that despite this, surveys conducted in various countries show the existence of mental rejection of sexual equality (even in developed countries). The excuse for giving priority to men for political appointments or positions with heavy responsibilities is usually justified by arguing that offering these responsibilities to women will decrease their motivations in regard to their responsibilities toward their families.

Mental Health

Although there are several definitions of mental health, the focus in general is on integrity and unity of personality. Goldstein defines mental health as balance between the person and the environment for achieving self-actualization.[4] Chauhann defines mental health as condition of mental maturity that is maximum effectiveness and contentedness emanating from interaction between the individual and society which include emotions and positive feedback toward the self and society.[5]

In recent years, (Canadian Association of Mental Health) has defined mental health in three categories:[6]

First category, Feedbacks concerning self which include:

1. Control over one's emotions;
2. Awareness of one's weaknesses;
3. Being content about one's (achievements? Happiness?)

Second category feedbacks concerning others including:

1. Interest in long term and cordial relations;
2. Feeling of belonging to a group;
3. Feeling responsible toward human and material environment.

Third Category, feedbacks concerning life including:

1. Accepting responsibility;

---

3. United Nation Development Program 16 October 2008, http// content. undp .org/go/news room/ 2008/October
4. www.hegmataneh.org
5. Chauhann, S.S, Mental Hygiene, New Delhi: Alied publisher, 1991.
6. Gangi, Hamzeh,Behdasht Ravani,Tehran: Arasbaran,1997.

2. Enthusiasm? Toward development of one's opportunities and interests;
3. Ability to make decision;
4. Enthusiasm for working well?

Chauhann mentions five behavioral patterns in regard to mental health including:[7]

1. Feeling responsible: a person who enjoys mental health is sensitive to the needs of other people and works toward satisfaction of their needs and providing comfort for them.
2. The feeling of self-confidence: the person who is mentally healthy is confident about self and his abilities. He views challenges as temporary phenomena which will be resolved. Therefore, obstacles do not influence his morale.
3. Being Goal-Oriented: the individual has a clear definition about his goals. Therefore, he mobilizes all his power and creativity toward the achievement of his goals.
4. Personal Values? Such person has a philosophy in life emanating from his beliefs, ideas and goals which will contribute to the happiness and success of the person or his associates. He is also in favor of social participation.
5. Individuality? A mentally healthy person recognizes his distinctiveness from the others and tries to develop his own feedbacks and behavioral patterns in a way that he is neither the victim of blind and unconscious complacency with desires and requirements of other people neither is he isolated from the others.

Indicators of Mental Health

L.W. Vent is recognizes seven indicators of mental health which are:[8]

1. Proper social behavior;
2. Freedom from anxiety? And guilt;
3. Absence of mental sickness?
4. Personal capabilities and self-control?
5. Self-acceptance and self-actualization?
6. Integrity and personal organization?
7. Openness and flexibility.

As was mentioned before, one of the indicators of economic and social development is the expansion of workforce which includes women as well. Despite revisions in outlooks toward women's work, in many societies, negative outlook

7. http://fa.parsiteb.com
8. Ventis, L.W , "The relationships between religion and Mental health" Journal of social issues, 1995, Vol 51, No. 2, pp.33–48

toward this issue persists. The Iranian sociologist, Gholam Abbas Tavasoli believes that factors such as each society's traditions and cultures affect women's employment. Different cultures have different views concerning women's employment. Altogether, views about women fall within the following categories:

1. Positive view
2. Negative view
3. A view which supports women's employment under certain conditions.

The Industrial Revolution played a crucial role in providing conditions for the inclusion of women in workforce. In this process women were able to go to school which in turn allowed them to strengthen their position in society by utilizing their knowledge and expertise. Needless to say that the differences in the rate and scale of women's employment in each given society are not just the byproduct of agreements or disagreements about this issue. Many factors impact this phenomenon. An Iranian sociologist in a comparison study of women employment in Iran and Western societies indicates that in last four decades women in Iran have constantly constituted 10 to 15 per cent of the workforces, while this ratio for the women in Western societies has been 30 to 40 per cent. The difference in the above example is not simply because of the opposition of traditionalists to women employment. There are other factors involved in this phenomenon that we now turn to.

Supporters of women employment argue that since the society at large shoulders the expenses of educating its youth (both men and women), if women are prevented from entering the job market, because of their gender, at least 50 per cent of the money invested on education is wasted.

Opponents of women's inclusion in workforce base their opposition on the following factors:

1. Religious codes
2. Customs and Traditions
3. Negative impact of women employment on the family

In some societies, religious codes are interpreted in a way to conclude that women's employment is contrary to the religious principles. Customs and traditions are yet other factors preventing women from joining the workforce.

Interestingly enough in advanced societies, opposition to women employment are justified on the third category above. Supporters of this view argue that women's work outside home would prevent them performing their role in the family and would be detrimental to their children upbringing and even their marital relation. They believe that women's employment has resulted in the mushrooming of daycare centers hence creating distance between children and their mothers.

The last view is very interesting in that, it supports women work under certain conditions. It is not an all or nothing approach, but has shady areas in this regard. Although it has negative outlook toward women's role in workforce in general, but allows it when it is deemed necessary. This view shared by some of the Arab countries of Persian Gulf including Saudi Arabia, indicates that when the work environment is completely female, interaction with men is not necessary in any aspect of work process, or the employment in certain industries (*i.e.*, women apparel) have traditionally been female, employment of women is allowed.

The Impact of Employment on Women's Mental Health

Anxiety and other mental disorders are on the rise throughout the world. 5 out of 10 incidents of (Natavani?) throughout the world are attributed to issues emanating from mental disorders. Both rich and poor countries are affected by this phenomenon. Women are more prone to mental disorders. Since employment provides economic stability, it might be a contributing factor to reducing mental disorder for both men and women. Employment provides mental health in following ways:

1. Time Structure
2. Social Contacts
3. Collective efforts
4. Social identity
5. Regular Activity

Of the above mentioned categories, social contacts and social identity affect women's mental health to a great extent. Establishing goal oriented social contacts and social identity emanating from employment play crucial role in women's mental health. It is worth mentioning that among women living in rural areas, it is collective efforts and not social contacts or social identity which affects their mental health positively.

References

1. Apter (1993): Working Women Don't has wives: Professional success in the 1990's. New York; St Martin Press, cited in Elgar K. and Chester a: The Maternal Health implications of maternal employment: Working verses at – home mothering identities. Advances in Mental Health. 2007, Vol 6, (1): 47–55.

Chapter 11

The Effect of Hygiene and Nutrition on Women's Empowerment

Maryam Ghadimi[1] *and Kobra Ghadimi*[2]

[1]*General Physician, Iran*
[2]*General Surgeon, Iran*

ABSTRACT

All humans have a right to be healthy, especially women, because they have an important role in providing hygiene and health in society. A major criterion for health is access to adequate nutrition. At all stages of life-from infancy until the post menopausal and old age, women's lives are affected by lack of hygiene and malnutrition. Malnutrition is a barrier for women's efficiency and productivity. It increases their susceptibility to infections, debilitating and fatal diseases. The cumulative effects of a lifetime of nutritional deprivation, excessive workload, continuous procreation and low self steam of women make them physically and psychologically fragile and vulnerable. The goal of this paper is to present a proper model of hygiene and nutrition for women in order to empower them in various fields of life. In primary hygiene care, there are two vital factors; public involvement and cooperation between various health sectors.

Keyword: *Woman, Nutrition, Empowerment, Health.*

Introduction

Health is a something that can be measured and defined. It is one of the major factors in achieving welfare, well being and improvement of in the quality of life. "Health" in all its aspects is among the primary human rights. In the view of WHO, it is a state when not only is the individual free from any particular suffering and diseases, but also, he/she is enjoying full physical, mental and social comfort. In their approach, women's health is the safest way to achieve the general goals of health and improvement of life quality for the whole world. Unfortunately, in most societies, unless the woman becomes unable to fulfill her assigned duties, she will be considered as healthy, while, many of them suffer from anemia, malnutrition, chronic fatigue, pelvic infections, etc. Emphasis on improving women's health in different societies has many realistic justifications. Women are the first healthcareers in the families that ultimately lead to improvement of health and welfare of family and society. They are the heart of progress of a society. The close relationship between women's health and improvement the quality of life (Q.O.L) could be explained in many terms. First, their role in giving birth to healthy children, second, their special role in raising children and providing necessary education to children, family and even the entire society, third, their role in meeting the mental and physical needs of the family as a mother and wife, four, the special duties and responsibilities which are entrusted to women in many societies, such as working outside the home in key sectors such as medical care, education or agriculture. In order to study the status of women's health, there should be some indexes and these should be in a way that can be used universally. In recent years, organizations and relevant centers have made some comments and suggestions which have been used, and one of the most complete indexes is the general index used by the United Nations to evaluate countries.

Indexes of women's health status are as follows:

1. Vital and demographic events
   - A. Birth and fertility
   - B. Death
   - C. Life expectancy
   - D. Marriage and divorce
   - E. Social groups
2. Indexes of susceptibility to diseases (commonness and epidemics)
   - A. Physical health
   - B. Psychological and social health
3. Welfare Indexes
   - A. Quality of life
   - B. Satisfaction
   - C. Life Style
   - D. Social consequences of diseases

Factors which Affect Women's Health

1. Stress and using resources and services:
   - A. Education and informative services
   - B. Job opportunities and income earning

   C. Family resources
   D. Social, political and legal resources
   E. Health Services
2. Participation and decision making:
   A. At an individual level
   B. At the family level
   C. At the social level

Since human force is one of the major pillars in the process of development and women, as half of the human population have a prominent place; therefore, social justice requires that there should be no discrimination and all groups of society should benefit equally from the results of development. In this approach, on the one hand, the status of men and women is not balanced, and as history shows, women have always been one step behind men. On the other hand, men and women have different needs. Therefore, the necessity of considering gender based views in planning appear, first due to the historical backwardness of women compared to men, second, due to differences in needs, and third, because of biological differences of men and women. Planning for promoting women's health has a high importance because it directly affects the health of 75 per cent of the population (women and children) and indirectly, it affects the remaining 25 per cent of society (men). Therefore; if health is the core of sustained development, woman is the core of health.

Nutrition and Health

Lifestyle and physical health are one of the indices of women's health, as they comprise an important item in achieving health and improvement in the nutritional status of women. Correction of both end of the spectrum of nutrition. that is, malnutrition and overweight, is an important and even vital subject. Unhealthy nutrition means not using accessible foodstuffs properly. It is one of the difficulties of the world at present. Woman is the main element of nutrition in many families. Although often men have a main role in providing a family's needs, it is the women who manage the nutrition of family. However, is it sufficient to have the entire efforts of women as the main element in a family's nutrition as criteria in achieving desirable nutrition?

This is a key role. However, one should not forget that the responsibility for a family's nutrition is shared by different sectors of the state; that is, Ministries dealing with production and importation of foods, policy-makers in foodstuffs, authorities for market regulation and prices, academic societies, and the media as a factor in culture development. Although it seems that selecting raw foods for a family and changing it into food at the table is often done by a woman; it is the opinions and attitudes of officials and authorities of foods, and nutritional policy-makers in a country that reveal the relationship between physical and mental capabilities, suitable nutrition and the importance of the ages of growing children, that need growth and the effects of suitable nutrition on the health of families, society and development of a country that paves the way for better nutrition of families.

Obesity, diabetics, cardiac inefficiency, heart infarctions, hypertension and consequences, brain stroke and the damage caused by it, skeletal diseases and many cancers could be prevented by improving nutrition.

Effects of Nutrition in Improving Capabilities

Health is considered as a positive value and it is usually expressed in the best wishes of people for themselves and others. Health is both a tool and a goal. Health is a tool to reach the dreams and ideals of life, to achieve success in work and life. At the same time, it is an aim, because all human efforts and activities combine to achieve a life of health and happiness. One of the essential factors in achieving health is to have a healthy nutrition. Nutrition is a key factor in that, if is slightly changed, it could be a factor in reducing the incidence of many diseases. In today's world, there is general agreement that any individual should have sufficient knowledge about nutrition in order to follow the diet plans suggested at international level. On this subject, the teaching of nutrition as one of the components of health services demands more attention. Effective projects for teaching nutrition in society should be accompanied by an understanding of the knowledge and the perspective of the people on nutrition. The positive effects of teaching women, on their own and their children's nutrition status could be achieved through their role in providing nutrition to their families. One of the main ways to improve the nutritional status of women is teaching them. The role of educating women in improving their health and the nutritional status of themselves and their families has already been discussed at length. Education is the key to improving the abilities, health, better nutrition, social and economic progress and promotion and protection of women against social hazards such as different inequalities.

Practically, it has been shown that improvement in the health status of women depends on improving and promoting the general, social and economic conditions of women. This issue should be clarified for people through necessary advertising, and it should be taught that discrimination in nutrition will be followed by lower social status for the whole society. The biological and social factors affect women's health in the course of their lives, and are followed by accumulated effects. Therefore, in studying the causes and consequences of poor health in women, it is necessary to pay attention to their life style in general terms. For example, young girls who lack good nutrition in childhood might face a low growth rate that might lead to more risks in childbirth.

Malnutrition, in addition to poverty, illiteracy and ignorance, is a serious problem particularly in developing countries and has a large effect on the welfare and health of women at all stages of life. There are several factors involved in malnutrition, ranging from an insufficient amount of food, and eating disorders, to the physiologic loss of body reserves in frequent pregnancies and labor. However, unequal distribution of food among family members is also a key sector with a major role. In many developing countries, reasons such as poverty, lack of knowledge particularly of the nutrition needs of women and girls and giving less value to girls, than boys, lead to giving more food and the best parts of foods to boys, and girls and women using the remaining foods or left overs. The statistical data gained from research conducted across the world showed that the more significant amount of malnutrition in women rather than in men is the result of selective nutrition of family members. In a study conducted in Bahrain, Oman and Tunisia, it was shown that the duration of lactation for male infants was longer than for girls. Studies in Latin America showed that supplementary nutrition was started earlier for boys than girls.

The nutritional needs of girls in the early teenage years increase during the growth spurt and the start of puberty. Unsuitable diet during this period could put the health and physical growth of girls at risk and cause consequences for menstruation throughout lives. Anemia due to iron insufficiency is common, especially in young girls. Their skeletal growth man slow down and stop. A low rate of growth in the pelvis may cause serious risks in their labor and becomes a barrier in labor. This inadequate or low growth skeletal development leads to longer labor. More than 50 percent of pregnant women in developing countries suffer from iron deficiency. Anemia increases the risk of fatal labor in women by up to five times (WHO, 1992) because women with anemia are more vulnerable to infections, bleeding or other pregnancy and delivery complication. The effective factors on this malnutrition include insufficient intake of foodstuffs, unequal (unjust) distribution of foods at the family level, unsuitable methods of storing and preparing foods, and the existence of taboos in connection with withdrawal of consuming some special foods, and the lack of knowledge on rich foods. Between 20 to 40 percent of women of childbearing age in developing countries do not have the required intake of 2250 Calories as suggested by WHO. In a general assessment, more than 500 million people in the world were found to suffer from malnutrition.

At the other end of this spectrum is disordered nutrition, obesity, overweight and fatness. As an example, the general problem in the USA is overweight people, 61 percent, and fat people, 14 percent. Fatness has undesirable consequences for the healthcare system and the economy of the society. Overweight people are more vulnerable to health problems and diseases such as diabetes type 2, cardiac diseases, and hypertension and brain stroke. Fatness might accompany a high rate of special types of cancers. Fatness has roles in psychological and mood problems, because many of these people become isolated, ashamed and depressed. Overweight in women has special importance. In women of childbear age, weight often increases, and around the menopause, reaches its maximum. The fact that overweight and fatness has increased more in women than men is an alarming problem. In general, an overweight condition in women increases risks of physical and mental or psychological diseases. Eating patterns and low mobility lifestyles, and also social and economic stresses are effective factors in becoming overweight. Withdrawal from eating fatty and high calorie foods, a suitable balance in eating foods, and an increase in fibers and vegetables in the diet are very effective in preventing such problems. Physical activities will have desirable results. Evidence shows that even a 5 to 10 percent reduction of weight, and maintaining that weight would cause desirable effects on an individual's health. Limiting intake of calories, adjusting behavior and taking exercises are the main basis for treatment. Major barriers that could affect treatment, in addition to lack of training and insufficient knowledge, include low income, limited time and lack of professional teaching.

Nutrition affects health in many aspects. Imbalance of nutrients in the body, whether in the form of insufficiency or over-consumption, affects individual's health and disorders the normal function of body. In third world countries, many problems and cultural traditions lead to an increase in malnutrition and anemia among women, and some other lead to unwanted pregnancy and pre-term death.

On the other hand, the trend to use fast foods and replace traditional foods with them are among the factors that threaten individuals' health, particularly that of women. Of course, along with nutrition, one should cite lack of sufficient physical activities and the low amount of sunshine that intensifies women's problems, particularly among Iranian women. Low physical movement as a result of old age, overweight the menopause and little physical activities might lead to osteoporosis.

Conclusion

Although in past decades, infectious diseases and malnutrition were among the major factors causing death and disabilities in many developing countries, at the present time, by controlling those diseases, people enjoy longer lives. However, the non-contagious diseases, so-called "modernity-related diseases" have overtaken populations and after developed countries, those diseases are increasing in the developing countries. This happens while developing countries still face the challenge of their traditional problems and now, both problems come hand-in-hand. These diseases are diabetics, hypertension, cardiovascular diseases, osteoporosis and other such cases that have direct and close relationship with the lifestyle of people. Using saturated fats in foods, using high amounts of salt, using low-volume and high-calorie foods, a lowered intake of fiber, smoking, and alcohol, insufficient physical activities, gains in weight and obesity are the most harmful factors in society's health in general, and women's health in particular. In order to prevent such diseases, it is required to change lifestyle and ensure sufficient physical activities, and balanced nutrition, and giving up smoking should be practiced at the society level. Women's health is affected by biological, psychological, social, emotional, economic, cultural and environmental factors, and the outcome of such factors is a phenomenon that starts in the embryo's development period. Each stage afterwards (lactating infant, childhood, adolescence, youth, fertile years and old age) are all built on the previous stages. Therefore; the primary healthcare plan should include the following:

1. Efforts to correct nutrition status in women and girls.
2. Birth control to delay the first pregnancy, the time between pregnancies, limit the number of pregnancies; and prevent unwanted pregnancies and pregnancy in old age.
3. Taking the necessary measures to prevent violence and other forms of physical harm.

Women are both recipients and main providers of healthcare. However, there are many steps that should be taken in promoting their capabilities, capacities and abilities to lead health affairs in societies. Before the time when women become a source of making decisions in all healthcare, the issue of women's health will be neglected, and services provided will lack sufficiency and usefulness.

References

1. World Health Organization. Overview of WHO. URL:www.who.int/about/en.
2. Women's Health. WHO position paper, Geneva. World Health Organization, 1995.
3. WHO Kobe Centre. Women and Health: Better Health and Welfare Systems: Women's Perspectives. Proceeding of WHO Kobe centre International Meeting, Awaji Island, Japan, 5-7 April 2000.
4. WHO Kobe Centre. Women and Health. Maximizing women's capacities and leadership, Proceeding of WHO Kobe Centre, Second International Meeting, Canberra, Australia, 4-6 April 2001.
5. Health, Population and Development. WHO Position Paper, Geneva: World Health Organization, 1994, Prepared for the International Conference on Population and Development, Cairo, 1994.
6. Manderson, L. (2001). Global Priorities, local sensibilities: Maximizing women's capacities in health development. Proceeding of WHO Kobe Centre, Second International Meeting, Canberra, Australia, 2001, pp. 28-32.
7. Sivard, R.L. (1995). Women: A world survey. New York: Carnegie Corporation, 2nd edition.
8. Wellman, N.S. and Friedberg, B. (2002). Causes and consequences of adult obesity: Health, social and economic impacts in the United States. Asia Pac J. Clin. Nutr., 11(Suppl.): S705-9.
9. Bowers, D. (1997). Excess body weight in women. Prim. Care Update ob/gyns 4(6): 224-227.
10. Cogswell, M.E., Perry, G.S., Schieve, L.A. and Dietz, W.H. (2001). Obesity in women of childbearing age: Risks, prevention, and treatment. Prim. Care Update ob/Gyns, 8(3): 89-105.
11. Smyke, P. (1991). Women and Health. Zed Books Ltd., London and New Jersey.
12. World Health Organization (2002). WHO calls for strong focus on health promotion for women. Note for the press no. 3. URL:www.who, int/inf/en/note2002-03.Html.
13. World Health Organization. Physical inactivity a leading cause of disease and disability, WHO", URL:www.who.int/mediacentre/relases/release23/en/.
14. The World Bank (1994). A New Agenda for Women's Health and Nutrition. Washington D.C.

Chapter 12

Health of Women in Iran

Ziba Nikaeen[1] *and Zinat Nikaien*[2]

[1]*Biomechanical Engineering (Master of Philosophy)*
Faculty of Irost, Iran
[2]*Master of Science of Management in*
Sport Faculty of Asad University, Iran
E-mail: [1]*znikaeen@gmail.com,* [2]*z.nikaien@gmail.com*

ABSTRACT

The health of women is important to a community and can have impact on the health and behavior of a family and the country at large. Regular physical exercises are very important. The women must get opportunities for participating in many scientific and economic activities. Physical exercise and good nutrition decreases stress and improves self confidence. It is advisable that during pregnancy, women should have balanced diets and physical exercises.

***Keywords:** Women health, Feeding, Sport, Pregnancy, Iran.*

Introduction

Women have diverse roles in life from the time she is a girl not yet married, to the time when she is a mother and wife. In order to enable her to effectively accomplish her roles, she must be in a perfect health.

Feeding

Focus on good feeding for a girl child should be emphasized right from childhood, through adolescence to adulthood. In Iran, The Ministry of Education has put in place a number of programs for the girl child, for example providing milk to schools, regular medical check-ups and vitamin/iron supplementation for the girl child in schools. The ministry also encourages physical exercises in schools and homes.

After marriage she will counter with many harmonic and nervous changes. In the pregnancy period, she needs good feeding and well healthcare. She must do especial sports in these times. She needs more kindness and more considerations. She must be at rest completely, because she is not alone and all of her behaviors transform to her baby. Weight of baby depends on feeding of mother and getting away from stresses and tensions and healthcare in these times is too important and after that she must milk her baby. Breastfeeding too is complete and necessary for child and vitamins will be added to his foods. Sports in pregnancy period and after delivery are too important.

The mother should have good feedings and she must do biomechanical movements. When she wants to lift any things she must sit and lift it. She mustn't lift any weighty things and standard skeleton curves of the body must be considered to be in good situations. The muscles must be reinforced till can bear the whole weight without changes in the curvatures. She must check her breast after monthly period and she must check her cervix for preventing from cancer. In Iran in healthy centers all of these are done freely. She must control her teeth and check her blood every 6 months and then if there is not any important problem, every 1 year is advised. The baby must be vaccinated and controlled and checked.If mother can't milk the baby, help- milk is added to its feeding and baby is checked and vaccinated till he goes elder. All of these are done freely in IRAN till he is 18 years old.

In Iran gender disparities in primary and secondary education are eliminated and in our universities most of girls are studying and they are more than boys and in many courses in engineering and medical, women are working. The women have 6 months rest after delivery for milking and they have their salary at these times. In IRAN the women train how to married, how to milk, and care themselves and their babies and for preventing of unwanted pregnancy. They consult with doctors and them advice to use many ways for contraception.

In Iran we use meat, rice and bread more than usual rates. We must restricted eating of them and we must use to eat less salt and sugar for preventing of diabetes mellitus and heart diseases. We must accustom our children for eating of healthy foods and fruits. We do these in schools. As the women are multi - dimensional, they do all of those very well.

Methods

Sports and healthy nutrition decrease stresses, help the body to act successfully in controlling of nervous systems, self-confidence, good working, Some persons with good, healthy nutrition are placed less than the other one under critical nervous situations. Long activities of body in comparison with short times sports have more effects on decreasing cholesterol of blood. For developing and expanding of women's sports, in addition to healthy, safe places for sport is needed. We must consider utilization of scientific applications of sport in all of women's life, so that we increase qualities, quantities of participating of women, make awareness in them. In Iran we have parks for women in every place near their residence, where they can do sport. They can go swimming, walking. In many courses of sports competitions, they have active presence (*e.g.* Boating, swimming, volleyball, basketball, shooting), where it needs concentration, sharpness, tenderness, cleverness, the women are also there.

Overall, regular exercise stretches muscles, Stretches ease back pain, walking improves your circulation, and swimming can strengthen your abdominal muscles. Weight gain during pregnancy helps your baby grow. Gaining weight at a steady rate within recommended boundaries can also lower your chances of having hemorrhoids, varicose veins, stretch marks, backache, fatigue, indigestion, and shortness of breath during pregnancy. The extra weight you gain during pregnancy provides nourishment to your developing baby and is also stored for breastfeeding to your baby after delivery.

Where does all the extra weight in pregnancy period go? [1]

Here is an approximate breakdown of your weight gain:

- ☆ Baby: 7-8 pounds
- ☆ Placenta: 1-2 pounds
- ☆ Amniotic fluid: 2 pounds
- ☆ Uterus: 2 pounds
- ☆ Maternal breast tissue: 2 pounds
- ☆ Maternal blood: 4 pounds
- ☆ Fluids in maternal tissue: 4 pounds
- ☆ Maternal fat and nutrient stores: 7 pounds

Healthy Eating During Pregnancy

A sensible meal plan that is rich in vitamins and minerals is essential for a developing baby. You may want to ask your healthcare provider for food recommendations, or seek the help of an area. Women who are underweight during pregnancy tend to eat low calorie foods and not enough protein.

The following are ways to get more calories:

- ☆ Eat breakfast every day. Peanut butter or a slice of cheese on toast can give you an extra protein boost.
- ☆ Snack between meals; yogurt and dried fruits can provide protein, calcium, and minerals.
- ☆ Try to eat more foods that are high in good fats such as nuts, fatty fish, avocados, and olive oil.
- ☆ Drink juices that are high in vitamin C or beta carotene, such as grapefruit juice, orange juice, papaya nectar, apricot nectar, and carrot juice.
- ☆ Avoid junk food.
- ☆ Consult your healthcare provider about taking prenatal vitamins.

Can Gaining Too Much Weight be Harmful?

The following are potential problems with gaining too much weight:

- ☆ Gestational diabetes
  - Backaches
  - Leg pain
  - Increased fatigue
  - Varicose veins
  - Increased risk of cesarean delivery
  - High blood pressure

The following self-care tips can help you make your pregnancy a healthy one for you and your baby:

- ☆ Avoid pregnancy risks such as alcohol and smoking.
  - Try not to gain too much weight; your healthcare provider will provide recommended weight gain.
  - Be selective about your food choices; choose food sources that contain vitamins, minerals, and protein.

Body Activities and Sports in Pregnancy Women

Regular exercises in pregnancy period cause improvement in their sleep, increasing of their self-confidence, decreasing of intensity backache or appearing of pain, varicose veins preventing of increasing of weight, protection of readiness, fitness of their, decreasing blood pressure, heartbeat, fat percentage, increasing of respiratory capacity, reinforcement of skeletal, preventing of atherosclerosis.Consideration of pregnancy age is of extreme importance. Not less than 18, no more than 35 years old. For pregnancy, it is advised not to have more than 3. The women should not smoke, don't drink alcoholic liquor. In Iran because of Islam religion, we don't use these, so we have healthy women. In spite of doing their jobs, they have healthy babies.

Conclusions

Empowering women's thorugh better healthcare is very important, because they are the most important key in feeding of family and health of them. Especially for health of children, the governments must encourage woman to take care of health of children.

The women need more consideration for:

- ☆ Free of cost kindergarten for taking care of their babies.
  - Free and regular healthy schedules in accordance with their age.
  - Free and healthy places for swimming, exercising.
  - Free hospital for therapy and testing, healing, etc.

All the governments must have some strategies for these; In Iran we do most of them by assurance.

Some of Solutions are:

- ☆ Improvement of health condition like fertility healthcare.
- ☆ AIDS preventing and curing.
- ☆ Development of awareness among women about laws. Elimination of every kind of discrimination against women. Increasing of women's partnership in political determinations.
- ☆ Women's partnership in civil society.
- ☆ Access of women to total credits.
- ☆ Preventing of coarseness treatment.
- ☆ Increasing of economical opportunity
- ☆ Increasing of women's partnership in making peace.

References

1. http://www.hawzah.net '1381 esfand
2. Iranian association of women's studies N 19 Aban 1385
3. N132 women report
4. Reviewed by the BabyCenter Medical Advisory board last updated: November 2006
5. Seven great benefits of pregnancy exercise

Chapter 13

Empowering Women through Better Healthcare and Nutrition: The Case of Kenya

Catherine W. Mutie[1] *and Florence M. Kyallo*[2]

[1]*Assistant Director–Research,*
Ministry of Higher Education, Science and Technology,
Directorate of Research Management and Development, Kenya
[2]*Lecturer, Jomo Kenyatta University of Agriculture and Technology,*
Department of Food Science and Nutrition, Kenya
E-mail: [1]*c.mutie@scienceandtechnology.go.ke,* [2]*florencemuthiani@yahoo.com*

ABSTRACT

The United Nations Children Fund (UNICEF) conceptual framework on malnutrition identifies the underlying causes of child malnutrition as insufficient food access, inadequate maternal and child care practices as well as inadequate maternal health services. The Government of Kenya has consistently worked to ensure equitable allocation of resources so as to reduce disparities in health status. Various strategies have been proposed in a number of policy documents such as 2nd National Health Sector Strategic Plan 2005-2010 (NHSSP II), Kenya National HIV/AIDS Strategic Plan (2005/06-2009/10), Child Survival and Development Strategy 2008-2015, Kenya Vision 2030. These strategies contribute immensely to the efforts of both the public and private sector in ensuring women and children get adequate health services. To accelerate promotion of good nutrition within the health sector in the Sub-Saharan Africa, a five step process has been proposed which includes; advocating for action in maternal health and nutrition at all levels, integration of essential maternal health and nutrition actions into existing health delivery system, proper management to assure quality services are offered, measurement of changes made in maternal health, nutrition and mortality, and development of capacity in nutrition and maternal health issues. These processes have been discussed in this paper using findings of the Kenya Demographic

Health Survey (KDHS) 2008-09 and other Kenya health sector policy documents. Use of lifecycle approach to women's nutrition and health issues in the Kenya Health sector is a good strategy and it is hoped that women will be better empowered as they get specialized attention at all health sector levels. A concerted effort however, is still required at the budgetary, policy and implementation levels to ensure good health and nutrition status among women and children.

Keywords: Empowering women, Maternal healthcare, Nutrition, Related to health sector.

Introduction

The United Nations Children Fund (UNICEF) conceptual framework on malnutrition identifies the underlying causes of child malnutrition as insufficient food access, inadequate maternal and child care practices as well as inadequate maternal health services (UNICEF 1990). With the recognition that good health enhances human capital development, the Government of Kenya has consistently worked to ensure accessible, equitable and affordable allocation of resources so as to reduce disparities in health status caused either by region, age or sex. The country's new development blueprint, the "*Kenya Vision 2030*" aims at transforming Kenya into a newly industrializing, "middle-income country providing a high quality life to all its citizens by the year 2030". To achieve this, the National Health Sector Strategic Plan 2005-2010 (NHSSP II) outlines the Government's strategy and emphasis on provision of an integrated and high quality, promotive, preventive, curative and rehabilitative healthcare service (MOH 2005). This will be done through a two-pronged approach: (*i*) devolution of funds and management of healthcare to the communities and district medical officers; and (*ii*) shifting the bias of the national health bill from curative to preventive care. It is hoped that this would contribute immensely to the efforts of both the public and private sector in ensuring women and children get adequate health services.

This paper will focus on the current status of women's health and nutrition and related policies in Kenya. Reference will be made to the findings of both 2003 and 2008 Kenya Demographic Health Survey (KDHS) (CBS, MOH *et al.*, 2004; KNBS, NACC *et al.*, 2009) and other policy documents such as the Kenya Vision 2030, National Health Sector Strategic Plan 2005-2010 (NHSSP II), Child Survival and Development Strategy 2008-2015 and Kenya National HIV/AIDS Strategic Plan (2005/06-2009/10) (MOH 2005; NACC 2005; GOK 2007; MOPHS 2008). It is recognized that proper maternal healthcare during pregnancy, delivery and postnatal care are important for the health of both the mother and the baby. Attempt will be made to identify areas of weakness, obstacles and challenges in providing adequate healthcare and nutrition for women in Kenya.

Promotion of Good Maternal Health and Nutrition within the Health Sector

Mwadime (2001) proposes a five step process for accelerating promotion of good nutrition within the health sector in the Sub-Saharan Africa region. This will be adopted and modified to include maternal health and nutrition (Figure 13.1).

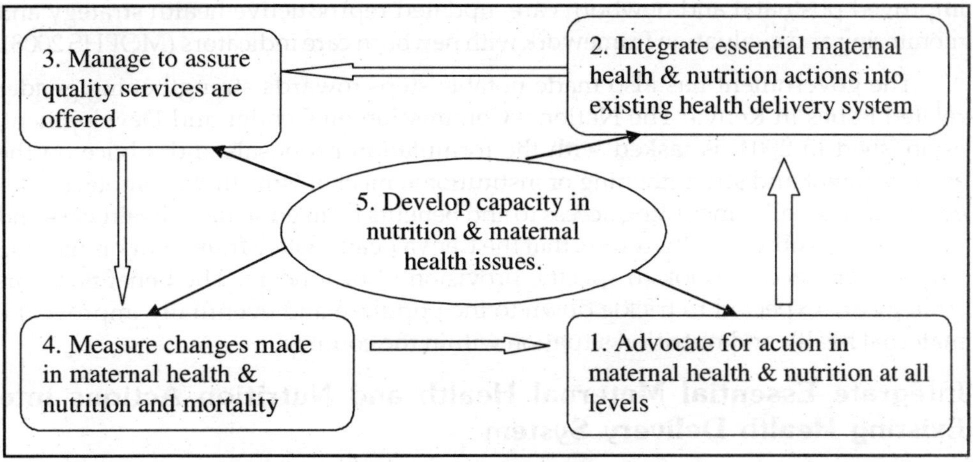

Figure 13.1: Components of Maternal and Child Nutrition Strategy in Africa

Advocate for Action in Maternal Health and Nutrition at All Levels

The goal of NHSSP II is to reduce health inequalities and to reverse the downward trend in health related outcome and impact indicators. To achieve this goal, a sector-wide approach has been adopted and key intervention areas in service delivery identified. NHSSP II is implemented through the *Kenya Essential Package for Health* (KEPH) approach. The KEPH approach reduces fragmentation and improves continuity of care by emphasizing the inter-connectedness of the various phases in human development (MOH 2005). Targeted interventions are defined using life-cycle cohorts as illustrated in the Figure 13.2.

The Child Survival and Development Strategy 2008-2015 (CSDS) recognizes the need to increase use of quality focused ante-natal care, skilled care at delivery and

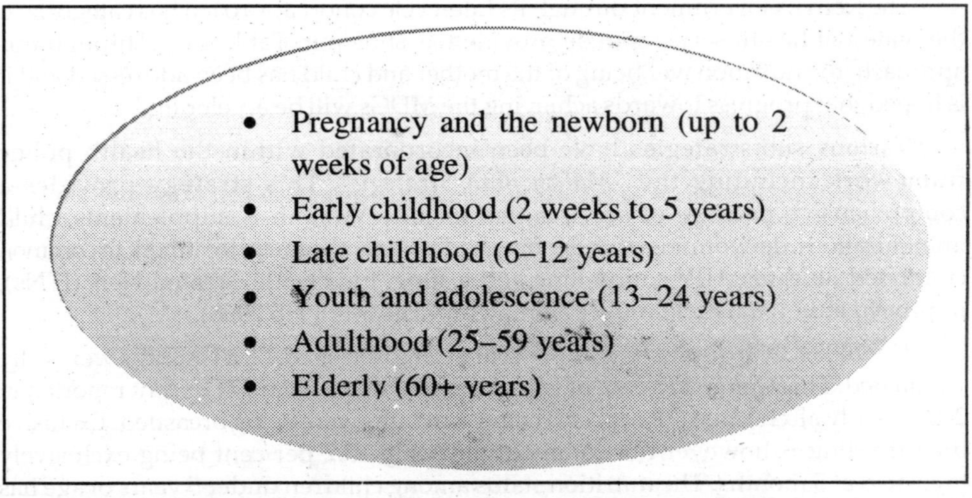

Figure 13.2: Life-Cycle Cohorts as Classified In NHSSP II

improved postnatal and newborn care, updated reproductive health strategy and monitoring and evaluation framework with newborn care indicators (MOPHS 2008).

The government has also made notable steps towards strengthening gender related issues in Kenya. The National Commission on Gender and Development, established in 2004, is tasked with the formulation proposals and advice on the establishment and strengthening of institutional mechanisms that promote gender equity and equality including access to and benefits from education, healthcare and nutrition. It is observed therefore, that the Kenya heath policy framework is moving from generalized outlook to specific provision of healthcare. The benefits of this strategy are expected to trickle down to the populace and eventually improve the maternal health and nutrition situation within the country.

Integrate Essential Maternal Health and Nutrition Actions into Existing Health Delivery System

Maternal malnutrition results in lost lives, lost health, lost opportunity and lost income (Linkages 2001). The progress towards achieving the Millennium Development Goals (MDGs) on maternal and child nutrition has been rated as insufficient in the latest progress report by UNICEF (UNICEF 2009). It is therefore paramount that health sector actions address the most critical nutrition problems of women in an efficient manner. This would contribute greatly to the achievement of MDGs and nutrition related outcomes as outlined under the Essential Nutrition Actions strategy including:

1. Adequate food intake during pregnancy and lactation
2. Adequate micronutrient intake during pregnancy and lactation
3. Reduction of malaria infection in pregnant women in endemic areas
4. Reduction of hookworm infection in pregnant women in endemic areas
5. Birth spacing of three years or longer

The Kenya Government through its Life-cycle cohort approach has categorized the maternal health services to be provided as shown in Table 13.1. Through this approach, the nutrition wellbeing of the mother and child has been addressed and it is hoped that progress towards achieving the MDGs will be accelerated.

Various sub-strategies have been incorporated within the health policy framework including the *"Malezi Bora Strategy"*. This strategy provides a comprehensive package of services that include Vitamin A supplements, child immunizations, de-worming of under fives and pregnant women, treatment of common childhood illnesses, HIV counselling and testing, Insecticide Treated Nets (ITNs), improved ante-natal and family planning services (MOPHS 2008).

The 2008 KDHS found that 77 per cent of children aged 12-23 months were fully vaccinated. This was an increase of vaccination coverage from 57 per cent reported in 2003. Nearly all children (99 per cent) below 6 months were being breastfed. Exclusive breastfeeding is however not common with only 13.2 per cent being exclusively breastfed at 5 months. The nutrition status among children under 5 years of age has not changed significantly over the last five years with slightly more than a third of the

Table 13.1: Maternal and Child Health Services Identified in the Kenya's NHSSP II

Life Cycle Cohort	*Services Needed*	
	Promotive/Preventive	*Curative*
Pregnancy and the newborn (up to 2 weeks of age)	1. Ante-natal and nutritional care 2. Intermittent prophylactic treatment (for malaria) (IPT) and ITN promotion and use 3. Tetanus Toxoid vaccination (TT2) 4. Use of skilled births attendants, clean delivery, BCG and Post natal care 5. Breast feeding support and Supplementary feeding 6. Family planning services. 7. Prevention of Mother to Child transmission (PMTCT). 8. Micro-nutrient supplements (iron) 9. Hygiene, water and sanitation	1. Adequate and timely referral system, 2. Transport (Ambulance) system. 3. Basic and comprehensive emergency obstetric care (BEOC). 4. Newborn resuscitation.
Early childhood (2 weeks to 5 years)	1. Community Integrated Management of childhood Illness (IMCI) + ITN. 2. Appropriate nutrition & Extended breast feeding 3. Growth monitoring 4. Expanded Program of Immunization 5. Provision of vitamin A/zinc 6. Psychological stimulation 7. Physical/cognitive development 8. Exercise and recreation	1. Clinical IMCI. 2. Oral rehydration salts for diarrhoea 3. Antibiotics, anti-malarial & Anti-retroviral therapy drugs.

children (35 per cent) being stunted and 7 per cent being wasted (KNBS, NACC *et al.*, 2009).

The proportion of children and pregnant women who slept under an ITN the night prior to the interview increased greatly from 15 per cent and 4.4 per cent to 46 per cent and 48 per cent respectively. This could be attributed partly to the provision of ITNs during the *"Malezi Bora weeks"* among other Promotive strategies. The proportion of mothers reporting they received antenatal care from health professionals has increased slightly from 88 per cent in 2003 to 92 per cent in 2008 (Table 13.2).

Table 13.2: Comparisons of Key Maternal Care Indicators from the 2003 and 2008 KDHS

Background Characteristic	*Sample Size (n) 2003/2008**	*Per cent with ANC from Health Professional*	*Per cent whose Last Live Birth was Protected Against Neonatal Tetanus*	*Per cent Delivered by a Health Professional*	*Per cent Delivered in a Health Facility*
Mothers age at birth					
<20	647/564	84/89	50/65	47/48	46/47
20-34	2821/2883	90/93	54/75	42/44	41/43
35+	584/526	82/85	46/67	29/37	28/36

* The first figure indicates 2003 findings while the second represents 2008 KDHS findings (CBS, MOH *et al.*, 2004; KNBS, NACC *et al.*, 2009).

Integration of family planning (FP) services into ANC has resulted in an improvement in uptake of FP. In 2003 only 39 per cent of surveyed women were using some contraceptive, as compared to 46 per cent in 2008. Though still lagging behind, contraceptive use in rural areas increased from 29 per cent in 2003 to 43 per cent in 2008, while in urban areas, it improved from 40 per cent to 53 per cent in the same period. It is therefore not surprising that at 5.2 births, TFR in rural areas is significantly higher than in urban areas (2.9 per cent). Education level of women was associated with contraceptive use, with the later increasing with education levels in both surveys.

The Kenya National HIV/AIDS Strategic Plan (KNASP) and the National Health Sector Strategic Plan (2005-2010) underlined the need to effectively address malnutrition among people living with HIV infection and those affected by the pandemic. With support from the President's Emergency Fund for AIDS Relief (PEPFAR), Kenya has initiated programs such as Food by Prescription (FBP) in collaboration with the National AIDS and STI Control Programme (NASCOP) and Insta Products Ltd. (Kenya) in 2006. The program provides fortified blended flour (FBF) by prescription to malnourished adults living with HIV (PLHIV), HIV-positive pregnant and postpartum women (P/PP) and orphans and vulnerable children (OVC) who are either clinically malnourished or at risk of malnutrition (FANTA-2 2009). The strategy for mainstreaming gender in KNASP provides a framework for integrating gender sensitivity into the HIV/AIDS response and this would contribute greatly to women empowerment (NACC 2005).

Despite the progress made in integrating maternal health in primary healthcare, other emerging reproductive health issues affecting women need urgent attention. In Kenya, over 10 million women aged 15 years and above are at risk of developing cervical cancer. At 13.2 per 100,000 women, the crude mortality rate due to cervical cancer in Kenya is higher than world rate of 8.9 (WHO and ICO 2010).

Manage to Assure Quality Services are Offered

NHSSP II is grounded in a fundamental respect for human rights and community participation and acknowledgement of what is doable during the target period. To strengthen the quality of services provided, a shift from disease burden (curative and vertical) to a human capital development approach by focusing on health promotion while at the same time stimulating a human rights approach in all interventions has been adopted. Other strategies adopted include capacity development of community-owned resource persons (CORPs) and health workers at grassroots levels, definition of ownership of service delivery at district and health facility levels, establishing Health Stakeholder Forums to monitor performance and improving resource allocation and financial targeting to underserved and poor areas. The Government has also made efforts to make health insurance accessible to all Kenyans. The National Hospital Insurance Fund (NHIF), originally tailored for salaried individuals, has been revised to accommodate unemployed Kenyans as well as those in casual employment. It is hoped that women, who form the bulk of the unemployed majority, will benefit from this revised legislation.

The Kenya *Economic Recovery Strategy for Wealth and Employment Creation* (ERS) stresses the need to shift health resources away from curative provision to preventive and promotive healthcare (GOK 2003). This has provided for an increasing trend of promotive and preventive finance allocation from 17.8 per cent in 2005/06 to 18.6 per cent in 2006/07 and finally 21 per cent in 2007/08. However real allocation in the health sector declined or remained constant over the past decade and yet it is a key sub-sector in the social sector (Ochieng and Gachambi 2008).

The per capita total health spending stands at about Ksh500 (or US$6.2), showing that health spending remains far below the WHO recommended level of US$34 per capita. This low allocation of resources makes it difficult for the health sector to achieve both the local and international policy targets. It also falls short of the Kenya government's commitment to spend 15 per cent of the total budget on health, as agreed in the Abuja Declaration (MOH 2005; Ochieng and Gachambi 2008). A study done in 2006 showed that budget allocations and actual expenditures in part go against policy objectives and the tread of weak policy implementation in the Kenyan health sector has not been significantly reversed (Glenngård and Maina 2007). The gender-insensitive budgeting process in Kenya has also been faulted by development partners, with the ADB pointing the non-inclusion of gender concerns in the budgeting process as one of the challenges in implementing policies (ADB 2007).

Measure Changes Made in Maternal Health and Nutrition and Mortality

Policies, even when they have been adopted, do not automatically translate into quality services at the local level. According to the Maternal and Neonatal Program

Index (MNPI 2002), Kenya's ratings for maternal and neonatal health services in some key areas lag behind the global average. The largest disparities between ratings for the global assessment and Kenya were found in budget resources (48 vs. 26 respectively) and provision of emergency obstetric care (55 vs. 35). Highest ratings for Kenya were for encouraging breastfeeding (79), immunization (71), and maternal health policy (63). This trend is expected to change with the implementation of the focused approach of health sector actions addressing maternal health and nutrition issues.

The CSDS through its focused approach to improve child survival and development has linked its targets to the Millennium Development Goals. Monitoring and evaluation has been proposed to be carried out as part of the annual health sector reviews and Health Management Information Systems (MOPHS 2008). The table below show selected performance indicators and targets as outlined in the CSDS (Table 13.3).

Table 13.3: Selected Child Survival Strategy Performance Indicators and Targets

Indicators	*KDHS 2003/ Baseline*	*Preliminary KDHS 2000*	*Target by 2015*
Maternal mortality ratio	414	–	147
Per cent deliveries conducted by skilled staff	42	44	90
Per cent receiving ANC care from a health professional	88	92	90
Per cent WRA receiving FP method	39	46	–
Per cent pregnant women receiving iron and folate supplements	47	–	50
Per cent postpartum mothers who received Vitamin A within 4 weeks after delivery	14.2	–	60
Infants exclusively breastfed for 6 months	2.6	13.2	60

–: Indicates missing data/information either in the KDHS or CSDS

For these targets to be achieved, the proportion of health budget allocated to maternal nutrition and child health services must be substantially increased. Increased advocacy and communication on nutrition and maternal health issues is required at the grassroots especially to address cultural barriers such as those hindering exclusive breast feeding, PMTCT and family planning.

Develop Capacity in Nutrition and Maternal Health Issues

This strategy identifies three areas in which the government should develop human capacity. This includes

- ☆ Developing nutrition leadership
- ☆ Improving coordination and integration
- ☆ Stronger and wider networking among professionals (Mwadime 2001).

The NHSSP II and CSDS recognize that human resource is an important factor in providing better health services to the mothers. Among the strategies proposed include:

1. Strengthening and integrating maternal nutrition and Child health (MNCH) components within pre-service and in-service training
2. Review of human resource policy to support adequate staffing
3. Participation in curriculum development to reflect Ministry of health needs
4. Advocating for increased resources to training institutions.

Full implementation of the above strategies has however been slowed down by low budget allocation and stop gap policies that have reduced further recruitment of staff in the Ministries concerned.

The health sector in partnership with other organizations such as UNICEF has made efforts to standardize methods of collection, analysis and interpretation of the nutrition and mortality data for the whole country. The development of *"Guidelines for Nutrition Assessment" (2008)* by Ministry of Health and Kenya National Bureau of Statistics is a good example of this effort (MOH and KNBS 2008). Nutrition information system as a key strategy for nutrition policy is continually being developed through the Food Nutrition Planning Unit in the Ministry of State for Planning, National Development and Vision 2030 and the Inter-ministerial Committee of Food and Nutrition.

Conclusion

Use of lifecycle approach to women's nutrition and health issues has been proposed as a good strategy by other stakeholders in maternal health and nutrition programmes. It is therefore a positive action for the Kenya Health sector to have adopted this approach in its policy. The findings of the 2008 KDHS show that a concerted effort is still required at the budgetary, policy and implementation levels to ensure good health and nutrition status among women and children. Continual improvement and support for coordination and implementation of essential maternal health and nutrition actions with other sectors such as education and agriculture is encouraged for maximum effect for women empowerment.

References

1. ADB (2007). Kenya Country Gender Profile 2006, African Development Bank, Human Development Department (OSHD).
2. CBS, MOH, *et al.* (2004). Kenya Demographic Health Survey: 2003, CBS, MOH, ORC Macro, Calverton, Maryland USA.
3. FANTA-2 (2009). Review of Kenya's Food by Prescription Program., Food and Nutrition Technical Assistance II Project (FANTA-2). Academy for Educational Development, Washington, DC.
4. Glenngård, A. H. and T. M. Maina (2007). "Reversing the Trend of Weak Policy Implementation in the Kenyan Health Sector? – A Study of Budget Allocation

and Spending of Health Resources Versus Set Priorities." Health Research Policy and Systems **5**(3).

5. GOK (2003). Economic Recovery Strategy for Wealth and Employment Creation 2003–2007 (ERSWEC). Ministry of Planning and National Development, Nairobi.
6. GOK (2007). The Kenya Vision 2030, National Economic and Social Council of Kenya, (NESC) and Ministry of Planning and National Development.
7. KNBS, NACC, *et al.* (2009). Kenya Demographic Health Survey: 2008-09: Preliminary Report, KNBS and Measure DHS, Calverton, Maryland, USA.
8. Linkages (2001). Essential Health Sector Actions to Improve Maternal Nutrition in Africa: (Summary), LINKAGES: Breastfeeding, LAM and Related Complementary Feeding and Maternal Nutrition Program.
9. MNPI (2002). Maternal and Neonatal Program Effort Index: Kenya, Policy project, The Maternal Health Study.
10. MOH (2005). Reversing the Trends: The Second National Health Sector Strategic Plan of Kenya - NHSSP II 2005–2010., Ministry of Health, Health Sector Reform Secretariat, Kenya.
11. MOH and KNBS (2008). Guidelines for Nutrition Assessment, Ministry of Health and Kenya National Bureau of Statistics, Kenya.
12. MOPHS (2008). Child Survival and Development Strategy 2008-2015, Ministry of Public Health and Sanitation, Kenya.
13. Mwadime, R. K. N. (2001). "Health Sector Actions to Improve Nutrition: Challenges and Opportunities in Sub-Saharan Africa." African Journal of Food and Nutritional Sciences **1**(1).
14. NACC (2005). Kenya National HIV/AIDS Strategic Plan 2005/6-2009/2010 (KNASP), National Aids Control Council, Kenya.
15. Ochieng, S. and B. Gachambi (2008). Health Sector: Budget Performance 2003-08 and Emerging Policy Issues. Issue no 16. May 2008, IEA Budget Information Programme.
16. UNICEF (1990). Strategy for Improved Nutrition of Children and Women in Developing Countries., UNICEF, New York.
17. UNICEF (2009). Tracking Progress On Child And Maternal Nutrition: A Survival and Development Priority, UNICEF: Communication Division, New York.
18. WHO and ICO (2010). Human Papillomavirus and Related Cancers. Summary Report Update, January 2010., apps.who.int/hpvcentre/statistics/dynamic/ico/methodologies.

Chapter 14

HIV/AIDS and Low Births Weight in Kenya: Experiences, Challenges and Effective Interventions

Wambui Lydia Kimani

Ministry of Public Health and Sanitation,
Provincial General Hospital, Nakuru, P.O. Box 14844, Nakuru, Kenya
E-mail: lydiashikhalis@yahoo.com

ABSTRACT

The birth weight of an infant is the single most important determinant of its chances of survival and healthy growth and development. According to the World Health Organization, Low Birth Weight (LBW) is defined as a birth weight of less than 2,500g. An estimated 22 million babies are born each year with LBW; the majority of them in developing countries (McCormick *et al.*, 1990). Low Birth Weight can be caused either by pre- mature delivery (short gestation) or by fetal growth retardation. Known factors associated with LBW include low maternal food intake, cigarette smoking, high parity, close birth spacing and high HIV infections (Klingenberg *et al*, 2003; Renqvist *et al.*, 1994; UNAIDS, 1999). The increase in survival rates of LBW infants leads to increasing healthcare costs due to extensive hospital stays. The reduction of low birth weight is an immediate and urgent concern in developing countries where interventions are required. This paper focuses on the nutritional interventions against low birth weight among women infected with HIV/AIDS in Kenya. The paper recognizes that maternal nutrition is important for health and reproductive performance of women as well as the survival and development of their children. Specifically, this paper discusses in detail the interventions against low birth weight among HIV-infected women. The interventions include: Adequate food and micronutrient intake; Nutrition education and counseling; Food safety and hygiene; Management of diet-related HIV problems; safer sex and reproductive health practices; Psychosocial support and Antenatal care (Lwanga and Piwoz, 2001; Huffman, 2001). Further, the paper identifies issues and challenges for the above interventions (Lwanga, 2001; UNAIDS, 2001). First, most women do not know their HIV status until later. Secondly, stigma and discrimination continue to be a challenge, especially for women who for social and cultural reasons may have less access to care and support services. Also, access to food is one of the challenges often compromising women's ability to choose safer and healthier life strategies. The paper also singles out the gender challenges of HIV, including women's vulnerable social status and legal rights and its influence on food security and risk of malnutrition. Finally, on the basis of the field experiences, the paper recommends feasible interventions aimed at reducing low birth weight babies. These include: need for accessible counseling and testing services; addressing of stigma, gender and cultural issues and changes in women's rights and empowerment.

Keywords: *Low birth weight, Pregnancy, Risk factors, Malnutrition, HIV.*

Introduction

More than 20 million infants worldwide, representing 15.5 per cent of all births are born with low birth weight, 95.6 per cent of them in developing countries. The level of low birth weight in developing countries (16.5 per cent) is more than double the level in developed regions (7 per cent). Half of all low birth weight babies are born in South-central Asia, where more than a quarter (27 per cent) of all infants weigh less than 2,500 g at low birth weight levels in sub-Saharan Africa are around 15 per cent. World-wide, about 16 per cent of live births, or some 20 million infants per year, are born with less than 2500g of weight and 90 per cent of them are born in developing countries (McCormick *et al.*, 1990). The prevalence of low birth weight (LBW) varies between and within geographical regions.Almost a quarter of all babies born worldwide are low birth weight, 8.2 per cent being in USA. Babies born in developing countries are susceptible to complications and infections in developing countries, chronic malnutrition, and poor weight gain during pregnancy contribute to low birth weight.

In Africa, the estimated percentages of LBW infants for 1982 is 14.0 per cent, 1 per cent lower than that for 1979. This decrease is largely due to changes in Northern and Southern Africa, where more recent data have changed the estimates for a number of countries, including Egypt and Lesotho. There is no evidence of substantive changes in Eastern and Western Africa, with the possible exception of Kenya which has improved, and Rwanda and the United Republic of Tanzania which have deteriorated. New information is available for a number of countries in these regions, but national rates are all between 10 per cent and 20 per cent.

Birth weight is a powerful predictor of infant growth and survival. Infants born with low birth weights begin life immediately disadvantaged and face extremely poor survival rates. In most developing countries it was approximated that every ten seconds an infant dies from a disease or infection that can be attributed to low birth weight. Many of those infants who survive suffer cognitive and neurological impairment, increased risk of high blood pressure, obstructive lung disease, cholesterol, renal damage, acute diarrhea, impaired immune function and poor cognitive development (Fonseca *et al.*, 1990; McLachlan, 1999; Podja and Kelley, 2000; Jurjus, 1995). Generally the risk of neonatal mortality for LBW infants is 25 to 30 times greater than for infants with birth weight exceeding 2500g, and it increases sharply as birth weight decreases (Podja and Kelley, 2000). The increase in survival rates of LBW infants leads to increasing healthcare costs due to extensive hospital stays. It is estimated that extremely LBW babies are up to six times as costly as normal weight babies (Chang, 2003; Klingenberg *et al*; 2003).

One of the goals of the 1990 World Summit for Children was to reduce the prevalence of low birth weight to less than 10 per cent by the year 2000 (Boerma *et al.*,1996; Podja and Kelly, 2000). However, this remains a formidable challenge to-date. It is therefore encouraging that the international public health community has begun to increase its attention toward these four million infants who die each year and the many more that survive with a diminished quality of life. Low birth weight is a reasonable well-defined problem caused by factors that are potentially modifiable and the costs of preventing them are well within reach, even in poor countries like Tanzania. It is therefore imperative to identify risk factors for LBW in various communities in the country in order to come up with feasible intervention strategies to minimize the problem.

Literature Review

Causes of Low Birth Weight

According to the World Health Organization, Low Birth Weight (LBW) is defined as a birth weight of less than 2,500g. Low birth weight can be caused either by premature delivery (short gestation) or by foetal growth retardation. The primary cause of low birth weight is premature birth (born before 37 weeks gestation). Another cause of low birth weight is intrauterine growth restriction (IUGR). This is when the baby does not grow well during pregnancy because of several factors that include; problems with placenta that can lead to poor blood flow and nutrients to the fetus, mother's health *e.g.* sick with malaria, or birth defects of the baby that are more likely to restrict growth because of genetic conditions and structural abnormalities.

Known factors for pre-term delivery and fetal growth retardation which are associated with LBW include low maternal food intake that may be caused by illness or food insecurity, hard physical work during pregnancy, and illness, especially infections (Klingenberg *et al*, 2003; Renqvist *et al.*, 1994). Other factors that can also contribute to the risk of low birth weight include; Age (< 15 years have higher risk), multiple births (10 per cent of twins and one-third of triplets are low birth weight) and mother's health (smoking, drug abuse, socioeconomic status, inadequate prenatal care, and pregnancy complications), high parity and close birth spacing (Bang *et al.*, 1999).

Birth weight is affected to a great extent by the mother's own fetal growth and her diet from birth to pregnancy, and thus, her body composition at conception. In those settings, the infant's low birth weight stems primarily from the mother's poor nutrition and health over a long period of time, including during pregnancy, the high prevalence of specific and non-specific infections, or from pregnancy complications.

A very large number of studies have shown the relationship between cigarette smoking and reduction in birth weight. Smoking reduces appetite, reduces oxygen supply due to carbon monoxide as more likely explanation. In Kenya men smoke in the house even when their women are pregnant and this could be a contributing factor to low birth weight babies.

Physically demanding work during pregnancy also contributes to poor fetal growth. Richard Naeye tried to analyze women engaged in hard labor in Ethiopia during pregnancy and birth weight of offspring's – offspring's were lower compared to those in less active mothers. Most of the women do not compensate the hard labor with sufficient eating. A recent study in Tanzania showed that the risk of giving birth to a low birth weight babies increased with severity of HIV infection in pregnant women (Dreyfuss *et al.*, 2001).

About 70 per cent of total population is at risk of malaria infection. It is a major cause of maternal and neonatal mortality and morbidity. Malaria may cause upto 30 per cent of preventable low birth weight and 3-5 per cent of neonatal deaths. Malaria increases the risk of premature labor, spontaneous abortion and still births. Malaria and febrile illness is also responsible for increasing cases of anemia among pregnant women.

Nutrition and Low Birth Weight among HIV Infected Women

Nutritional status has greater implications on women or adolescent girls who are at greater risk of delivering premature or low birth weight infants and malnutrition. Good maternal nutrition during pregnancy is vital for survival and wellbeing of the development of infants. Well nourished mothers have healthier babies and lower rate of mortality and morbidity. Physiological changes that occur during pregnancy require extra nutrients and energy to meet the demand of: Expanding blood supply, growth of maternal tissue, developing fetus, loss of maternal tissue at birth and preparation for lactation. Pregnancy related health and malnutrition problems have an effect on the quality of life and life of newborns.

In all pregnant women, malnutrition increases maternal mortality and morbidity and birth outcomes. For HIV infected women, HIV infection cause nutrient losses and increase nutritional requirements and risk of malnutrition which increases the risk of Mother-to-Child Transmission of HIV and high chances of getting low birth weight babies. Anemia affects half of all pregnant women in Africa and is common in HIV infected women. It is a risk factor for pre-term delivery and low birth weight. Increased energy requirements during lactation may also increase weight loss. This can lead to low birth weight if the mother did not practice family planning.

Nutritional status have greater implications for HIV infected women or adolescent girl who is at greater risk of delivering premature or low birth weight infants and malnutrition. Malnutrition and HIV work in tandem. Malnutrition weakens the immune system increasing vulnerability to infection. HIV compromise nutritional status increasing vulnerability to infection. Consequently the nutritional status of HIV infected woman or adolescent girl before and during pregnancy or after may influence her own status as birth outcomes.

Nutrition, Teenage Pregnancy and Low Birth Weight

A young age (11-18 yrs) increases nutrient needs above the ordinary demands of pregnancy due to adolescence growth and fetal growth and development. For HIV infected pregnant adolescent, the nutrients requirement are even higher as a result of HIV infection. Thus, the requirements for energy, protein and other nutrients increase overall to ensure continued growth of adolescent mother, fetus and fulfillment of increased demands of the body by HIV infection. Such adolescent is at increased risk of malnutrition.

A teenager is a maturing individual whose eating habits may be at their worst. The emotional stress that teenage pregnancy imposes on both girl and family may further interfere with sound nutritional practice. On realizing that the teenage is HIV positive is like dropping a bombshell. Meal skipping and the teenage preference for snacks foods low in nutritional value add to the difficulties in meeting the increased nutritional needs of pregnant adolescent. As may be expected many teenagers have difficulty establishing sound eating habits for their off-springs, since they have not yet done so far for themselves.

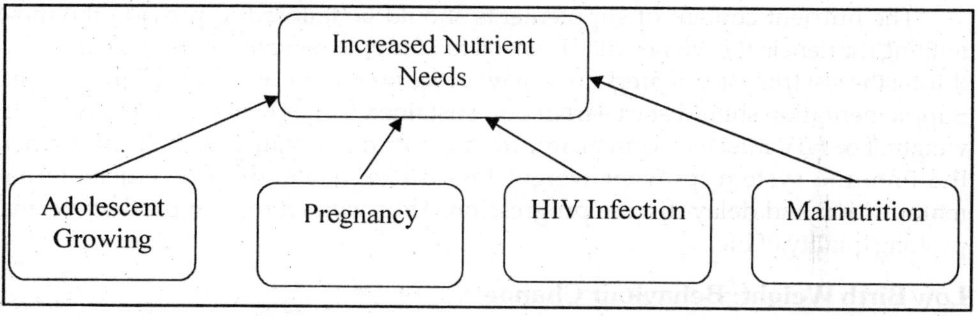

Figure 14.1: Relationship Between HIV, Malnutrition and Pregnancy

Recommended Interventions against Low Birth Weight

Low Birth Weight: The Role of Nutrition

Intervention at any point has the potential to break the cycle of intergenerational under-nutrition and low birth weight. Where resources are scarce, programmers designed to increase pre-pregnant weight and weight gain during pregnancy should be given priority. In many populations, food supply and birth weights are seasonal, so it is especially important to target interventions during hungry or wet seasons. During the last two trimesters of pregnancy, a woman should gain at least 1 kg per month for a total of 6 kg. Lack of weight gain during these last two trimesters, or weight loss is very detrimental to the fetus and/or mother and requires immediate action.

Good nutrition throughout the lifecycle is critical. Breastfeeding, appropriate complementary feeding, and adequate micronutrient status are especially important during infancy and early childhood. It is less clear what can be done during the adolescent period to promote growth, particularly in height. Adolescents, however, should receive dietary counseling, especially if they are pregnant.

Mothers with protein-energy malnutrition or appropriate food supplementation during pregnancy can improve incidence of low birth weight. The effect of birth weight is greater in population with moderate to severe malnutrition a detected through anthropometric, simple, social scales, choose accessibility to health services, literacy and environmental sanitation, dietary surveys or through monitoring food availability at family level.

Low Birth Weight: The Role of Micronutrient Supplementation

Good micronutrient status is important to birth outcome. Micronutrient supplementation may cause an increase in maternal appetite, which may lead to increased food intake and/or reduced morbidity. Deficiency in one or more micronutrients may be due to inadequate food intake, poor dietary quality, or when micronutrients are not readily released from foods, not absorbed efficiently, or a combination of these factors. Prenatal supplementation in combination with post-natal supplementation and with availability of healthcare services is associated with improved survival, physical growth and mental development of off-springs.

The nutrient content of supplements should be tailored to provide the most limiting nutrient in the women diet. Prenatal food supplementation or food deprivation during the last trimester of pregnancy may suffice to produce an effect on birth weight. Supplementation should start earlier and sustained through gestation to give birth weight. For HIV infected women, improving nutritional status can help strengthen the immune system, prevent weight loss during lactation, prevent maternal malnutrition and delay disease progression. Thus women remain productive and prolong quality of life.

Low Birth Weight: Behaviour Change

It is widely recognized that cultural beliefs and practices play a role in the successful delivery of nutrition messages to the community. Communication is a central aspect of directed behaviour change, and communication, by definition, involves multiple parties. An important question is Whose cultural beliefs and practices will constrain or facilitate the implementation of interventions? The multiple parties involve not only the recipients of the interventions " the women in the communities where low birth weight is endemic and their husbands, mothers, mothers-in-law, neighbors and community leaders " but the cultural beliefs of public health and nutrition professionals at different levels of the system must also be examined and understood.

Some general principles as to how information on cultural beliefs and practices can be used in the design of interventions to prevent low birth weight include: (1) Work with local people to adapt dietary recommendations for locally available foods, identify appropriate analogies (an analogy that links a new idea with one that is already present in the culture helps to make this new information understandable and at least potentially actionable), and develop educational messages built on local concepts. (2) Avoid making recommendations that are *head-on collisions* with local cultural beliefs. Frame recommendations in terms of the cultural beliefs of the community. In addition to the challenges of obtaining information on local beliefs quickly and inexpensively, the concept of *non-shared assumptions* must be considered.

This means health professionals engaging in cross-cultural communication which may run counter to their own beliefs and can present a major hurdle.

Low Birth Weight: The 'Packages'

Little has been implemented to date that translates existing information and recommendations into effective programmes for improving maternal nutrition and preventing low birth weight. Programmes to prevent low birth weight call for "packages" of interventions at various stages of the lifecycle. At minimum, low birth weight prevention programmes should have three components: (1) case management which increases the coverage of antenatal care and helps prevent repeated pregnancies in quick succession, (2) behavioural change communication strategies including those that defer pregnancy until after adolescence and to improve nutrition, and (3) linkages between existing healthcare facilities and the community.

It is crucial to develop and implement intervention packages for low birth weight prevention and particularly for safe motherhood and reproductive health programmes, and for Integrated Management of Childhood Illness (IMCI) programmes.

Low Birth Weight: Safe Sex and Reproductive Health Practices

Extending birth spacing and giving women longer non-pregnant, non-lactating intervals provides them the time they need to replenish their energy and micronutrient stores. As well as improving maternal nutrition, longer birth intervals improve child survival and health. An inter-pregnancy interval of 39 months allows for six months of exclusive breastfeeding, followed by at least 18 months of breastfeeding and complementary feeding, and at least six months of neither pregnancy nor lactation.

Prenatal care is a key factor in preventing preterm births and low birth weight babies. At prenatal visits, the health of both mother and fetus can be checked. Because maternal nutrition and weight gain are linked with fetal weight gain and birth weight, eating a healthy diet and gaining proper amount in pregnancy are essential. Mothers should also avoid alcohol, cigarettes.

Low Birth Weight: Antenatal Care

The essential healthcare sector actions aim at ensuring for pregnant or lactating women. ANC contacts with mothers can be used for VCTs to determine early in pregnancy whether a mother is HIV positive. ANCs can be used for nutritional assessments to assess whether early patterns provide adequate nutrient intake and allow early interventions (Monitor weight gain during pregnancy, support infant feeding).

Management of secondary infections is important to minimize their impact on the mother's nutritional status. This includes: promoting the treatment of opportunistic infections Management of common HIV symptoms that are diet-related *e.g.* Nausea, Vomiting, Diarrhoea, fever, anorexia, Heartburn, taste changes, mouth sore, constipation, bloating. These conditions can have serious impact on the HIV infected pregnant women's nutritional status because they reduce food intake and absorption.

Low Birth Weight among HIV Infected Women in Kenya

A Case Study of Rift Valley Provincial General Hospital, Nakuru (Kenya)

Background Information

Rift Valley Provincial General Hospital, Nakuru is a teaching and referral Hospital located 150 km away from Nairobi (Kenya's capital city). It is a government hospital that caters for patients from Nakuru Municipality and those referred from other district hospitals and health centers. It provides medications for all types of ailments and conditions both for in patients and outpatients.

Interventions Against Low Birth Weight on HIV Pregnant Women

At the Rift Valley Provincial General Hospital Nakuru, there is a progamme known as PMTCT standing for prevention of mother to child transmission of HIV that is incorporated in antenatal clinic Antenatal clinic, comprehensive care center which is an outpatient clinic for persons living with HIV and AIDS, and also in the maternity services. The services offered at this levels if followed to the letter can help mothers to prevent HIV transmission to their children before and during delivery and also prevent them from being borne with low birth weights. HIV infection to the fetus can lead to low birth weight.

Antenatal Clinic (ANC)

The following services are provided at the ANC:

- Nutrition assessment and counseling which includes taking the weights of the mothers to asses monthly weight gain
- Blood pressure assessment
- Hemoglobin level assessment for anemia
- TB screening and referral
- Tetanus immunization
- Iron supplementation
- Folic Acid supplementation
- Malaria prophylaxis
- HIV counseling and testing

Those who turn positive are given ARV and Cotrimoxazole prophylaxis for the mother and children to prevent mother-to-child transmission of HIV and other opportunistic infections. There is also partner testing for HIV and HIV positive women are referred to a Mothers' Support Group.

Mothers Support Group

This is a support group that was started in 2005 by hospital staff and a few HIV positive mothers after realizing that women were becoming very withdrawn and felt hopeless after knowing their status. Its main objectives were to help them fight self stigma and discrimination, to have quality life and to choose appropriate infant feeding options for their children. They have been meeting on monthly basis with the support of hospital staff and they have been sharing experiences and are counseled/ educated on health/nutrition issues during and after pregnancy by the hospital staffs. They are also referred to comprehensive care centre for further HIV care

The Comprehensive Care Centre (CCC)

This is an outpatient clinic for HIV positive persons. The following services are offered:

- ✰ Voluntary counseling and testing of HIV
- ✰ Persons are assessed and started on anti retroviral (ARV) therapy once they are eligible which is given at no cost
- ✰ They are also treated for opportunistic infections connected to HIV *e.g.* TB, herpis zoster, Karposis sarcoma, skin infection, sexually transmitted infections. In this case there is a pharmacy specifically that is meant for CCC client that gives drugs free of charge
- ✰ They also receive nutrition services that involve nutrition assessment, counseling and food and micronutrient supplementation. United States aids agency (USAID) through the government of Kenya provides food supplement in form of porridge floor to HIV positive children and adults including pregnant women with poor nutritional status. The supplementation is supplied until the nutritional status of individual client is improved. For pregnant HIV positive women with poor weight gain or a mid upper arm circumference of less than 22 cm, they are provided with the porridge flour until they are 6 months postpartum. Rift valley provincial general hospital is a beneficially of this program.
- ✰ Children born to HIV positive mothers are also given free services at CCC and also tested for the HIV virus
- ✰ They also receive spiritual support. Every morning at CCC waiting bay they receive pastoral services for 15 minutes. This helps them psychologically. They also come for free medical check up on regular basis

The Maternity

All women who come for maternity services are counseled and tested for HIV after or before delivery. Those who turn to be HIV positive are referred to CCC for care and also to mothers club for psychosocial support. They are also given ARV prophylaxis for the mother and children to prevent mother to child transmission of HIV. They also receive nutrition counseling on infant feeding options from the counselors

Case Study

A case study was carried at the hospital to determine the extent of low birth weight babies within the hospital in relation to the services being offered.

Methodology

Secondary data was used where clients' information was gathered from maternity registers, Antenatal care clinic register, HIV clinic nutrition register and mothers' support group records. This information was retrieved for the last 6 months for the Antenatal data, HIV nutrition information, mothers' Club and 4 months for maternity data. The following data was captured to determine the extent of low birth weight namely: Age, Parity, HIV status, Baby's birth weight, multiple pregnancy and gestation period (full or preterm).

Results and Discussions

Data on Antenatal clinic (ANC) was analyzed and summarized in Table 14.1.

Table 14.1: Antenatal Attendance Data (July–December 2009)

Month	*Total Attendance n*	*Tested for HIV n (per cent)*	*HIV Positive n (per cent)*	*Tested with Partner n (per cent)*	*Revisit n (per cent)*
July	527	476 (90.3)	40 (8.4)	27 (5.67)	68(12.9)
August	508	469 (92.3)	16 (3.41)	17 (3.02)	90 (17.7)
September	532	507 (95.3)	33 (6.5)	23 (4.53)	45 (4.32)
October	627	567 (90.4)	28 (4.93)	32 (5.64)	63 (10.04)
November	574	520 (90.5)	27 (5.19)	30 (5.76)	66 (12.69)
December	656	580 (88.4)	14 (2.4)	16 (9.28)	82 (12.5)

Source: Unpublished Data, Nakuru PGH, 2010.

Table 14.2: Maternity Data for the Months of November 2009 to February 2010

	Nov N (per cent)	*Dec N (per cent)*	*Jan N (per cent)*	*Feb N (per cent)*
Total Deliveries	692	868	740	675
Total LBW	63 (9.1)	96 (11.05)	73 (9.86)	39 (5.7)
HIV Positive	23 (3.3)	42 (43.8)	26 (35.6)	25 (64.1)
HIV +ve LBW	3 (13.04)	6 (14.3)	2 (7.7)	3 (12.0)
Pre-term LBW	26 (41.2)	25 (26.0)	44 (60.2)	28 (71.7)
Still birth LBW	6 (9.52)	3 (3.12)	21 (28.8)	7 (17.9)
Multiple Pregnancy	7 (11.1)	7 (7.3)	7 (9.6)	8 (20.5)
Adolescence pregnancy (18 years and above)	42 (6.1)	67 (7.7)	31(4.2)	10 (1.5)
Had lost a baby before (baby died)	4 (1.5)	4 (1.5)	7 (2.6)	10 (3.7)

Source: Unpublished Data, Nakuru RVPGH, 2010.

From Table 14.1, out of 3119 women tested from July to December 2009, 158 (5.07 per cent) were positive. Only 145(4.6 per cent) of women were tested with their partners during that period. Over 90 per cent of those who attended the clinic were tested for HIV.

Analysis of delivery information from the Hospital Maternity section was analyzed to assess the proportion of low birth weight and the predisposing factors in the last 4 months. According to data (Table 14.2), the following observations can be made:

From the month of November 2009 to February 2010 there were 2975 deliveries out of which 271(9.1 per cent) were born with low or very low birthweights.116(3.8 per cent) of the mothers were HIV positive and out of this 14(12 per cent) mothers gave birth to low birth weight. 123(45 per cent) of the total deliveries were preterm. Out of total deliveries 37(13.6 per cent) babies were stillbirths. Out of the total low birth weight babies 29(10.7 per cent) were bone from multiple pregnancies. Out of the total deliveries 150 (5.0 per cent) were born to adolescent mothers

Table 14.3: Mothers Support Group Attendance (July 2009–Dec 2009)

Month	*Attendance*	*Pregnant HIV Positive*
July	35	7
August	37	4
September	9	1
October	13	1
November	12	2
December	21	5
Total	**127**	**21**

Source: Unpublished Data, Nakuru RVPGH, 2010.

Out of 127 HIV positive women that attended the mothers support group only 21 were pregnant in the course of the 6 months as opposed to 158 HIV positive mothers that were referred from ANC clinic

Table 14.4: Data on Food by Prescription at CCC for HIV Positive Mothers

Month	*Total Attendance*	*No. of Women given Food*
July	35	2
August	37	3
Sep	9	1
October	13	1
November	12	1
December	21	2
Total		**10**

On the basis of Table 14.4, In the course of 6 months only 10 women received food by prescription.

Summary Findings

On the basis of the data analysis and results given in Tables 14.1–14.4, the following deductions can be made:

- ☆ HIV testing and counseling rate is very high. This could be attributed to the PMTCT clinic being more or less mandatory for visiting patients.
- ☆ The HIV positive women visiting the clinic account for between 2-8 per cent of the total women tested for HIV.
- ☆ Most women who turn positive are often reluctant to go for HIV comprehensive care because they fear consequences of their partners knowing their status. Furthermore, some women who are malnourished refuse food supplementation since they are not sure of their husbands' reaction.
- ☆ The proportion of women turning up for testing accompanied with their partners is very low (4-9 per cent). This in turn is likely to affect the support given by their partners. This situation also encourages re-infection by un-tested partner, because in the African society, the woman lacks bargaining power to convince the man to use a condom.
- ☆ Some women even after being counseled on good nutrition, they cannot implement since they are not *"bread winners"* within the households.

Regardless of the hospital good interventions to help pregnant mothers carry on pregnancy well and give birth to health, term with normal weight babies there were still high rates of babies bone with low and very low birth weight babies 5.7 per cent of total deliveries. Out of the total low birth weight babies 12 per cent were borne to HIV positive mothers. This could have been contributed to stigma and lack of treatment seeking for the HIV positive mothers and lack of adherence to counseling. Also some of those who came to deliver were either attending ANC care else where or did not attend at all

Issues/Gaps and Challenges

This paper recognizes the vital role of nutritional care and support plays in overall care of pregnant or lactating women or adolescent girls living with HIV and prevention of low birth weight. In view of the existing interventions at the Rift Valley General hospital, this paper has identified a number of issues/gaps and challenges.

- ☆ Although HIV testing rates among the women visiting the ANC clinic are generally very high, majority of the women remain untested and only attend hospital during delivery. This implies that most women do not know they are HIV-infected until they have advanced disease or choose to be tested at ANC. This implies a need for more accessible counseling and testing services to capture the many pregnant women who remain untested in the villages, or attend other local health centers or attend private hospitals
- ☆ It is apparent that stigma and discrimination continue to be problematic, especially for women who for social and cultural reasons may have less

access to care and support services then men. For instance, families are more likely to buy medicine and care for ill males than females.

- Access to food is one of the main challenges facing people living with HIV/AIDS in Africa. Improving food security for all including HIV infected pregnant and lactating mothers or adolescent girls is a challenge to policy-makers. Food insecurity increases vulnerability of women and young girls to HIV infection as social status is diminished, thus compromising their ability to choose safer and healthier life strategies. The burden of women who must care for HIV infected children and a family member is great and increases food insecurity. Lack of adequate food and nutrition significantly complicate the management of HIV/AIDS.
- The gender challenges of HIV, including women's vulnerable social status and legal rights must be addressed. In several countries (including Kenya), rural women whose husbands died of AIDS were forced into commercial sex to survive insecurity because they had no legal rights to their husband property. This increases food insecurity and risk of malnutrition. Reversing the spread of HIV will require changes in women's rights and empowerment.
- HIV is said to have the face of a woman in Africa. This notwithstanding, the planting of food crops is the responsibility of women. AIDS-affected households may plant less food or replace labour intensive but nutritious crops with less nutritious and profitable crops. This contributes to household food insecurity and may increase malnutrition, particularly in nutritionally vulnerable pregnant and lactating women and children.
- One of the major challenges in measuring the incidence of low birth weight is the fact that more than half of infants in the developing world (Kenya included) are not weighed. Low birth weight data, if available are based on data compiled from health facilities. These estimates are biased for most developing countries because the majority of newborns are not delivered in facilities, and those who are represent only a selected sample of all births.

Recommendations

Based on the case study the government has done tremendous efforts to help pregnant women but it seems the issue of low birth weight persists. This paper recommends the following measures to address the problem of low birth weight in Kenya:

- The government to strengthen support groups by giving the mothers some motivations such as providing snacks during the meetings and also motivate the facilitators who come to talk to mothers. More support groups should also be started and supported in residential areas and villages.
- Community health workers should be sensitized on the issues of low birth weight and also be paid for their work. At times the community health workers work on voluntary basis but they have monetary needs and they cannot continue working on voluntary basis.

- ✰ The government should also employ more nutritionist to cater for the growing population among other staffs.
- ✰ Women should be empowered on their rights so that they can be able to make independent decision on matters of sex and family planning. Men should also be sensitized on the importance of discussing family planning issues and sex with their partners. For a long family planning has been seen as a woman responsibility.
- ✰ School feeding programmes should be strengthened to ensure they provide balanced diet and adequate to provide for the needs of adolescent girls that might get pregnant
- ✰ Parents should be encouraged to support their adolescent girls who get pregnant rather than stigmatize them
- ✰ Looking at the ANC data 90 per cent of those who visit the clinic are tested for HIV. But what happens to the people in the village who only rush to this hospital when in labor. The government should advocate for door-to-door campaign of HIV testing and nutrition counseling.

Conclusions

Low birth weight has multiple etiologies, however, intrauterine growth retardation accounts for the majority of Low birth-weight in developing countries (Kenya included). This paper has attempted to highlight issues related to low birth weight especially among HIV-infected women and adolescent girls. This paper has also illustrated the interventions adopted by Kenya and the various challenges encountered.

This paper conclusively appreciates that there is an urgent need to intensify studies on the problem of low birth weight and adopt sustainable practices to improve women's nutritional status prior to pregnancy, and their weight gain during pregnancy. This paper notes that these practices require behavioural change within households, and behavioural change and communication strategies have been a weak link in many programmes trying to address this issue. This paper thus concludes that low birth weight solutions require packages of interventions, and that these need to be incorporated into all antenatal healthcare programmes and that both the number and coverage of these existing programmes be expanded. Care for women should be the foundation upon which all low birth weight prevention/reduction programmes are based.

In summary, improving pre-pregnancy weight and weight gain during pregnancy are effective strategies which reduce and prevent LBW. Good nutrition throughout the lifecycle, however, is critical. Breastfeeding, appropriate complementary feeding, and adequate micronutrient status are especially important during infancy and early childhood. Improved dietary intake should be promoted among adolescents, particularly among pregnant adolescents. Food supplements need to reach undernourished pregnant women. Reducing and preventing LBW requires a commitment to implement long-term strategies.

Acknowledgements

The author wishes to acknowledge the Ministry of Public Health and Sanitation (Kenya), through the Department of Nutrition for their facilitation to attend the seminar. Credit goes to the Provincial General Hospital Nakuru (Kenya) for permission to access the data and permission attend the seminar. At personal level, the author would thank to Mrs. Ngaruro (Chief Nutritionist, Department of Clinical Nutrition) for her tireless logistical support. Thanks go to Dr. Mbuthia, Head of Nutrition Department (Egerton University) for her contribution.

References

1. Huffman, S (2001). Essential Health Sector Actions to improve Maternal Nutrition in Kenya. Washington.
2. Institute of Medicine, National academy of Sciences (1990). Nutrition during Pregnancy. Washington DC, National Academy Press
3. Klingenberg, C., Olomi, R., Oneko, M., Sam, N. and Langeland, N. (2003). Neonatal Morbidity and Mortality in a Tanzanian Tertiary Care Referral Hospital. *Annals Paediatrics* 23, 293-299.
4. Lwanga, D (2001). Clinical Care of HIV-Infected Women in Resource-Poor Settings: Nutritional Care and Support. Baltimore.
5. Lwanga, D and E, Piwoz (2001). Nutritional Care and Support for Women Living with HIV / AIDS in West Africa. Washington DC. FANTA Project.
6. McCormick, M.C. (1985) The Contribution of Low Birth Weight to Infant Mortality And Childhood Morbidity. *New England Journal of Medicine* 312, 82-90.
7. Renqvist, R., Kardjati, S. and Kusin, J.A. (1994) Martenal Body Mass Index: The Functional Significancy During Reproduction. *European Journal of Clinical Nutrition* 48, Suppl 3556-3567.
8. UNAIDS (2001). Fact Sheet: Gender and HIV / AIDS. United Nations Special Sessions on HIV / AIDS. Geneva.
9. UNAIDS (1999) AIDS Epidemic Update. Geneva: United Nations Administrative Committee on Coordination Sub Committee on Nutrition (2000).Low Birth Weight. *Nutrition PolicyPaper No 18.*

Chapter 15

Women in Politics and Public Life (Modern Russia)

Vitalina Lobach

Philosophy Department, Moscow State University, Moscow, Russian Federation

E-mail: vitalina_odissi@yahoo.com

ABSTRACT

The population of our planet Earth is about 7 billion at present with about 53 per cent women and the remaining, men. But at the same time not only women, but politicians, scientists and demographers alike speak about women as being a discriminated majority. Legally men and women have equal rights in Russia. But there is a patriarchal standard which welcomes one code of conduct for a boy and another for a girl. Secondly, the private property in the country is divided so that 92 per cent is registered with men and only an insignificant part lies with women. Thirdly, almost no woman is in the echelons of power and directors. In labor and employment in Russia women face a diminished level of wages; rejection in hiring women with young children; dismissal of pregnant women accompanied by examples of the prohibitions of pregnancy when hiring; and formal regulation of labor, where women are working at weekends and on days without additional charges. Many employers are straight faced in telling that under equal conditions men will give a free job sooner than women. And although they know that the quality factor of the sex of a person executed in most cases does not significantly affect, stereotypes for many years, are stronger than logic. Therefore all traditionally the most highly paid and prestigious jobs accrue to men. In terms of women's education Russia consistently has one of the first places in the world, with the proportion of women with higher education higher than that of men. There is a tremendous potential of social development and personal development of women as a social group. At the same time educational resource of women is not sufficiently effective. Even among educated women the wages are barely 2/3rd of men's wages. Women constitute the majority of university students and assistants, senior lecturers and assistant professors.

But their number is way too smaller among the professors, doctors and other senior professionals. At higher levels of education very few women are represented. The last 17 years have witnessed a mode of depopulation in Russia. During this period the number of Russians has decreased by more than 6 million. If the figures for Russia and Europe are compared, it may be easily deduced that the child mortality in Russia is almost double of the European average and maternal mortality is even more, at above 2-3 times. According to the World Health Organization (WHO), the mortality rate of children below one year, and maternal mortality are crucial to assess not only the health but also the state of development of society as a whole. In modern Russia there are about 1 million, six hundred thousand abortions a year, which far exceeds the number of births. Each year abortion increases the number of infertile women by at least 160-170 thousand people. As a consequence the infertile women in Russia currently are about 5.5-6 million. Talking about the problems of women's health in Russia is necessary not only in terms of gynecological problems or reproductive problems, but in terms of the notion of women's health in general. For example, currently 65 per cent mortality among women in Russia is due to cardiovascular diseases, and the second place is taken by cancer. There is a critical need to promote healthy lifestyles as a policy. Adolescent girls must actively engage in health pursuit, because this is the time when during pregnancy the diseases begin to manifest several complications. Substantial funds should be allocated for spending on improving reproductive health and women's health in general, on children's allowances, payments to working and non-working mothers, etc. In fact, in modern day Russia, women do not actually have the capacity to act with an independent intellectual, moral and political authority, because such notion is exclusively in male domain and is outright rejected. At each Party Congress in Russia one can see in the hall 4/5th delegates being the men. This necessitates the gender imbalance in the political life of society to be aligned in favor of women. Meanwhile, in today's Russia there are no women party leaders, only as clerical functionaries. The positive changes are however occurring slowly, and the movement for the better can be noticed. For example, there are two women now in the government in powerful positions. One of them is a woman governor of St. Petersburg, Valentina Matvienko, which is the second largest region of Russia. In Soviet cinema, a large number of films, *viz.* "Shining Path", "Moscow does not believe in tears", etc. tell how a woman becomes a leader in the public sphere like the chief of an industrial plant or a parliamentarian ('deputy' in Russia) such that she becomes a leader in her own right. It was a sign of success for the women in Soviet times. She made a career for herself through her own efforts and stimulus and not through a man. On the contrary, a creative man appears as a result of success, not as a path to success. That was a fundamentally different approach with the woman having shown much more independence and confidence in strength at least at the level of declarations. Yes, it was an ideology, not more than propaganda, but these are the images that give the society a model for imitation. Such images are not visible in modern Russia's cinema and literature. All stories as a rule reflect only the real success of men. A male model of social career does not understand that people must somehow resolve the question of where to leave the children during working hours and a number of other domestic problems. The issues identified in the present report clearly point out to the disappointing findings about the existence of social discrimination against women in contemporary Russia. All the societies are based on national history and national character. The Russian women were given the right to vote, right to abortion and right to work at very early stages of the formation of Russia. However it remains another issue that they have lived 70 years in a totalitarian society and even till date poorly comprehend the idea of liberal values and the significance of fighting for their rights. Rights and privileges are not given; these have to be taken and acquired. Therefore women should cease to tolerate the status quo, which is forced upon them in the modern Russia. They must begin to actively defend their positions and their case; express their views; and forcefully state their views. When it succeeds, there will be a qualitative leap. And, of course, a comprehensive solution of all the existing problems of women in Russia should take place at the state level and receive the full support of the society.

Keywords: *Women in politics, Women power in Russia.*

Introduction

The tendency to strengthen the role of women in politics up to electing them presidents and prime ministers is gradually becoming a symbol of the time in the world. This happens because modern type of society imposes higher demands on the reproduction and development of human capital, which in turn redistributes the usual functions of the State from the traditional, mainly related to the repressive and regulating functions, to modern ones.

What are these advanced features related to? Firstly, these are linked to the policy of the State in such important areas as education, health, social security and fundamental science. Gradual reformatting problems of the modern State involves more strict requirements to restore the gender balance in the leadership of the State and to create more efficient mechanism of governance at all levels.

That is why the promotion of women into the power is considered as a tool for sustainable, humane and stable society as the real equality between men and women changes the priorities of State policy and the life of the country as a whole.

The statistics shows that the States with less than 25-30 per cent of women in their parliaments and governments poorly tackle the problems of maternal and child health, child rights and social protection. It means that these States do not allow due respect and ensure human rights in accordance with basic democratic requirements. Consequently, the struggle for genuine democracy involves an important component-the full equality of women having parity with men in government, parliament and all state institutions to ensure social justice and social stability.

Representation of Women in Power in Russia and Other Parts of the World

According to the Russian Statistics Agency Russia has more than 77 million women, almost 10 million more than men, and the entire world has more than 3 billion women. On average, in many countries women make up half or slightly more than half the population. Moreover, in most countries women were allowed to participate in the ballot process much later than men. For example, in the USA men got the voting right in 1870 and women after lapse of 50 years, in 1920; In Japan men got this right in 1925 and women only in 1945.

In Russia women won the right to vote on April 15, 1917 by the order of the Provisional Government on the production of transparent elections city councils and urban district offices. Accordingly, the voting rights were vested to all citizens over 20 years old, regardless of their nationality and religion. On June 20, 1917 the Provisional Government adopted the provision on the election of the Constituent

Assembly, the supreme legislative body, which came into force on September 11, 1917. It clearly stated the "'universal suffrage' without distinction of sex". Subsequently, the first election of the Constituent Assembly was held In September 1917 in which women were able to participate fully.

The data show that many countries have made women's representation in parliament at the level of one third or more of the total number of deputies. During the second half of the twentieth century the percentage of women in legislatures in countries with parliaments, has grown by 4 times. According to statistics, IPU, Russia shares the 84 place with Guinea-Bissau, Cameroon ranking at 85, comprising 14 per cent of women in the lower house of the Parliament and 4.7 per cent in the Senate. In terms of the participation of women in the highest organs of representative government not only the European CIS countries but also Tajikistan (17.5 per cent), Uzbekistan (17.5 per cent), Turkmenistan (16 per cent), Kazakhstan (15.9 per cent) have left Russia far behind in this respect. The main reason is the weakness of civil society institutions, low political involvement of women by themselves, low levels of democracy, and insufficient legal and regulatory framework. But, I believe that the main factor significantly hindering the advancement of women in Russia in politics and power is sustainable conservation of the socio-cultural patriarchal traditions and stereotypes.

A unique research was conducted by a leading expert S.G. Aivazova, the chief researcher at the Institute of Sociology RAS on "Russian Elections: A Gender Reading". She assessed the electoral law, its changes and election campaigns for 10 years. It made it possible to evaluate the general trends of the evolution of the electoral process in Russia from a gender perspective. Questions were raised about how deeply men and women with different age and educational characteristics and natives, both from the mega-cities and the villages and towns are involved in the electoral process and what are the chances of obtaining a parliamentary mandate.

In modern Russia, the interest of women in politics, and consequently, their participation in politics has significantly declined in recent years. During the perestroika (transition period in Russian politics of 1990s) a lot of women have entered politics and in some cases even have taken key positions in the supreme power, and furthermore they had their representation in parliament as an independent faction called "Women of Russia". Notwithstanding this, currently their positions in government, both at the center and in the field, are much weaker. Studies have shown that women themselves answer these questions quite clearly.

On the one hand, many of them do not consider themselves harmed in terms of their social and political self-realization. Moreover, 45.8 per cent of women as against 29.3 per cent believe that over the past ten years the ability of women to realize themselves in business, social activities and politics has increased significantly. On the other hand, approximately the same proportion (52.7 per cent to 24.9 per cent) of respondents indicated that men still possess greater rights and opportunities for political activity than women.

Most women believe that today there are no serious constraints to full social and political life of women and accordingly, there is no political discrimination based on sex. Simultaneously, women face such a number of problems in everyday life that politics and social activities recede into the background for them. For almost half the women interviewed (44.0 per cent), political and public career, either now or in the future, is not among their vital plans. Only 5.5 per cent claimed that they had made a serious career in this area. All the rest believe that either they can achieve this if they want (25.7 per cent), or cannot achieve, even if they wanted (23.5 per cent). Thus a group of politically active women is slightly less than a third of all respondents. It should be borne in mind that many women find it possible and even necessary to take part in so-called social work and to strengthen the role of women's organizations in society. Therefore under certain conditions the number of women involved in this activity can actually increase. Moreover, attention is drawn to the fact that the opportunities of this kind of participation are viewed by women as rather optimistic: 47.4 per cent of them stated that men and women have equal opportunities to participate in public life, and only 27.3 per cent believe that men have more rights.

The connection between the estimates of new opportunities for political and social self-realization on the one hand and evaluating a person's own capabilities on the other can be traced. Thus the Russian women, who have already managed to achieve something, or hope to do so in the near future, estimate these possibilities more positively (Table 15.1).

Table 15.1: Assessment of New Opportunities for Self-Realization of Women in Business, Politics and Social Activities According to their Own Success (in per cent)

Evaluation of the Success Already Achieved in Professional, Political and Public Career	*Change in Opportunities in Past 10 Years*		
	It was Easier	*It was Harder*	*Not Changed*
Already achieved success	7.7	4.2	3.5
Not yet achieved, but I think that I can do it	31.8	19.3	23.3
It would be desirable but is unlikely to be able.	19.7	30.4	23.6
In my life plans have not been	40.8	46.2	49.6

The greatest career is achieved by women in older age groups: 12.4 per cent with 5.6 per cent on average. But in this age group there is the highest percentage of those women (56.9 per cent), who did not see any prospects for personal fulfillment. It is also interesting that women of the youngest age group (17-25 years) are most optimistic about their opportunities. As for the middle-aged women (31-40 years), they are dominated by skepticism: 53.3 per cent of them declare that they have no plans to make public and political career, and 24.0 per cent say that even if they wanted, then they are unlikely to succeed.

The factor of education also affects the ability of self-realization: it increases involvement and gives confidence that these opportunities could arise. For comparison, the share of those who are optimistic about their career prospects are twice as many among women with higher education than among those with incomplete secondary or secondary education. With regard to social characteristics, the "proactive" model of thinking is mostly held by those women who assess their financial and marital status, social status and degree of satisfaction of life in a more positive way (Table 15.2).

Table 15.2: Assessment of Professional, Political and Social Self-Realization Depending on the Level of Material Security, Family Relations and Social Status (in per cent)

Various Contentment Aspects of Life	*Make a Professional, Political and Public Career*			
	Already has	*Not Yet Achieved, but I think that I can do it*	*Would be Desirable, but is unlikely to be able to achieve*	*In my life plans that do not*
Material Security				
Well	12,4	38,7	13,1	35,8
Satisfactory	6,0	29,1	23,4	41,5
Bad	3,1	17,4	27,4	52,1
Relationships in the Family				
Well	6,8	29,9	22,2	41,0
Satisfactory	4,2	21,1	24,8	49,8
Bad	4,2	23,2	30,5	42,1
Status and Position in Society				
Well	15,0	37,3	11,6	36,1
Satisfactory	3,3	24,1	26,1	46,4
Bad	–	15,3	34,2	50,5
In General Growth in Life				
Well	9,9	43,1	16,7	30,3
Satisfactory	4,9	22,0	24,6	48,5
Bad	–	10,6	35,0	54,4

This shows that the lowest differentiation in this capacity is correlated with the relationships in the family. Do the mere presence/absence of the family, its composition and distribution of family roles affect the political socialization of women? As demonstrated by this study, if affected at all, it is not as significant as might be supposed. Married women are somewhat more successful, but the unmarried are more optimistic in their forecasts for the future. As for the distribution of family roles in terms of material contributions of the spouses, survey did not record any significant differentiation. In other words, the question of who is the main "breadwinner" in the family is not vital for assessment of the possibility of participation/non-participation in social and political life.

As for the priority opportunities for men to participate in political life, this view is shared by most of the women surveyed, regardless of marital status, age and other social characteristics. Against this background, only women who positively evaluate their material and social status can be distinguished. This part of the Russian women often has the opinion that they have equal opportunities and rights with men (Table 15.3).

Table 15.3: Assessment of the Degree of Equality Between Men and Women to Participate in Political Life, Depending on the Level of Satisfaction of Women Various Aspects of Life (in per cent)

Evaluation of the Success Already Achieved in Professional, Political and Public Career	*As a Changed Opportunity in the Past 10 Years*		
	Become Easier	*Become Harder*	*Not Changed*
Already succeeded	7.7	4.2	3.5
Not yet achieved, but I think that I can do it	31.8	19.3	23.3
It would be desirable but is unlikely to be able to	19.7	30.4	23.6
In my life plans have not been	40.8	46.2	49.6

Politics in Contemporary Russia largely involves the use of power, financial and administrative resources. They are mostly concentrated in the hands of men, so this makes women to assess men's opportunities much higher. Inequality of resources, in turn, places women in an unequal position in the competitive political struggle. That perhaps attributes to the fact, why those few women who managed to win this fight often show not the best personal and professional qualities. That is why many women are extremely wary of women - professional politicians. In particular, the majority of Russian women are very skeptical about the possibility that a woman could be elected the President of Russia. This opportunity is seen as desirable only by 36.8 per cent of women, while 61.2 per cent would prefer to see a man as the President of Russia. Another aspect is the local political level associated with specific social problems, where the role of women is seen somewhat more preferable than men. Thus 51.8 per cent would prefer to solve their personal problems contacting local female politicians and administrators and 45.7 per cent would like to see men in those positions. Apparently, women officials at the middle and grassroots level are considered by the women themselves as possessing certain qualities more suitable for this work that include patience, attention, less corruption, and most importantly, the understanding of those everyday problems that concern women, and that is not always easy and possible to discuss with men. It is most clearly seen in the estimates of the most affluent and least affluent. Those who have serious problems in family relations and material security would rather turn to female officials.

It can be concluded that most women throughout the country consider the politics as a joint activity, or as an activity which is predominated by males. Extraction of a "feminine" aspect does not seem productive. It is not accidental that the fraction "Women of Russia", which set out to find their electorate and to formulate their own "women's" agenda, has not managed to acquire an independent political entity and a foothold in the next elected parliament. This is largely due to the fact that the ideological and political sympathies of representatives of both sexes tend to indicate a lack of significant differences by sex: they can be divided into right and left, centrists, and radicals in the same proportion. From this perspective it seems justified that the current legislation does not allow creating the party of sex, nationality or religious beliefs. At the same time, there remain opportunities to participate in politics within the existing party-political spectrum, as well as self-organization of women for social and humanitarian problems, than what is currently available and at the same time is in great need.

It should be emphasized that the "successful women" are more willing to delegate political rights and responsibilities of men. For example, among those women who managed to create a happy family, respectively, 65.9 per cent and 33.0 per cent would like to see a man and woman as president, while these figures are respectively 54.1 per cent and 43.2 per cent for those who did not build a happy family. Approximately the same is true with regard to the material factor, although at first glance, this contradicts the fact that women from highly affluent groups are active in the political sense, and seem to trust female politicians, including the prospect of election to the highest office – the President of the Russian Federation - to a greater degree. However, this does not happen. Women from high-yielding groups are 2 times more likely to prefer to see men as president, whereas among the poor, the gap is not so significant, although it also occurs. This is because a woman having a normal and happy family as well as sustainable sources of material wealth is accustomed to trust the man, rather than less prosperous and materially underprivileged women. Another interesting fact is that women do not agree that it is better not to participate in social and political life. This view is shared by only 30.3 per cent of all women surveyed, while 41.6 per cent strongly disagreed. At the same time, women want to have such a redistribution of roles within the family, so that everybody was able to combine the care of home and family with full participation in social and political life. The overwhelming majority of Russian women (68.0 per cent to 10.5 per cent) insist on this, regardless of their marital status. In other words, women need a strong family support. And if they have it there are no problems with social activities for them. And most importantly, in this case women do not require any special privileges from the state and society.

For example, among those who evaluate relationships in the family as "good", almost half the respondents did not support a quota of seats in the Duma (Russian Parliament) by sex (43.7 per cent to 23.0 per cent who believed that at least half the seats should be given to women). This idea is supported among those who evaluate the relations within the family as poor, at a ratio of 38.1 per cent against 32.0 per cent. Only about a third of women who assess their family situation as unsatisfactory stated the necessity to have the government "women's sections at the level of at least 50 per cent of its composition".

In evaluating the idea of quotas, many women may consider the practice of Soviet times, when there were unspoken rules of women representation in all elected bodies, except perhaps in the Soviet Politburo. Some of the women apparently believe that this practice is fully justified and worthy in the new circumstances, while others consider it flawed and therefore oppose it.

Contradictory attitudes among Russian women to women's participation in politics and public life quite clearly manifested the role and place of public organizations of women. Many women do not tend to see some fundamental differences between the interests of men and women and therefore in their view, the fact about who protects them and submits to the authorities at central and local levels is less important. On the other hand, about the same number of Russian women is convinced that women can represent and protect the interests of women better. Perhaps this suggests that today in society there are no effective mechanisms for representation and protection of the interests of women. They are protected neither by men nor by women themselves, in any case, within those organizations that operate in the country today. Women are interested in the effectiveness of such activities, but at this stage the implementer is not relevant for them. But at the same time they believe it is important to develop women's associations in the future.

The study found that the higher the welfare level of the respondents, the less they are convinced that their interests can be understood and protected only by women, and the more tolerant they relate to social and political activities of men. The lower the levels of the income of the women interviewed are, the more strongly they are convinced to have their interests represented and defended by women. And for this, from their point of view, new women's associations must be established and the existing ones further reinforced.

It should be noted, however, that most women do not pay attention to the sphere of activities of such organization as well as the very existence of many of them. Thus despite the fact that over the past 10 years a large number of women's social organizations claiming to represent the various interests of women have popped up in the country, 70.6 per cent of Russian women know nothing about their existence in the city, province, region or republic. Among those who know about their activities, more than half believe that they personally do not need these associations. And only 8.8 per cent of the respondents have positive attitude to this activity. Among these, 5.1 per cent would like to participate in the work of such organizations; 2.5 per cent are treated in such organizations for helping solve their problems and 1.2 per cent is personally involved in the activities of a women's NGO.

According to the survey, women's organizations, even if they exist, are concentrated mainly in large industrial centers and metropolitan areas. As for small towns and villages, the survey revealed a consistent pattern: the smaller the town, the less information about the work of such organizations its residents possess. Thus 62.5 per cent did not know about the work of women's groups in metropolitan areas, and 76.2 per cent in rural settlements. Substantial variations among these indicators depend on the region of residence. Thus the most informed about the activities of women's associations are the residents of Novgorod (57.1 per cent) and St. Petersburg (50/0 per cent), and among the least informed are Voronezh (17,1 per cent) and Kemerovo - (12,9 per cent).

The above data indicate that the currently existing women's social and political organizations have not yet become an important factor in Russian politics and the emerging civil society. Perhaps this is due to the fact that so far women's organizations have failed to meet the interests of different groups of women. Meanwhile, as shown by this study, "women's agenda" does not look unexpected and extraordinary. The Russian citizens see the priorities, which should be implemented by such women's organizations, as follows:

- ☆ 54.4 per cent - providing psychological assistance to women in difficult life situations;
- ☆ 45.7 per cent - assistance in finding a job;
- ☆ 42.3 per cent - protecting the interests of children (from organization of children's leisure activities to Soldiers' Mothers Committees);
- ☆ 41.4 per cent - providing material assistance to women who are in a quandary;
- ☆ 26.8 per cent - the fight against such phenomena as drug addiction, alcoholism, prostitution, etc.;
- ☆ 24.0 per cent - the fight against all forms of discrimination against women;
- ☆ 18.3 per cent - protection from domestic violence;
- ☆ 9,4 per cent - support in establishing their own business;
- ☆ 8,0 per cent - a political struggle for women's rights;
- ☆ 5,4 per cent - the organization of leisure for women.

The first position associated with the necessity of psychological rehabilitation of women, ahead of such forms of activities, such as income support, combating discrimination against women, etc. looks unexpected. This is probably due to the socio-psychological stress, from which women have suffered in the last decade. On the other hand, this aspect of women's organizations, as a rule, is not the first priority today. Apparently, women require not only the specific material and social assistance, but also they are in need of sympathy, attention and friendly advice.

It is also curious that the number of those who believe that women need more help with employment than direct material support is higher, although not much. Quite a lot of Russian women (24.0 per cent) also believe that women's organizations have to fight discrimination against women in all its forms and manifestations. As for political issues, then it is considered important only by 8.0 per cent of the respondents. The Russian women, having problems with work, would like to see women's organizations assist them in locating employment (61.1 per cent). Those who are malnourished would like to receive material assistance (51.5 per cent). If a family member has bad habits, a woman needs protection from domestic violence (29.0 per cent). And if respondents have no opportunity to help their children, they are convinced that women's organizations primarily have to protect the interests of the children (50.8 per cent). In addition, they also believe that their activities should focus on the fight against drug addiction, alcoholism and prostitution (38.1 per cent). Single Russian women are especially in dire need of psychological care (61.3 per cent). They dream of escape from their loneliness and are determined to expand the circle of acquaintances. Therefore, more than any other group of respondents they are interested in the fact that the activities of women's organizations help in establishing their own business and leisure.

Thus the desired directions of women's public organizations largely depend on the disorders in the life of Russian women. As for the influence of the fears and concerns of women in their perceptions of the priorities of women's organizations, the psychological support is especially needed by women who suffer from loneliness, the threat of old age, those who are afraid of bitterness, loss of mutual understanding between people, and the prospect of losing health by them or their relatives. It would seem that it is mainly the problem of the older generation, but in reality it is the problem of younger women. Interestingly enough, in this regard 61.0 per cent of 17-18-year-old girls facing the problem of adaptation in the "adult" life would like to receive psychological care.

So after the return to free elections Russia undergoes a return to patriarchal values and stereotypes. And it takes time for new democratic values and practices to mature. In 2001, Russia adopted an amendment to the law "On political parties", under which political parties were obliged to "create equal opportunities for representation in the governing bodies of political parties, list candidates and other elected positions in government agencies and local government for men and women, citizens of Russia of different nationalities and members of political parties. However, this rule is purely advisory in nature and does not provide penalties for its violation.

Experience shows that in many countries around the world, for promotion of women in power the regulating system at all levels is an important means of public policy. In Russia, however, a further substantial government support, connected with the expansion of the system of measures promoting women in power is not prominent. Global trends so far bypass Russia. However, one cannot say that some work in this direction in Russia is not conducted. Since the early 1990's, a number of legal acts improving the status of women in post-Soviet Russia were adopted by the President and the Government of Russia. But these documents, unfortunately, have not been supported by the necessary procedures for implementation and financial support, so a real mechanism for the advancement of women in power cannot be based on them.

In 2003, the State Duma held a first reading of bill on 'State Guarantees of Equal Rights and Freedoms of Men and Women and Equal Opportunities for Their Realization'. Over a third of the State Duma deputies supported the idea of a legislative rule that would allow women to dispose law eligibility, that is, the right to be elected to the bodies of representative power. However, specific rules of representation of women and the sanctions for their violation have not been adopted. It is possible to agree with the general conclusion of the well-known expert and researcher of women's equality issues, S.G. Aivazova that, "the main obstacle to the integration of women into the political process is that the gender equality principle is not properly executed in the relevant specific provisions of the electoral law".

In general, discussions on mechanisms for the promotion of Russian women into the power bare some uncertainty: no one says either "yes" or "no". On the one hand, the development of democracy in Russia requires recognition of this rule, and decision how to implement it in practice. On the other hand however a tendency can be observed to defer specific decisions, not to take any immediate legal action and not to assume legal obligations, which would force parties to seriously prepare women candidates for the election at all the levels of the government. Quotas and standardization of participation of women in elected bodies is not the same thing:

quotas come down from above and "They give". Standards are the result of the social contract as enshrined in the law with interest groups seeking for their adoption.

The idea of introducing the standards and ensuring gender balance in the lists of candidates in the power structures has provoked rejection in Russian political circles for a long time. Today it has become fashionable to talk about the crisis of family, the demographic crisis. Or, perhaps, the problem is primarily in the need for full and guaranteed rights for women and men. Quite a number of surveys, unfortunately, have consistently shown that the gender imbalance in power affects the daily lives of Russian women – namely their salaries, pensions and children allowances. And this situation persists.

Poor women's participation in politics will reproduce traditionalist - not civil and democratic - and "poddannicheskoy" political culture. And political life for most women will remain a minor, alien to their everyday life and activity. But, being the bearer of "poddannicheskoy" culture, they will definitely play it in the process of educating the younger generation, handing their children the "poddannicheskiy" way of thinking. Given this far-reaching consequences, one can legitimately argue that gender inequality in politics is one of the most significant obstacles to the democratic transformation of Russia.

Immediately after his election President D.A. Medvedev had said that legal nihilism is one of the most acute problems of Russia. In this context it is appropriate to recall that, contrary to many international treaties signed by Russia, there are no national mechanisms and procedures which will not only legally, but actually guarantee the constitutional principle of gender equality, including in the electoral process. And if the political parties should follow the principles of equal opportunities for political participation of all citizens regardless of gender in their activities, addressing parity representation of women in power structures should be seen as a vital indicator of social justice and equality in society.

Conclusion

Experiences shows that in many countries around the world, for promotion of women in power the regulating system at all levels is an important means of public policy. In Russia, however, a further substantial government support, connected with the expansion of the system of measures promoting women in power is not prominent. Gödel trends so far bye pass Russia. However, one cannot say that some work in this direction in Russia is not conducted. Since the early 1990's a number of legal acts improving the status of women in post–Soviet Russia were adopted by the President and the Government of Russia. But these documents unfortunately have not been supported by the necessary procedures for implementation and financial support, so real mechanism for the advancement of women in power cannot base on them.

References

Aivazova, S.G. (2008). Russian elections: gender reading. Moscow.

Aivazova, S.G. (2004). We choose, choose us. Gender analysis of parliamentary and presidential elections, 2003-2004, in Russia. M. (in collaboration).

Consortium of Women's Non-governmental Organizations on April 17, 2003 Moscow Center for Gender Studies.

The bill in the State Duma of the Russian Federation "On state guarantees of equal rights and freedoms of women and men and equal guarantees of their realization." Document to Duma (Russian parliament).

Korbut, L., and Polenina, S. (1997). International conventions and declarations on the rights of women and children. Collection of universal and regional international instruments. M: IC – Garant.

Chapter 16

Maternal Health and Low Birth Weight Problems in Tanzania: Possible Reasons and Potential Remedies

Judith Francis

Research Officer, Tanzania Commission for Science and Technology, Ali Hassan Mwinyi Road, P.O. Box 4302, Dar-es-salaam, Tanzania E-mail: jkadege@costech.or.tz, barautj@aol.com

ABSTRACT

Tanzania being among the Least Developed Countries (LDCs) faces many challenges, in terms of health and nutrition issues, which at the end contribute in a large quantity to the problem of high number of Low birth weight cases. Likewise, in other developing countries and in Africa as a continent low birth weights "the devil" and under-nutrition matters are still among the most fundamental challenges for improved human development. One of the major reason for this problem being that of a limited time and capacities of the healthcaregiver, as a result many mothers and children (the vulnerable) are unable to access and effectively use at all times the food and health services they need for a healthy life. Women's health, nutrition, social and cultural challenges that Tanzania has been facing for decades (though improvement was observed during the last decade) have highly contributed to the increase of low birth weights cases; infant and under -five mortality crisis. These problems have affected women (pregnant mothers and their children) both directly and indirectly, most common ones being (mentioning a few); infections and maternal risk factors for example diseases such as Malaria, HIV/AIDS, TB, Pneumonia, Diarrhoea, Malnutrition etc; poor maternal health and education; and low social economic status (ability to afford/acquire a well balanced diet). Mothers and children form a large group in Tanzania, whereby nearly 75 per cent of the populations are mothers (from child-bearing age) and children. On the other hand, low birth weight infant delivery has been a major health problem associated with high morbidity and mortality rates in the country. As a result, this group being the most vulnerable in the country is highly and badly affected as issues such as inadequate health services and malnutrition are concerned. Similarly to other countries, Tanzanian women play a big role in the economy and development of the country. Women contribute vastly in different sectors of health, education, agriculture, industries, businesses, gender, human rights, good governance and food systems (security) for the entire household etc. Despite the fact that, women form a backbone of the development of the country, still challenges exist, such as a large number of women and their children have unequal access to resources, quality health services, education, income; they participate less in decision-making, affected by hunger and under-nutrition; and also violation of their basic rights etc. This country report to be presented focuses on the low birth weight matters and engagement/ role of a woman in tackling or reducing the problem of the low birth weight in Tanzania. The status of low birth weight cases, efforts done by the government (concerned Ministries), NGO's etc in reducing such cases in relation to engaging (empower)women in combating such crisis of pre term low birth weight in babies, its causes and associated factors that lead to the problem, despite the challenges that they face as women. Also, the recommendations/ solutions and suggestions will be discussed.

Keywords: *Maternal health, Low birth weight, Empowering women, Least developing countries, Health related issues.*

Introduction

Tanzania is situated on the Eastern Coast of Africa. Agriculture is a key sector of Tanzania's economy, with almost 80 per cent of its total population depending on it for their livelihood. Tanzania is categorised as a least developed and low-income food-deficit country. Poverty remains widespread with almost over 58 per cent of the population living on less than $1 per day. More than 80 per cent of the population of TanzaniaShortly after independence in 1961, Tanganyika and Zanzibar merged to form the nation of Tanzania in 1964. One-party rule came to an end in 1995 with the first democratic elections held in the country since the 1970s.

Tanzania totally has an area of 364,900 square miles, with estimated population of approximately 36million people, out of which 54 per cent are in the working age group and 46 per cent are dependent population, where around 3 per cent of the population being over 65 years of age and 45 per cent under 15 years of age. (UN Report 2003). The migration rate is very high, where by the in-migration number is higher than the out-migration.

The ethnic composition in Tanzania mainland consists mainly of - native African 99 per cent (of which 95 per cent are *Bantu* consisting of more than 130 tribes), others 1 per cent (consisting of Asian, European, and Arab). Tanzania has a huge tribal population with various beliefs that are mostly local. It has as many as 25 per cent of population that have indigenous beliefs. Apart from that 35 per cent of the population is Muslims and 40 per cent follows Christianity. However in the territory of Zanzibar approximately 98 per cent of the people are Muslims. Official language in Tanzania is Swahili; however English is also used as a second language for international transactions/communications.

Health and Nutritional Issues in Tanzania

Health Issues

The United Republic of Tanzania was the first African country to pioneer the health centre as a local point of delivering primary healthcare back in the 1970s. After independence, in 1961, healthcare facilities were re-directed towards rural areas and free medical health services were introduced.

However, after a series of major economic and social changes, the Government adopted a different approach to the role of private sector. New policies were developed that looked favourably on the role of the private sector. The importance of the private sector in healthcare delivery was further recognized with an amendment to the Private Hospitals (Regulatory) Act, 1977 which resulted into the establishment of the Private Hospitals (Regulation) (Amendment) Act, 1991. Following this Act, individual qualified medical practitioners and dentists could now manage private – hospitals, with the approval of the Ministry of Health.

For a period of almost forty years, health issues and health services delivery has been mainly a prerogative of the state, only a limited number of private-for-profit health services were provided in major towns of the country.

The distribution of Health Facilities has a heavy rural emphasis because more than 70 per cent of the population live in rural areas. Plans for the establishment of health facilities have in the past taken into consideration the facility/population ratio, but with time this has in some areas been seriously overtaken by the high population growth-rate.

Table 16.1: Health Facilities–Upto year 2000

Facility	*Agency*				
	Govt.	*Parastatal*	*Vol/Rel*	*Private*	*Others*
Consultancy/Specialized Hospitals	4	2	2	0	-
Regional Hospitals	17	0	0	0	-
District Hospitals	55	0	13	0	-
Other Hospitals	2	6	56	20	2
Health Centres	409	6	48	16	-
Dispensaries	2450	202	612	663	28
Specialized Clinics	75	0	4	22	-
Nursing Homes	0	0	0	6	-
Private Laboratories	18	3	9	184	-
Private X-Ray Units	5	3	2	16	1

Source: Ministry of Health Statistical Abstract.

Health Sector Reforms

In 1994, the Ministry of Health appraised the health sector performance with the intention of raising strategies to improve quality of health services and increase equity in health accessibility and utilization. This appraisal came up in the report named "Proposals for Health Reforms, Ministry of Health, 1994 (HSR)". The reforms were in the following dimensions: decentralization of health services; financial reforms, such as enhancement of user-charges in government hospitals, introduction of health insurance and community health funds and public/private mix reforms such as encouragement of private sector to complement public health services. They also include organisational reforms such as integration of vertical health programmes into the general health services; health research reforms such as establishment of a health research users fund and propagation of demand oriented researches in the health sector.

Nutritional Issues

Generally, good nutrition is both a desired outcome for ensuring optimal human health, as well as a key determinant of development, for the individual and for the society as a whole. Tanzania has been at the forefront internationally in promoting a conceptual framework for nutrition through its national institution, the Tanzania Food and Nutrition Centre (TFNC).

TFNC was established in order to provide expert guidance to key players at various levels through research, advocacy, education and training, for the provision of quality nutrition services to the Tanzania community in the prevention and control of all forms of malnutrition. The Center's main responsibilities among others are:

- ✰ To plan, coordinate and implement food and nutrition programmes for the benefit of the people of the United Republic of Tanzania;
- ✰ Carrying out research in matters relating to food and nutrition;
- ✰ Advising the Government, training institutions and other public organizations on matters relating to food and nutrition and to stimulate the public;
- ✰ Creating awareness of the importance of good nutrition and dangers of malnutrition.

Women Health and Low Birth Weight Problems

Being among the Least Developed Countries (LDCs), Tanzania, faces many challenges, in terms of health and nutritional issues, which at the end contribute in a large quantity to the problem of high number of poor maternal health and that of Low birth weight cases.

Likewise, in other developing countries and in Africa as a continent, mothers' health, low birth weight babies and malnourishment problems are still among the most fundamental challenges for improved human development. One of the major reasons for these problems being that of a limited time and capacities of the healthcaregivers; health services and facilities as a result many mothers and children (the vulnerable) are unable to access and effectively use at all times the food and health services they need for a healthy life.

Major Health and Nutritional Challenges

Women and Children Health

Women and children health is an important element in the development of the economy of any society. Tanzania being among such nations; women, children issues (health, rights etc) and gender equality are of a major concern for the national health system. Nevertheless, Tanzania for decades has been facing a high rate of health problems which associate with women and children health as well as healthcare services.

Major health problems among children include malaria, low birth weight, acute respiratory infections, fever and diarrhea. Nevertheless, immunization coverage of young children is high. According to the TDHS, in 2004-2005, 71 per cent of children age 12-23 months were fully immunized (BCG, measles, and three doses each of DPT-HB and polio vaccine - excluding polio vaccine given at birth) (NBS and ORC Macro, 2005).

The Tanzania Demographic and Health Survey (TDHS) 2004-2005 indicate a significant decline in infant mortality rate from 100 per cent in 1995-99 to 68 per cent in 2000-2004.

Maternal mortality ratio has remained high during the last decade[1]. 53 per cent of pregnancies are delivered at home (mostly in rural areas), and very few of these deliver with the help of skilled personnel. However, the maternal mortality estimates are subject to large sampling errors. Although the 2004-2005 maternal mortality ratios are higher than the 1996 estimate, the difference between the two figures is not statistically significant. Thus, it is impossible to conclude that there has been any change in maternal mortality ratio in Tanzania during the last decade.

Tanzania also has one of the highest adolescent pregnancy rates in the world[2]. Pregnancy in very young girls is always associated with high risk for mother and child. Early entry into reproductive life increases the risk of health threats such as anaemia, low birth weight, malnutrition and sexually transmitted diseases, including HIV and the risk of obstructed labour and vesico-vaginal fistula (VVF).

Malnutrition is the most widespread health disorder in Tanzania alongside vitamin A deficiency, iron deficiency anemia and iodine deficiency disorders. Malnutrition results from inadequate intake of food and/or frequent infections. Nutritional status of preschool children (below five years of age) is a proxy indicator for the economic and nutritional status of the population of a country. It is also a reflection of maternal nutritional status. During the last decade, three[3] national surveys

---

1. 529 per 100 000 live births for the period 1987-1996 and 578 per 100 000 live births for the period 1995-2004. (NBS and ORC Macro, 2005).
2. 29 per cent of rural girls age 15-19 have given birth or have been pregnant.
3. Tanzania Demographic and Health Survey (TDHS) 2004-2005, Tanzania Reproductive and Child Health Survey 1999 and TDHS 1996 (NBS and ORC Macro, 2005; NBS and Macro International Inc., 2000; BoS and Macro International Inc., 1997).

documented the prevalence of malnutrition among children less than five years. According to the most recent national survey conducted in 2004-2005, the proportion of children less than five years of age who were underweight was 22 per cent, while the prevalence of stunting was 38 per cent, and that of wasting was 3 per cent.

Comparison of the three national surveys of 1996, 1999 and 2004-2005 shows that the nutritional status of children less than five years of age has remained unchanged between 1996 and 1999, but has improved after this period. Between 1999 and 2004-2005, both the prevalence of stunting and wasting decreased. Most of the reduction in stunting prevalence took place in the rural sector (prevalence of stunting remained at 26 per cent in the urban areas) while the decrease in prevalence of wasting was observed in both the urban and rural sectors.

HIV/AIDS[4] is one of the leading causes of lost productivity in Tanzania with a highly negative impact on household savings and assets. High rates of HIV/AIDS infected population is among the vulnerable mostly being mothers and their children. In Tanzania the rate of HIV infection is high with adult transmission rate of 7 per cent (THIS, 2004). The epidemic continues to have a devastating effect. The main mode of transmission is heterosexual (90 per cent) and Mother to Child Transmission (MTCT) which contributes 5 per cent. MTCT in Tanzania is set to have a dramatic and deadly impact on child survival. The dimension of the epidemic and rising demand by persons living with HIV/AIDS for quality medical care and treatment makes the healthcare system respond to these demands.

HIV/AIDS care and treatment and support has reached a new era in terms of the accumulated knowledge of the disease and its management and availability of potent drugs not only for the treatment of opportunistic infections, but also antiretroviral drugs that slow the progression of the disease to AIDS allowing PLWA to live a much longer quality life.

Status of Low Birth Weight in Tanzania

According to the World Health Organization low birth weight (LBW) babies are those born with less than 2500g. Infants born with low birth weights begin life immediately disadvantaged and face extremely poor survival rates. Many of those infants who survive suffer cognitive and neurological impairment, increased risk of high blood pressure, obstructive lung disease, cholesterol, renal damage, acute diarrhea, impaired immune function and poor cognitive development.

Birth weight is a powerful predictor of infant growth and survival. Low birth weight (LBW) and poor maternal (women) health services remain significant public health problems in Tanzania as it is in many developing countries. Poor nutrition both before and during pregnancy is recognized as among the important causes of LBW.

There are has been a little improvement regarding the problem of Low birth weight in Tanzania, in the past few years. In 1999, Tanzania Reproductive and Child Health Survey (TRCHS) recorded that 9 per cent of babies who had been weighed at

4 Over 2.2 million people live with AIDS in Tanzania.

birth had weights under 2.5 kg. On the other hand, in the TDHS 2004/05, the corresponding figure was 7 per cent. Notably, about half of all births take place at home; hence, birth weights are recorded for only about half of all births. Besides, the majority of the neonates weighed at birth were born in a favorable environment, in urban areas and/or of mothers having a higher educational level. Therefore the prevalence of 7 per cent low birth weight is not representative of the true situation in the country.

Causes Pertaining to Poor Maternal Health and Low Birth Weight in Tanzania

Despite these little improvements, over the last five years rates of maternal death, low birth weight and infant mortality have been on the rise.

Causes of Low Birth Weight

Among many other causes of LBW in Tanzania, the common ones remain to be:

- ☆ Premature delivery (short gestation) or by foetal growth retardation.
- ☆ Poor maternal health and nutritional status during pregnancy.
- ☆ Deficiency of micronutrients among pregnant women
- ☆ Hard physical work during pregnancy
- ☆ Illness, especially infections *i.e.* Malaria, malnutrition[5], HIV infections.
- ☆ Maternal risk factors *i.e.* short maternal stature, very young age, grand multiparty, close birth spacing etc
- ☆ Cigarette smoking, genetic and environmental factors.

In Tanzania, poverty is still a big challenge and one of the major causes of LBW, especially in rural areas, where about 39 per cent of the population lives below the basic needs poverty line compared with 26 per cent in urban areas. There is a slow trend towards decrease in the prevalence of poverty. Poverty acts to limit access to care and the choice and amount of foods available to pregnant women. According to the 2007 Household Budget Survey (HBS), 12.9 million Tanzanians live below the poverty line as compared to 11.4 million in 2000 - 2001.

Causes of Poor Maternal Health

- ☆ Inadequate health facilities with unqualified staff
- ☆ Shortage of medical personnel
- ☆ Poor and/or low level of health education and awareness
- ☆ Lack of well equipped health centers
- ☆ Poor sanitation and care practices
- ☆ Low accessibility to adequate health services
- ☆ Mass poverty among societies.

---

5. There is evidence from a survey of low birth weight that adolescent mothers are more likely to be anemic and malnourished than their older peers (TFNC, UNICEF (Tanzania) and Centre for International Child Health, 2002

Other Public Health challenges in Tanzania include:

Access to Quality Health Services

Healthcare in Tanzania is provided by a mixture of government, private non-profit (*e.g.* Mission hospitals); private for-profit (including traditional healers); and company services. The government provides more than half of the facilities in the health sector and coverage is improving: 80 per cent of the population has physical access to health services and 90 per cent of households report living within ten (10) or more kilometers from a dispensary or health centre. However, there are still great disparities between urban and rural areas. Most of the health centers in rural areas have poor services and facilities, they lack enough qualified healthcare personnel etc.

As a result, the quality of healthcare is still low and poor, also due to the limited number of skilled staff at primary health facilities. Moreover, the introduction of user's fees at national, regional and district health facilities has made access more difficult.

Inadequate Accessibility to Clean and Safe Water

Access to clean and safe water is still a problem in many parts of the country, especially in rural areas and informal urban settlements. According to UNICEF, 62 per cent of the population have access to an improved drinking water source, and 47 per cent have access to proper sanitation (53 per cent in urban areas and 43 per cent in rural areas) (UNICEF, 2007).

Women Involvement in Health and Nutritional Issues

Women play a major and an important role in the development of a society. Similarly to other countries, Tanzanian women play a big role in the economy and development of the country, by contribute vastly in different sectors of health, education, agriculture, industries, businesses, gender, human rights, good governance and food systems (security) for the entire household etc.

In Tanzania, 75 per cent of the populations are mothers (from child-bearing age) and children. Despite the fact that, women form a backbone of the development of the country, still challenges exist, such as a large number of women and their children have unequal access to resources, quality health services, education, income, they participate less in decision-making, affected by hunger and malnourished and violation of their basic rights etc. Mothers and children form a large group in Tanzania, whereby nearly half of the agriculture labour force is made up of women. But, this group is the most vulnerable in the country as issues such as inadequate health services and infections are concerned.

Women health/wellbeing are an essential element of good health and human development. In order to attain both the MDG and National Strategy for Growth and Reduction of Poverty (NSGRP)[6], goals such as those concerned with women and

----

6. Kiswahili is known as Mkukuta 'Mkakati wa Kukuza Uchumi na Kupunguza Umaskini Tanzania

adolescent health, maternal and newborn health, HIV/AIDS and gender equality have to be given the upper hand.

Tanzania has witnessed a significant reduction in child mortality rates over the past two decades, but maternal health statistics have yet to improve. Poor women are 7 times more likely to give birth at home than the rich, and with little or no post-natal care both for the mother and the newborn. Huge differences in utilisation of services between pregnancy and delivery prevail with 99 per cent of women attending Antenatal Clinics (ANC) at least once, but only 46 per cent of births are attended by skilled personnel. Regardless of the little reduction in child mortality, Tanzania loses about 8,000 women every year to maternal health complications, a significant loss within the country's productive labour force.

Nevertheless, Tanzanian government continuously has been working with various organizations (both national and international) that deal with women and children health matters. Through these organizations different projects have been developed that have involved women directly and indirectly. Women have been highly encouraged to participate in various programmes that tend to empower them, their health and their communities. There has been an increase of community awareness around essential health interventions such as birth preparedness, ante-natal/post-natal support, low birth weight complications and prevention, diet during pregnancy and after, family planning, early identification of complications, vaccination during pregnancy and after delivery, Vitamins and micronutrients taking, management of childhood illnesses, HIV/AIDS infections etc, through health communication and education activities, advocacy, community mobilisation, mediation and lobbying where key actors/participants have been women.

Efforts and Plans Done by the Government

For many years, Tanzanian government has been in the front line in the formulation and developing new health strategies aiming at improving women health as well as reducing infant and child mortality.

The government's efforts and plans include the following:

- ☆ Developed strategies that aim at reducing infant mortality and child mortality, especially malaria-related morbidity and mortality. Programmes include improved vaccination coverage, availability of services including drugs at the time of need, Integrated Management of Childhood Illnesses (IMCI) rolled-over to all districts, efficient implementation of planned programmes; malaria control through use of mosquito nets particularly insecticide-treated nets (ITNs). Also, Intermittent Preventive Treatment (IPT) during pregnancy and immediate medical treatment of malaria for children under five years within the first 24 hours of the onset of symptoms.
- ☆ Programs aiming at improvement of maternal health, promotion of exclusive breastfeeding for the first six months of infancy; and effective management of childhood diarrhoea. A Road Map for accelerating the reduction of maternal, newborn and child morbidity and mortality: 2008 - 2015 was launched in 2008.

- ✰ Awareness programs and introduction of Vitamin A Supplementation (VAS), Prevention of Mother to Child Transmission (PMCT)
- ✰ The malaria Strategic Plan 2002-2007 has been reviewed and a new plan 2008-2013 is in place.
- ✰ In combating the HIV/AIDS epidemic, the Tanzania Commission for AIDS (TACAIDS) was established in 2001 to provide strategic leadership and to coordinate multi – sectarian responses.
- ✰ The National Family Planning Programme provided by various agencies[7] – and coordinated by the Reproductive and Child Health Unit of the Ministry of Health.

Also, with the help of public, private development partners, religious groups and NGO's efforts have been made to improve access to effective treatment for infections by strengthened healthcare services, through subsidised drugs, establishment of health learning institutions, social marketing campaigns to inform the population on various health problems and preventions *i.e.* Malaria Haikubaliki[8] campaigns, Tanzania Bila UKIMWI inawezekana[9], National Fistula program/ campaigns etc., training and supportive supervision of health personnel, the establishment of new health centres, drug stores etc.

Above all, the government's policy framework and in particular the Tanzanian Development Vision 2025 aims to eradicate poverty and improve quality of life (health) through the National Strategy for Growth and Poverty Reduction[10].

Possible Solutions, Recommendations and Conclusion

Surveys that have been conducted on low birth weight, women/maternal health and nutritional problems in Tanzania, have shown that poor nutritional status, poor maternal health and infectious diseases contribute to the burden of Low Birth Weight.

Following solutions and recommendations should be observed by the Ministry of Health and the government in reducing the overall prevalence of LBW. These are:

1. Importance of proper antenatal care should be more reemphasized to the community as whole. Pregnant mothers should attend antenatal care as regularly as required. Accurate records taking and keeping should be practiced as these are very important.
2. Strategies that combine nutrition-based interventions, such as improving food intakes and micronutrient status, especially iron status, with

7. For example: Marie-Stopes (TZ), AMREF, Women's Dignity, CARE, etc.

8. Fight Malaria

9. Tanzania without AIDS, We can.

10. This is the second national organizing framework for putting the focus on poverty reduction high on the country's development agenda. It is committed to the Millennium Development Goals (MDGs), as internationally agreed targets for reducing poverty, hunger, diseases, illiteracy, discrimination against women and environmental degradation by 2015.

approaches that improve women's status and reproductive health are needed to reduce LBW.

3. More effective and continuous education and awareness campaigns about nutrition and health matters are extremely important for maintaining the health of women (young girls/mothers) and their children. It is vital that women be educated about nutrition and health so that when they are pregnant they will eat foods that will provide more nutrition for themselves and the fetus; as well they will know their health status *i.e.* once they feel unwell, complications and have labour signs, it will be easy for them to take immediate steps.
4. Improvement of healthcare services and facilities especially maternal healthcare and facilities.
5. There is a need of enough and qualified human resource for health especially the medical doctor profession.
6. Establishment of quality and well equipped health centers in both rural and urban areas; more practicing hospitals and health learning institutions.
7. Promotion of care and support for pregnant women is very important. Thus, reduction of women workload by excusing pregnant mothers from heavy labour demanding activities, providing more time to rest especially during the last trimester of pregnancy, discourage gender based division of labour and traditions and customs that undermine women must be encouraged and highly considered when formulating health policies.
8. Support women's rights as well as child rights to survival, growth, development, participation, and protection.

While programs to support poverty reduction through economic growth[11] are undertaken by the government, social programs for the poor are limited or non-existing. Religious groups or non-governmental organizations are the main players involved in such programs supporting poor people. Thus, even though national policies to improve Maternal Newborn and Child Health (MNCH) exist, and interventions to prevent maternal, neonatal and child deaths are available in Tanzania, yet MNCH indicators remain unacceptably poor. Progress has been hindered by poor policy implementation and weak health systems, which do not engage with or respond to community needs. This results in poor access and utilisation of preventive and curative health services. However, some programs have been less successful because these interventions are expensive and difficult to manage *i.e.* food and micronutrients intakes during pregnancy where it depends on the status of a pregnant woman, in the sense that if she can afford to have a well balanced diet etc during that period etc.

In Tanzania, there is an improvement in issues relating to gender status. Women are beginning to stand up for themselves. Much of this progress is due to the effect that education has had on allowing women to broaden their horizons. It is necessary

11. Such as the National Strategy for Growth and Poverty Reduction (NSGPR)

that government continues to carefully support the education of women, especially in areas concerning health and nutrition. It is believed that, the education of women would hugely improve the status of the typical families in Tanzania. Children would be able to maintain better nutrition and better education as well. Infant and maternal mortality rates would decrease if women were educated on how to take care of themselves and their bodies before, during and after a pregnancy.

All in all, strong and constantly advocacy for women health, nutrition and effective coordination of interventions under national leadership are urgently required to raise the profile of nutrition, women and children health so that to improve maternal health and nutritional issues in Tanzania.

In general, as reported[12], Tanzania (through the National Strategy for Growth and Poverty Reduction) has (practically) achieved the MDG's for universal primary education already and significant progress has been made in reducing income poverty, malnutrition, child mortality and gender inequality in primary education. Despite this progress it may be more difficult to achieve all MDG targets by 2010 or even by 2015. Significant challenges remain in achieving health targets including the targets for child and maternal mortality and for combating diseases like HIV/AIDS and malaria and in achieving environmental sustainability. High economic growth and a commitment to improve public service such as healthcare services delivery remain crucial to keep Tanzania on a path towards achieving the MDG targets.

References

1. NBS. 2002. *Tanzanian Household Budget Survey (HBS), 2000/01*. National Bureau of Statistics. United Republic of Tanzania. (available at http://www.tanzania.go.tz)
2. NBS and Macro International Inc. 2000. *Tanzania Reproductive and Child Health Survey 1999*. National Bureau of Statistics, Tanzania, and Macro International Inc., Calverton, Maryland, USA. (available at www.measuredhs.com)
3. NBS and ORC Macro. 2005. *Tanzania Demographic and Health Survey, 2004-2005*. National Bureau of Statistics, Dar es Salaam. www.nbs.or.tz
4. Rikimaru, T. 2000. *Nutrition and poverty: study on food consumption patterns and nutritional economic value of common foods in Dar es Salaam*. Tanzania Food and Nutrition Centre.
5. UNICEF. 2007. *The State of the World's Children 2007*. United Nations Children's Fund. New York. USA. (available at http://www.unicef.org)

Electronics Sources

6. www.povertymonitoring.go.tz
7. www.siteresources.worldbank.org

---

12. Survey prepared by IMF and IDA National Strategy for Growth and Reduction of Poverty (NSGRP–MKUKUTA) Joint Staff Advisory Note, 2006.

Chapter 17

Healthcare and Nutrition in Myanmar

Mya Thandar Kyu[1] *and Aye Aye Thaw*[2]

[1]*Lecturer, Department of Technical and Vocational Education, Naypyitaw, Myanmar*

E-mail: [1]*myathandarkyu@gmail.com,* [2]*aayethaw@gmail.com*

ABSTRACT

In developing countries, health, social, political, technological, economic and human growths are the main factors. To become a developed country healthcare and nutrition play a major role. Myanmar's population is over 54 million and over half are women. Thus, women's population in Myanmar is over 27 million. Therefore, the nutritional status of women in Myanmar is alarming. The health of women is a critical factor in the health of children. Proper nutrition is a key determinant of health both in childhood and beyond. The nutritional status of girls is particularly important due to their future potential reproductive role and the intergenerational repercussions of poor female nutrition. Good nutrition plays an important role in maintaining the health of women. Myanmar has a policy of promoting food and nutrition program and providing comprehensive health services. In 1996, in partnership with the World Health Organization (WHO), the National Nutrition Centre embarked on a study of household food and nutrition security in Myanmar. A preliminary situation analysis revealed that transitional changes in the economic, demographic and social sectors have driven dramatic changes in people's lifestyles, behavior and practices and that these changes affect food and nutrition security and healthcare. The present paper describes healthcare and nutrition program in Myanmar. In addition, potential problems in implementing nutrition promotion and interventions are also discussed.

Keywords: *Nutrition, Healthcare, Myanmar healthcare system.*

Introduction

Myanmar is situated between South and Southeast Asia. It is bordered by India, Bangladesh and China to the north and west, and to the east by Thailand and Laos. It has an area of 676,578 square kilometers. Administratively, there are 14 states and divisions (with a further division into 17 states/divisions for the management of health programmes). The states/divisions are further subdivided into 63 districts, 324 townships and 65,148 villages. The total population of Myanmar is estimated at 57.504 million with a population growth rate of just over 1.75 percent (MOH, 2007).

In Myanmar, over 60 per cent of the total population is women and children. The population is made up of the Bamar ethnic majority, who live mostly in the lowlands and central part of the country, and some 135 different ethnic groups, mainly living in the highlands and eastern and western borders of Myanmar. More than 70 per cent of the total population lives in rural areas. The lowland delta and central dry zone are highly populated areas.

Nutrition is a highly complex science involving many interrelated factors and disciplines. Adequate nutrition is essential to maintain the immune system and sustain healthy levels of physical activity as for the quality of life. The under-nourishment in women that results in lack of breastfeeding exposes the infants to increasing risk of malnutrition and Life-threatening infectious diseases. Therefore, women's health is important not only to women themselves but also has an impact on the health and development of the next generation. Many of the main cause of women's morbidity and mortality in both rich and poor countries have their origins in societies' attitudes to women, which are reflected in the structures, and systems that set policies, determine service and create opportunities.

This document therefore, highlights Health Services in Myanmar, Maternal and Child Health, School and Adolescent Health and Nutrition Program. The Myanmar Government has a clear policy of improving the health, fitness and education of the entire nation and of striving for better conditions of food, clothing and shelter for its people. There is also a policy of self-reliance and self-sufficiency in terms of basic food within the country

The Ministry of Health has laid down the following objectives: to enable every citizen to attain full life expectancy and enjoy longevity of life, to ensure that there is freedom from diseases and to realize these objectives, all health activities are implemented in conformity with the following strategies.

1. Widespread disseminations of health information and education to reach the rural areas
2. Enhancing disease prevention activities
3. Providing effective treatment of prevailing diseases

Health Services in Myanmar

The Ministry of Health is providing comprehensive health services covering promotive, preventive, curative and rehabilitative aspects to raise the health status and prolong the lives of the citizens. With the objective of achieving Health for All goals, successive National Health Plans have been developed and implemented in accordance with the guidelines of the National Health Policy. The basic health staff down to the grass root level is providing promotive, preventive, curative and rehabilitative services through Primary Healthcare approach. Infrastructure for service delivery is based upon sub-rural health centre and rural health centre where Midwives, Lady Health Visitor and Health Assistant are assigned to provide primary healthcare to the rural community. Those who need special care are referred to Station Hospital, Township Hospital, and District Hospital and to Specialist Hospital successively. At the State/Divisional level, the State/Divisional Health Department is responsible for State/Divisional planning, coordination, training and technical support, close supervision, monitoring and evaluation of health services. At the peripheral level, *i.e.* the township level actual provision of health services to the community is undertaken. The Township Health Department forms the backbone for primary and secondary healthcare, covering 100,000 to 200,000 people.

The main areas of service delivery and support activities are presented here:

1. Health Service Delivery in the context of Primary Healthcare.
2. Services for the Target Population Group
3. Promoting Health, Ensuring Healthy Environment and Protecting Consumers
4. Controlling Communicable Diseases
5. Health in Natural Disaster

Maternal and Child Health

Maternal and Child Health including newborn care has been a priority issue in the National Health Plan, aiming at reducing the maternal, newborn, and infant and children morbidity and mortality. Approximately 1.3 million women give birth each year in Myanmar; thus, intensive efforts have been put to improve maternal and newborn health (MNH) services through various activities especially focusing on safe motherhood. The health system had focused only on the conventional maternal, newborn and childcare before 1988. After that period with the adoption of comprehensive reproductive healthcare in life cycle approach with emphasis on safe motherhood by ICPD (Cairo, 1994), Myanmar incorporated the comprehensive reproductive healthcare into the conventional maternal and child healthcare programme.

Maternal and child healthcare services are provided both in urban and rural settings and it is a crucial component of National Health Plan. The maternal and child healthcare, consisting of antenatal care, aseptic and safe delivery, postnatal care, newborn care, under-one infant care, immunization, growth monitoring of under-three children, nutritional education, control of diarrhea diseases and management of acute respiratory infections, has been provided by basic health workers with the assistance of voluntary health workers and the community throughout the country.

Ministry of Health is also collaborating with other related Ministries, INGOs and NNGOs in provision of comprehensive healthcare. They are Ministry of Social Welfare, Ministry of Education, Myanmar Women's Affairs Federation (MWAF), Myanmar Maternal and Child Welfare Association (MMCWA). MRCS (Myanmar Red Cross Society), Save the Children, World Vision International and JICA and other 25 international NGOs.

Some key approaches for attaining maternal and child health related MDGs.

1. Special emphasis to implement the Making Pregnancy Safer initiative, as a high priority component of reproductive health strategy
2. Introducing Voluntary Counseling and Testing (VCT) for prevention of mother to child transmission (PMCT) in routine AN Care
3. Strengthening collaboration between reproductive health programmes and other related key public health programmes such as immunization (utilization of safe delivery kits, improving TT2), nutrition (management of anemia in pregnancy, iron folate tablets, deworming in pregnancy), and malaria (prevention and management of malaria in pregnancy)
4. Development in progress of reproductive health five years strategic plan (2004-2008)
5. Strengthening the effective partnership among key stakeholders for promotion of reproductive health issues

Women and Child Health Development Project (WCHD)

Women and Child Health Development activities have been implemented since 2001 with the aim of achieving Millennium Development Goals and the following objectives; targeting health of mother, newborn, adolescent and children. With the general objective to provide quality healthcare services for women, children and adolescent in order to reduce under five mortality rate and maternal mortality rate and to promote health of the women, children and adolescent. The following were specific objectives; to reduce the under five mortality rate to achieve the Millennium Development Goal, to reduce the maternal mortality to achieve the Millennium Development Goal and to ensure quality health services for children, adolescent and women

WCHD strategies aim at ensuring that quality health services are accessible and affordable for women, children and adolescents and include four components: (1) women health development, (2) child health development, (3) adolescent health development and (4) newborn health development. In addition, WCHD have the following strategies:

1. Incorporating available strategies into the new program. IMCI for Child Health, Integrated Management of pregnancy and Childbirth (IMPAC) for Women Health and Life Skills Education for Health (LSEH) for adolescent Health.
2. Initiating coordination between departments, national/international agencies and organizations involved in health of women, children and adolescent.

3. Expanding WCHD activities in 12 new townships per year from 2006 to 2010.
4. Reinforcing IMMCI activities in areas where WCHD activities are not yet implemented.

School and Adolescent Health

Based on report by the Department of Education Planning and Training, student population in Myanmar is about 7.8 million. School Health Programme has been implemented with the objective of promoting the health standard of entire student youth through health promoting school programme. School health activities are being carried out by School Health Section of Department of Health in collaboration with international agencies like WHO, UNICEF and NGOs. Under the guidance of national health committee, various school health committees have been formed at each administrative level since 2000. The school health committees take the leadership roles and give guidance in implementing the school health programme systematically and efficiently.

School health strategies were based on the health objective under the national social objectives, the national health policy, national population policy and the primary healthcare approach aiming towards a successful implementation of the school health programme.

School Health Strategies

1. Conducting refresher training for teachers on the development of health promoting schools to promote the health standards of the entire student youth, the skills and knowledge needed for adopting a healthy life style at all levels.
2. Enhancing better quality and coverage of school healthcare by providing sufficient labor and supplies
3. Establishing school health committees at different levels for monitoring and evaluation mechanisms to ensure successful implementation
4. Conducting research on the impact of school health programme to promote existing school health activities
5. Promoting co-ordination and collaboration mechanisms with ministry of education and other related departments
6. Organizing resources for national school health programme through the involvement of local and international NGO's and international organizations.

With the objective to enhance health promoting school activities, the Ministry of Health, in collaboration with the Ministry of Education launched the School Health Week of 2008 in the 2nd week of August. The activities were held in all basic education schools of the country from August 11 to 17, 2008. As part of school deworming programme 6 million school age children and preschool age children from all States and Divisions were dewormed biannually during 2008 as an integrated approach with the support of WHO and UNICEF.

Ministry of Health has also attempted to improve coordination between a number of primary healthcare projects, and incorporate an adolescent health component into the health promoting schools strategy and transforming it into "School and Adolescent Health" in the 2001-2006 National Health Plan. Several ongoing collaborative programmes, through MOH, departments and other ministries (e.g. Education, Sports, Immigration and Population, Information, and Religious Affairs) have components that address the needs of young people. The national five-year adolescent health and development strategic plan (2009-2013) was developed to address the priority issues affecting the health of young people in the Union of Myanmar.

Moss De-Worming Campaign

As worm infestation is one of the causes of anemia. National Nutrition Centre launched Mass de-worming campaign in collaboration with Filarial Project and School Health Project All children aged between 2 years to 9 years, all primary school students, 2-9 years out of school children and pregnant women with at least 3 months gestation are targeted for de-won activity. This activity was implementing twice a year starting from January 2006.

Nutrition Program

The ultimate aim of the nutrition promotion activities in Myanmar is "Attainment of nutritional well- being of all citizens" as part of the overall social-economic development by means of health and nutrition activities together with the cooperative efforts by the food production sector. With the general objective to ensure that all citizens enjoy the nutritional state conducive to longevity and health, the nutrition promotion activities in Myanmar are implemented to control/eliminate all forms of nutritional deficiency; to promote healthy dietary habits and lifestyles among people; to prevent over-nutrition and diet-related chronic diseases. Myanmar has identified five major nutrition problems.

Protein Energy Malnutrition (PEM)

The overall nutrition status of children under-five has not significantly improved and malnutrition is still the main underlying cause of under-five deaths. However, the prevalence of under-weight among children below five years of age declined from 35.3 per cent in 2000 to 31.8 per cent in 2003 shown in Figure 17.1 (MICS Surveys, Dept. of Health Planning); MDG goal for under-weight prevalence is 19.3 per cent by 2015.

Table 17.1: Percentage of Under 5 Children with Sever and Moderate Malnutrition

	Urban	*Rural*
Severe	4.9	8.1
Moderate	25.3	33.5

Source: MICS 2003, DHP.

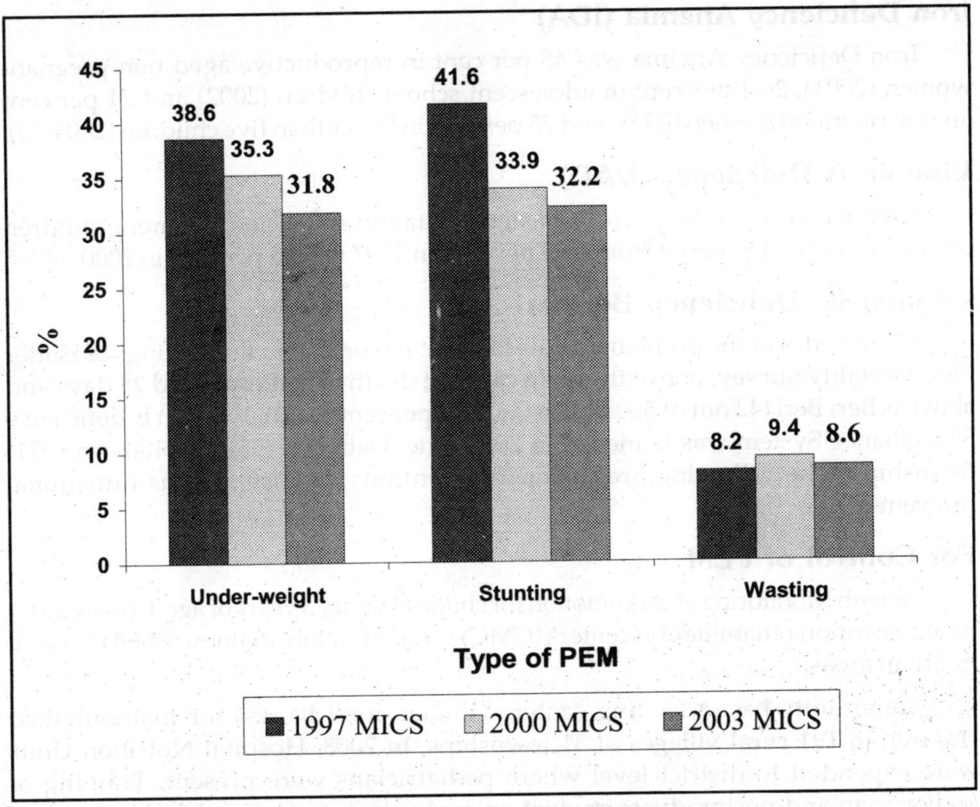

Figure 17.1: Prevalence of PEM among Fewer than 5 Children

Adequate nutrition is the key to a healthy and happy new generation. Table 17.1 shows the percentage of severe and moderate malnutrition in urban and rural areas which is more in rural arears. It may be due to the traditional beliefs and thus health education on nutrition. Community nutrition centers and village food banks are now established in many places to enhance the nutritional status of children. Distribution of pamphlets, poster, and flip charts about nutrition and video shows for the community is being done by NGOs.

Iodine Deficiency Disorders (IDD)

Iodine Deficiency Disorders are on the verge of virtual elimination. Visible Goiter Rate among 6-11 year old school children dropped from 12 per cent in 2000 to 5.5 per cent in 2003-04, (< 5 per cent in 2007 and 2 per cent in 2006 (Target < 5 per cent). Proportion of household consuming iodated salt was 86 per cent in 2003 and 87 per cent in 2007 Target>90 per cent). Median urinary iodine excretion for the whole country was 236mg/L in 2003-04, and 123mg/L in 2007 (Normal range 100-200 mg/L).

Iron Deficiency Anemia (IDA)

Iron Deficiency Anemia was 45 per cent in reproductive aged non-pregnant women (2001); 26.4 per cent in adolescent school children (2002) and 71 per cent among pregnant women (2003) and 75 per cent in fewer than five children (2004-05).

Vitamin A Deficiency (VAD)

Prevalence of Bitot's spot (ocular sign of vitamin A deficiency) among children under five years decreased from 0.23 per cent in 1997 to 0.03 per cent in 2000.

Vitamin B_1 Deficiency Beriberi

Magnitudes of the problems are as follows: According to the findings of Under Five Mortality Survey, one of the main cause of death in children aged 28 days and above is Beri Beri (42 out of 590 deaths, *i.e.* 7.12 per cent, 2003). Vitamin B_1 deficiency Surveillance System was launched in 2005 June. Data are, (55) hospitals and (21) townships. The following are major interventions against various nutritional problems:

For Control of PEM

Growth Monitoring and Promotion for children under 3 years of age. Community-based nutrition rehabilitation centers (CMC) for moderately malnourished children in urban areas.

Community-based feeding centers (Village food Banks) for malnourished children in 191 rural villages of 31 townships. In 2008, Hospital Nutrition Units were expended to district level where pediatricians were present. Training of pediatrician and postgraduate student on management of severely malnourished children were conducted.

For Elimination of IDD

Universal salt iodization (USI) is the major long-term intervention for elimination of iodine deficiency disorders. Quality of iodized salt was monitored by regular survey on iodine content of salt by titration and Urinary Iodine excretion

Conducted by National Nutrition Centre. At the State and Divisional level, salt quality was monitored as necessary by titration method. Public education program for iodized salt consumption to eliminate IDD was launched through radio, TV spot, videos with the voluntary assistance of popular movie stars. Ministry of Mine took a responsibility to check the iodine content of salt factory level, Yangon City Development Committee and Mandalay City Development Committee and Department of Developmental Affairs monitored the quality at retail level and basic health staff monitored at household level regularly. Laboratory of Nutrition Unit of Department of Health is responsible for regular assessment of Urinary excretion of iodine in school-age children every two years.

Myanmar Universal Salt Ionisation (USI) Programme

The 24th Meeting of National Health Committee in 1997 gave guidance to the Ministry of Mines and the Ministry of Health that all salt produced in Myanmar for human and animal consumption be iodized. Accordingly, the Ministry of Mines, in 1999, issued a regulation, which required that all factories licensed for production of salt for human and animal consumption only produced iodized salt with iodine level between 40 ppm and 60 ppm. Therefore, Iodized salt consumption increases the following years and ade. iodized decreases shown in Figure 17.2.

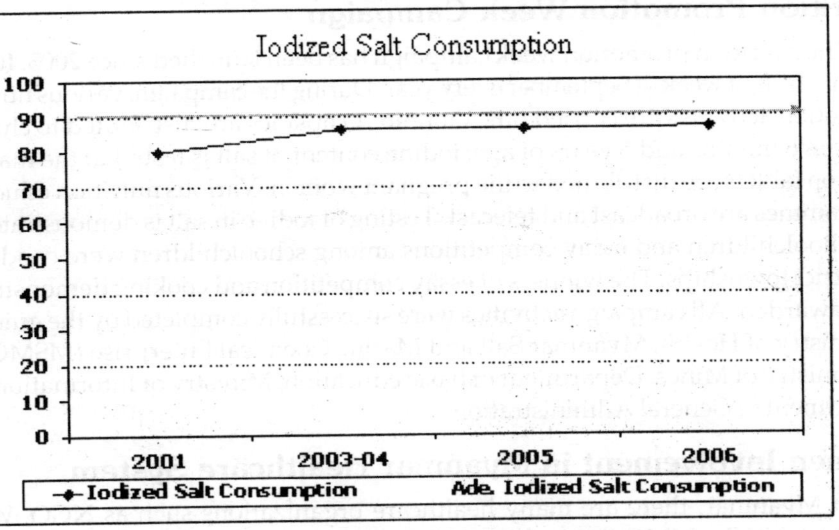

Figure 17.2: Iodized Salt Consumption by Year
***Source*: National Goiter Surve**

Virtual Elimination of IDD

Table 17.2: Virtual Elimination of IDD

Present Status	*Myanmar*	*Goal*
Total Goitre Prevalence Rate	2.0 per cent	< 5 per cent
Median urinary iodine excretion (ug/l)	123.0 mg/l	200 mg/l
Effectively iodized Salt Consumption	48.23 per cent	>90 per cent

Source: National HIE Survey, NNC, 2006

For Elimination of VAD

Biannual supplementation with high-potency vitamin A capsule is the main intervention against vitamin A deficiency among under-5 year old children. Lactating women receive one dose of vitamin A (200,000 IU) within one month after childbirth to ensure that the suckling baby gets sufficient vitamin A from the breast milk.

For Control of DA

Main intervention against anemia is iron fottate tablets supplementation for pregnant women throughout the country, for adolescent school girls in selected townships and children between 6 months and 3 years in selected growth monitoring sessions.

For Control of Vitamin B_1 Deficiency

Vitamin B_1 tablets were distributed to all townships for the risk groups especially to pregnant women one month before delivery and lactating mothers 3 months after delivery. Supply of Injection B_1 ampoules for treatment of Beriberi cases.

Nutrition Promotion Week Campaign

The nutrition promotion week campaign has been launched since 2003. It takes place in the first week of September every year. During the campaign, various nutrition promotion activities are carried out. Vitamin A capsules are distributed to children between 6 months and 5 years of age; iodine content of salt is tested in the markets; and iron tablets are distributed to the pregnant women. Various nutrition education programmes are broadcast and telecast. Testing of iodine in salt is demonstrated for the schoolchildren and essay competitions among schoolchildren were conducted in district townships. The winners of essay competition and cooking demonstration were awarded. All campaign activities were successfully completed by the guidance of Ministry of Health, Myanmar Salt and Marine Chemical Enterprise (MSMCE) of the Ministry of Mines, Department of basic education, Ministry of Information, and Department of General Administration

Women Involvement in Myanmar Healthcare System

In Myanmar, there are many healthcare organizations such as NGO, WHO, INGOs, NNGOs, MMCWA and MWAF. Among these, community based health activities are carried out through Myanmar Women's Affairs Federation (MWAF) and Maternal and Child Welfare Association (MMCWA). These organizations are the voluntary social organization that is working to help in healthcare activities, education and living standards of mother and children in Myanmar. The MMCWA carries out mothers and children care activities in order to ensure safe motherhood and safe childhood starting from pregnancy to birth. The maternity clinics are opened at many villages. They provide healthcare services for the reduction of maternal mortality, infant mortality and under-five mortality, which are included in the Millennium Development Goals. The maternity clinics provide access to reproductive healthcare services, care during pregnancy and safe delivery with professionals, postnatal care, health education, vaccination, birth spacing for the health of the mother and the child, breastfeeding, and the prevention of mother-to-child transmission of HIV/AIDS. In cooperation with the MoH and UNFPA, the MMCWA has carried out projects in reproductive health, behavioural change communication, and adolescent reproductive health and provided reproductive health education for young people with a special focus on HIV/AIDS and the prevention of narcotic drugs abuse.

Regarding the nutrition of children, the MMCWA is working to ensure under-five nutrition by conducting a survey of malnourished children, setting up village food banks in villages and townships, opening community nutrition centers, initiating a growth monitoring programme to ensure nutrition of children, carrying out education programmes for mothers on nutritious cooking and demonstration of cooking techniques, conducting training courses, and giving supplements for iodine deficiency, iron-deficiency, vitamin-A deficiency and other conditions caused by malnutrition. As a result of the endeavour's made by the Government health status has risen. The under-five mortality declines from 130 per 1000 live births in 1990 to 66.6 in 2005 while under-one mortality has decreased from 98 per 1000 live births in 1998 to 49.7 in 2003.

While the MCCWA is making special efforts to provide vocational training, assist in finding jobs and create income-generation opportunities with the aim of raising family incomes and living standards, the EU and the West imposed economic sanctions on our country, resulting in the closure of a number of factories, which greatly affected the working mothers. The Association redoubled its efforts for the benefit of mothers and families and has provided the necessary social support and assistance in the form of small loans, seed money or capital and assisted in finding employment. The MMCWA is also making efforts to promote health, education, economic and social activities for the benefit of mothers, children and families, it contributes on a continuous basis to activities that serve the fundamental interests of the nation. With the providing of these organizations, women and child health and nutrition, system is gradually increasing.

Conclusion and Discussion

People of Myanmar, as other people around the world, regard the mother's role as the most important role of women, rearing their children who are potential leaders of the country to become good citizens. Malnutrition is one of the most important health and welfare problems among infants and young children in Myanmar. Although there are five interventions against various problems, there are some problems still found in some cases. The most successful intervention is for elimination of IDD. In the PEM problem at the individual level, the pregnant and lactating mothers, infant, preschool children and adolescents were found to be groups most vulnerable to malnutrition, consuming much fewer calories and less protein than required. It was found that typical Myanmar families live in a strong cohesive community 50 per cent being extended families and most having only one breath winner. The poor housing environment and low levels of education point toward high health and nutrition risks.

A series of people's health plans and national health plans has made positive changes to health services in Myanmar. Various health facilities, from rural health centers to specialist hospitals, have increased in number over the years, with the result that the proportion of people having access to health services has increased. Nutrition promotion activities have moved from conventional education to behavioral modification approaches and have established a strong multicultural mechanism. The reasons for the continuing existence of malnutrition are to be found at the household and individual levels. While the National Nutrition Centre has reported finding more undernourished children in urban than rural areas, Myanmar's urban population is increasing. When the urban population increases, the food security of this population becomes increasingly risky because of increasing food prices.The decrease in the proportion of people working at home and the increased labor force participation of women are indications of the demand for women to work outside the home; 'traditionally', women were seen as caring mothers who stayed at home. More women in the workplace could lead to more dependent on street food, the quality and safety of which is still poor. Thus, the knowledge and practice (behavior) of the households in terms of health and nutrition becomes important for women. These findings point to the need to explore policy and programme requirements for the promotion of nutritional security in urban and rural households.

Women's empowerment, whether limited to household decision-making or extended to participation in other activities, such as income generation. Therefore, women's empowerment is very important in a family. In a family even if the mother has decision making authorities in some cases *i.e.* food sharing, food practices and food priority, the whole family will be healthy family. Therefore, women are very important person in healthcare and nutrition program. Social marketing will be used to promote the recommended approach. In Myanmar, the government and other organization support in finical help for healthcare and nutrition. In response to the felt need, it was decided to have a comprehensive document that embodies the national aspirations on reproductive health and child health development in the country, and the way to achieve it. The comprehensive document bringing together the strategic plans for reproductive health and child health, is a road map for maternal, newborn and child health, as well as for other essential components of reproductive health and for adolescent health strategic plan (under development), as well as to the existing disease specific strategic plans in the country. The strategic plans have the common programme approaches namely:

1. Improving skills of healthcare providers
2. Strengthening the health system to deliver child health services
3. Improving family and community practices
4. Improving the enabling environment
5. Improving the evidence-base for decision making.

Acknowledgment

I wish to express the deepest gratitude to Dr. Aye Aye Thaw, Deputy Director (Nutrition), Department of Health, for her kindly help, accomplished guidance, willingness to share ideas and helpful suggestions throughout the research. Her interest, patience and insightful comments and ideas solved many problems and helped guiding this paper. Especially, I would like to express my special thank to my parents for their noble support and encouragement.

References

1. Myanmar. Ministry of Health. Health in Myanmar 2004. Yangon: MOH, 2004.
2. Aye Thwin MPH (NUTRITION), DFs&N, MB, BS. National Nutrition Centre, Department of Health, Ministry of Health, Yangon, Myanmar, Promoting household food and nutrition security in Myanmar, Report of Asia Pacific J Clin Nutr (2001) 10(Suppl.): S34–S39

3. http://www.moh.gov.mm/
4. Myanmar. Ministry of Health. Myanmar reproductive health policy. Yangon: Department of Health, 2001.
5. Myanmar. Ministry of Health. National health plan 2003-06. Yangon: MOH, 2004.

Chapter 18

Women Economic Empowerment through Value Addition to Local Raw Materials:

The Role of Raw Materials Research and Development Council, Abuja, Nigeria

Maria N. Obi

Chief Scientific Officer,
Raw Materials Research and Development Council
No. 17 Aguiyi Ironsi Street Maitama District, Abuja – Nigeria
E-mail: mobi@rmrdc.gov.ng, emmaobiadp12@yahoo.ca

ABSTRACT

Women account for about 50 per cent of Nigeria's 140 million populations and contribute more than 65 per cent of labour resources to agricultural production, storage, processing and marketing of food crops in the country side. Several women of reproductive age in Nigeria face various challenges during pregnancy and childbirth as a result of not accessing maternal care from health facilities, deteriorating condition of health facilities, and lack of conscious care from husbands and immediate family members as well as poverty. Ability to access the good healthcare in the developing countries of the world by women is largely being determined by their financial/economic power. Indeed lack of access to various services, resources and opportunities may not be unconnected with poverty, food scarcity. Intact, poverty makes adequate nutrition impossible. The Raw Materials Research and Development Council (RMRDC) have created a gender development desk charged with the responsibility of integrating Nigerian women to tackle the challenges facing women in enterprises development. This paper discusses the role of Raw Materials Research and Development Council in ensuring that the Nigeria Women are economically empowered through processing of our agricultural raw materials for proper and good nutrition. It examines how RMRDC as a research organization embarks on researches that contribute towards the improvement of nutrition and healthcare of Nigeria women and of course the subsequent economic empowerment. Furthermore, it x-rays the activities of the Gender Development Desk created by the council to address the gender related issues for the well being of Nigeria women. Food processing in Nigeria is a major commercial focus for most women who are always ready to acquire knowledge and seek advice on healthy environment, techniques and mechanism that conform to International standard required to improve their efficiency.

Keywords: *Gender/women, Empowerment, Raw materials, Processing, Equipment, Capacity building, Technology.*

Introduction

About the Country–Nigeria

The Federal Republic of Nigeria is situated along the west coast of Africa, lies between latitudes 4º and 14º north of the equator and longitude 3º and 14º East of Greenwich meridian.

It shares borders with Benin in the West, Cameroon in the East, Niger and Chad in the North and the gulf of Guinea in the South. The longest distance being 1,126 kilometers East to West and 1,046 kilometers from North to South.

The land rises from the southern coast to hilly ranges in the North Central, North Western and Eastern parts of the country.

There are two major relief forms: - the high plateaus and the low lands. The main drainage system are formed by the Niger-Benue Rivers and Lake Chad and several other rivers which flow North-south to the coast.

The climate is tropical but differs sharply between the North, bordering the Sahara Desert and the South, bordering the Atlantic Ocean. There are two seasons, the dry (November –April) and the rainy (May- October).

Rainfall decreases from about 1,500 mm in the South to about 500mm in the North. The temperature ranges between 22º C and 41ºC.

There are four main vegetation belts. The Mangrove swamp on the coast, the rain forest, the wood land savannah, the guinea and Sudan savannah in the extreme north.

The population of Nigeria is estimated at 140 million with an annual growth rate of 3.4 per cent. About 47 per cent of this population is below 15 years of age and the urban population represents about 35 per cent of this 140 million. About 50 per cent of the total population is made up of women in various age brackets.

The country is divided into 36 states and the Federal Capital Territory (FCT) of Abuja which serves as the seat of the Government of the Federal Republic of Nigeria.

The 36 states are further grouped into 6 geo-political zones (GPZ) for administrative conveniences: *e.g.* North- East (GPZ), North- West (GPZ), North - Central (GPZ) South- East (GPZ) South- West (GPZ) South- South (GPZ)

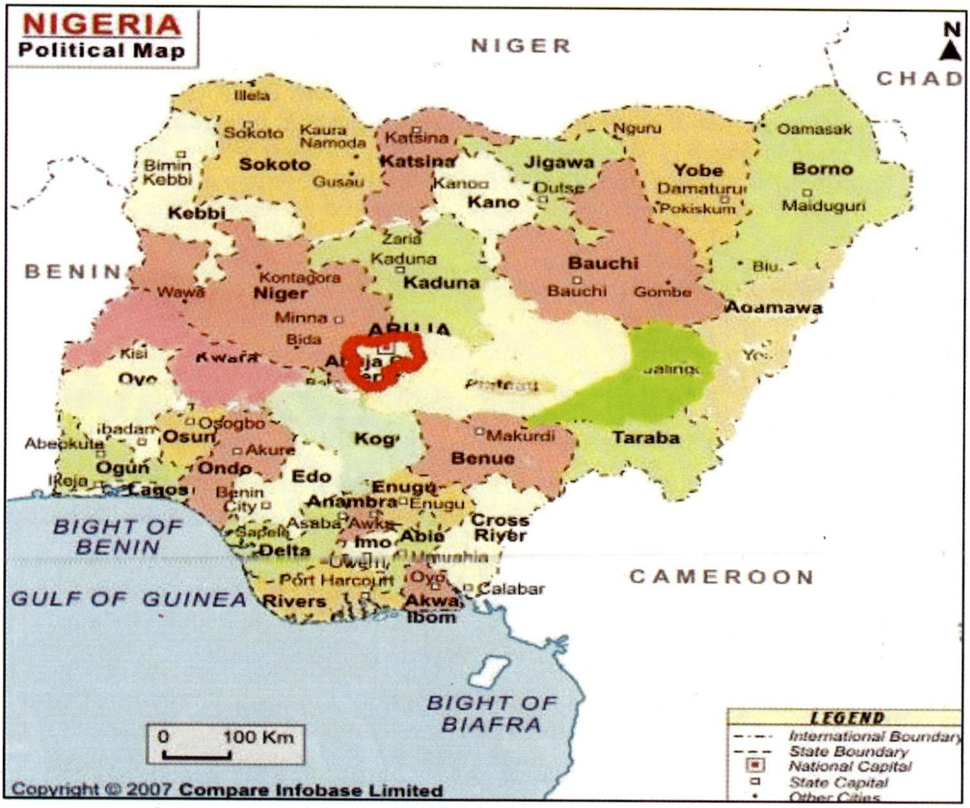

Figure 18.1: Map of Nigeria Showing 36 States and the Federal Capital Territory and its Borders

The country operates a presidential democratic system of government which comprises of a three-tier system of government: Federal, State and Local Government.

Natural Resource Endowment

The country is well endowed with abundant human and natural resources (mineral and agricultural). The mineral and agricultural resources are available in the rural areas where they are largely under-developed and not fully exploited. The country has a total land area of about 92.4 million hectares with about 67.5 million hectares suitable for the production of food and agricultural raw materials.

The major agricultural produce found in Nigeria include: cereals, legumes, roots, tubers, fruits, vegetables, tree crops, livestock, fishery and various wood species. There are also extensive mineral reserves such as Bitumen, Coal, Colum bite,Barite, kaolin, Talc, Limestone, Gypsum, Gold, Iron Ore, Galena, Gemstone etc. Although the country is a mono-economic one highly dependent on oil but the extensive mineral reserves and a strong agricultural base characterize the country's economic potentials. The major occupations of Nigerian women are:

- ☆ Farming
- ☆ Food Processing
- ☆ Petty Trading
- ☆ Hand Craft
- ☆ Tailoring and Fashion Designing
- ☆ Soap Making
- ☆ Weaving

In the hierarchy of man's needs, food occupies the highest position. Importantly, nations do recognize that food security, which is the first line security, is sine quo non for peace and peaceful co-existence and Nigeria cannot afford to do otherwise.

History has taught us that for a nation like Nigeria, which is well endowed with agricultural resources, the development of these resources is a pre-requisite, or at least corollary to the economic take-off of the nation. It is simply: if people are incompetent to develop their country by the use of its abundant natural resources, they cannot hope to do so on imported materials. Also with a population of over 100 million people, Nigeria cannot hope to afford to feed her people on imported food stuff as doing so would surely lead to budget crises and total collapse of the economy.

Agricultural development is also the basis for sustained economic development even for nations, which are obviously the most industrialized and developed.

Food processing in Nigeria is a major commercial focus for most women and they (Nigerian women) are always ready to go to any length to acquire knowledge and seek advice on new environment, techniques and mechanisms needed to improve their efficiency.

Women's Health

Women are described as the architects of the family and nation considering their functions as mothers, educationists, food producers and processors and the role models for their families and by extension the nation (Prof. B. E. P. Nwoke 2009). For this reason, they need to be in good state of health/well being to properly achieve these functions. Women's health is then the states of well being of women to enable them perform their roles in the society. Women's health has serious impact on these multi disciplinary task plus their double and triple work shifts in the formal and informal workforce. It is therefore obvious that a good health status is a pre-requisite for the good health of the whole family and by extension the community and the society. It then means that women's health is a societal issue and must be given priority by the global community. As mothers, educationists, food producers and processors women play a key role in determining the nutritional status of family members (World Bank, 1993). The millennium Development Goals (MDGs) and the Nigerian National Economic Empowerment Development Strategies (NEEDS) and States Economic Empowerment Development Strategies (SEEDS) program place strong emphasis on women development through economic empowerment and general improvement of women.

Factors Affecting the Health of the Women

Globally, the contribution of women to world economy and combating poverty through both remunerated and unremunerated work at home, in the community or at work place is highly acknowledged.

The factors that affect the health of women are determined by a complex of biological, socio-economic and cultural factors.

Sex discrimination had tended to be hidden within the general issue of poverty and under development which puts everyone (men and women and children) at risk.

In practice, women and girls are most vulnerable and suffer disproportionately because of their low status in society (Prof. P I K Onyeka 2009).

On the whole, the major factors affecting the health of women today includes:

- Poverty
- Education and ignorance
- Cultural and traditional practices
- Demographic factor
- Lack of personal and social status and opportunity
- Lack of access to healthcare.

Poverty and Other Economic Factors

Unemployment, marginalization and poverty are conditions that result in poor health and these are exacerbated and women face throughout their lives.

In virtually every society, women face discrimination in education, employment as well as social and economic status, all of which contribute to a heightened vulnerability to diseases (WHO, 1994b). Poverty often means that people exist on insufficient food or the wrong kind of food. It is a statement of fact that the majority of the 1.3 billion living today in extreme poverty are women and this is worst in the 10 per cent -27 per cent women headed families in the developing countries (WHO 1995). The poor women with their families live mainly in crowded urban periphery, squatter layouts or in their rural areas which are originally characterized by unsanitary environment with inadequate, or no water supply.

The consequent public health problems associated with these poor living conditions are very obvious, compounded by the fact that these women have little or no income earning capacity as well as very low purchasing power. The women have limited access even to free healthcare since they or their families cannot afford the cost of medication or transportation. Poverty is then addressed as the root course of malnutrition and poor healthcare in Nigeria women.

Education and Ignorance

In Nigeria teenage pregnancy is a major cause of school dropout among girls, increasing illiteracy and ignorance. Teenage mothers account for nearly 1 million births in Nigeria annually. Such young girls end up in marriages or pre-marital pregnancy with no knowledge or skills to protect or care for themselves. Their ignorance affects their access to healthcare, compared to the educated women of reproductive age who consciously access healthcare during pregnancy. Pregnant girls who are 15 years and under have maternal mortality ratio of 7 times higher them that of women 20-24 years.

Cultural and Traditional Practices

Traditionally, men seem to believe that pregnancy is the sole responsibility of the women and the men have little part to play. A vast majority of husbands pay more attention to the actual child delivery and ignore the risks associated with the issue of child bearing, and see it as part of life.

Demographic Factor

The following demographic factors are linked to

The health status of the population:

- ☆ Birth rate
- ☆ Growth rate
- ☆ Maturity
- ☆ Migration
- ☆ Aging
- ☆ Illness and
- ☆ Death rate

Demographic factors that affect women's health include:

- ☆ Marriage
- ☆ Childbearing
- ☆ Aging and its problems
- ☆ Women in refugee and
- ☆ Other displaced population

Lack of Personal and Social Status and Opportunity

This age long socio-economic practices has created a system whereby women are discriminated against *e.g.*

- ☆ Land ownership
- ☆ Inheritance
- ☆ Marriage
- ☆ Divorce
- ☆ In the developing country the society place value on their sons.

The pattern of family food distribution is in favour of the boys. Girls in poor families are likely to be malnourished.

In our society women with many daughters are under societal pressure to continue to bear children until they produce boys.

Lack of Access to Healthcare

Records show that women especially in developing countries tend to have less access to health inputs and service. They do not have the time needed to access the healthcare since they are burdened with house chores and always in all day long activity.

Nutrition

Nutrition can be defined as a process of nourishing or being nourished, provision of the materials necessary to support life. A good nutrition is the key to a healthier and longer life which consists of the following categories of food taken in right proportion and quantity: Fruits, Vegetables, Grains, Cereals, Oil seeds and nuts Roots and tubers and fibers

Food Processing

This is the conversion of edible food in another form more acceptable or more convenient to the consumer and still maintains the nutrients. It prevents spoilage of food, gives food longer life shelf without wasting the nutrients. Women generate income from food processing activities, and it is necessary for employment creation, industrial growth. The two major factors that affect nutritional requirements are *Quality* and *Quantity* of food.

The Raw Materials Research and Development Council (RMRDC)

The Raw Materials Research and Development Council (RMRDC) were established in 1987 and currently operate under the supervision of the Federal Ministry of Science and Technology. In addition to the headquarters in Abuja, the Council has a State Coordinating Office in every State Capital in Nigeria.

Mandate

The core mandates of the Council include:

- ☆ To draw up policy guidelines and action programmes on raw materials acquisition, exploitation and development;
- ☆ To view, from time to time, raw materials resources availability and utilization, with a view to advising the Federal Government on the strategic implications of depletion, conservation or stock-piling of such resources;
- ☆ To advise on adaptation of machinery and processes for raw materials utilization.
- ☆ To encourage publicity of research findings and dissemination of other information relevant to local sourcing of raw materials for industries.
- ☆ To encourage growth of implant research and development capacities.

- ☆ To advice and device award systems for industries that achieves any beak-through, make innovations or inventions.
- ☆ To organize workshops, symposia and seminars designed to enlighten people on new developments and solutions discovered from time to time.

RMRDC Renders the Following Services to their Clients

- ☆ Public policy advisory support.
- ☆ Upgrading of research facilities and promoting science and technology in Nigeria
- ☆ Provide industrial support services and promote new resource based investment using a net work of coordinating offices located in all state capitals in the federation.
- ☆ Servicing as Nigeria focal point for international collaboration on raw materials development
- ☆ Promoting industrial raw materials research innovations and utilization through merit award.
- ☆ Promoting investment in resource based industries.
- ☆ Promoting new resource based investment through joint venture projects and technical support services.

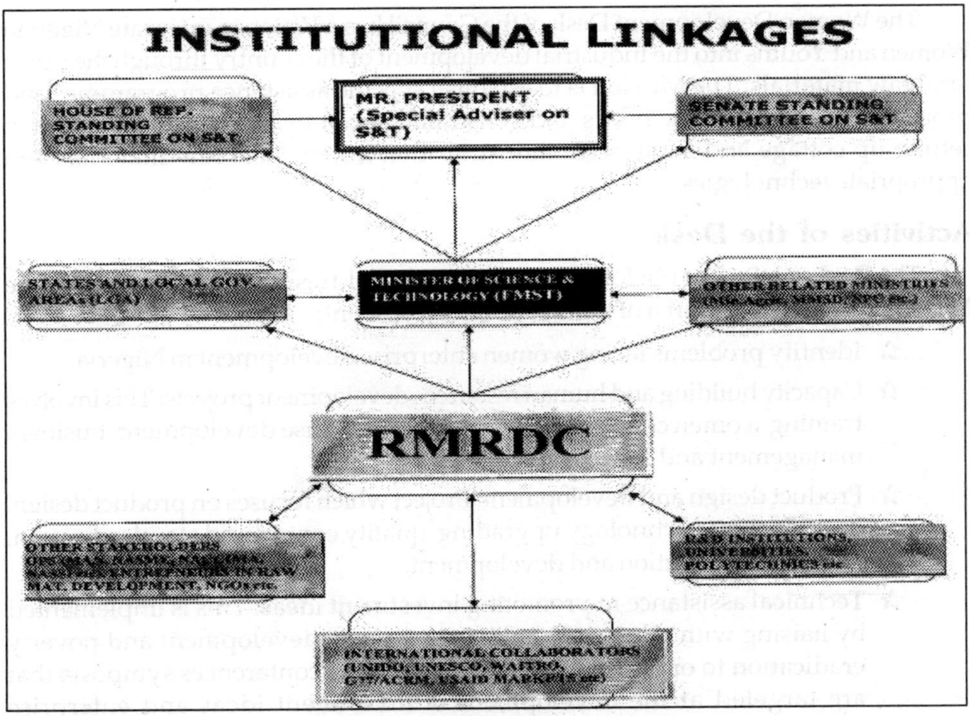

Figure 18.2

- ☆ Promoting advisory and technical support services to investors.
- ☆ Promoting the development of indigenous technology.
- ☆ Sponsoring Research and Development (R&D) activities for raw materials utilization and new products.
- ☆ Promoting local engineering capabilities in design and manufacture of plant/machinery for new materials processing.
- ☆ Review from time to time raw materials resources availability and utilization.
- ☆ Support agro-industrial raw materials production
- ☆ Publicizing, creating awareness and sensitization on raw materials resources potentials.

Creation of Women Development Desk

Raw Materials Research and Development Council (RMRDC) in fulfillment of the Council's mandate of optimal utilization of the nation's abundant agricultural and mineral resources, and in recognition of the immense contribution of Nigerian women towards downstream agricultural processing, the Women Development Desk was created for the following reasons: To address the constraints faced by women entrepreneurs in setting up cottage level enterprises and adding value to our agro raw materials, and to accommodate the needs of Nigerian women in promoting the use of local raw materials as industrial input.

The Women Development Desk of the Council has a Vision to integrate Nigerian Women and Youths into the Industrial development of the country through the use of local raw materials. The Mission is to establish specific assistance programmes and projects responding to the needs and constraints faced by Youths and Women in setting up cottage and small scale industries that utilize local raw materials and appropriate technologies.

Activities of the Desk

The Desk carries out the following activities to address the problems facing the Nigerian Women in the area of enterprises development;

- ☆ Identify problems facing women enterprise development in Nigeria.
- ☆ Capacity building and human resources development projects: This involves training women cooperative groups on enterprise development, business management and simple record keeping.
- ☆ Product design and development: Project which focuses on product design, development, technology upgrading, quality control and standardization, market identification and development.
- ☆ Technical assistance in promoting investment ideas: This is implemented by liaising with other stakeholders in women development and poverty eradication to organize workshops, seminars, conferences symposia that are targeted at the development of investment ideas and enterprise development.

- ☆ Business advisory and technical services: This entails provision of feasibility reports to women, assistance in raw materials and equipment sourcing business start-up, etc.

Identified Problems

- ☆ Inability to identify raw materials available in their localities and modern equipment to be used for processing of such raw materials, into intermediate or finished products.
- ☆ Lack of funds to procure equipment. Inability to maintain such equipment due to non availability of expert advice.
- ☆ Improper record keeping of business enterprises, which results into inadequate information on the progress and shortcomings of such businesses.
- ☆ Marketing of the products of such business as a result of inadequate monitoring and supervision.
- ☆ Production of sub-standard products that makes it difficult for such products to gain acceptance in the local and international market.
- ☆ Lack of continuity of such business enterprises which creates a bottleneck to enterprise development.
- ☆ Lack of government assistance through machinery/equipment provision.

Strategies Employed by the Desk to Address the Identified Problems

- ☆ Carry out needs assessment of industrial enterprises development of the youths and women.
- ☆ Organize sensitization workshops Seminars, symposia, roundtables in collaboration with the stakeholders in enterprise development.
- ☆ Assist/galvanize/organize the youth and women to forum production and processing cooperative societies to foster enterprises development through the use of local raw materials.
- ☆ Liaise with other stakeholders in women development and poverty eradication to organized programmes targeted at enterprises development and raw materials utilization.
- ☆ Technology intervention for the youths and women groups that produce process and utilize raw materials.
- ☆ Link the group to appropriate financial institutions (micro-credit) raw materials and the market.
- ☆ Provide general investment and enterprises support services to the women.

Results Achieved so far in Addressing the Problems Faced by the Nigeria Women

The Council has made a giant stride in ensuring that value is added to our local raw materials for good nutrition and healthy living in the following areas:

1. Boosting of agricultural raw materials
2. Development of agricultural implements, equipment and machineries
3. Development of tree plantations of indigenous economic species
4. Funding of research and development (R&D)
5. Development of process technology
6. Capacity building

The main successes recorded in above areas of intervention are:

- ☆ Through procurement, production and multiplication of improved seeds/ seedlings of high yielding varieties
- ☆ Procurement and distribution of improved premium quality of the following crops: groundnut, cotton, soyabean, maize, kenaf, tomatoes, pepper, mango citrus sugarcane, ginger, cassava, benniseed, castor, cabbage, onion, carrot, pineapple.
- ☆ The produced materials are distributed to Nigerian farmers for plantation establishment.
- ☆ The Council executes Research and Development (R&D) programmes to address the needs of manufacturing industries including Agro Allied Food Industries
- ☆ R&D is executed in collaboration with higher institutions research institutions cooperative societies, organized private sector (MAN NACCIMA NASSI and NASE, Non-Government Organizations and private entrepreneurs).
- ☆ Production of soya sauce a mixture of soya-bean and sweet potato extracts to produce food flavor
- ☆ Production of furfural Urea fertilizer from maize cobs.
- ☆ On-farm trials of alternative formulation of livestock feeds.
- ☆ Production and commercialization of dried mango chips using a locally fabricated multi-purpose dryer.

The Council executes Research and Development (R&D) programmes to address the needs of manufacturing industries including Agro Allied Food Industries.

R&D is executed in collaboration with higher institutions, research institutions, cooperative societies, organized private sector (MAN NACCIMA NASSI and NASE, Non-Government Organizations and private entrepreneurs).

Process Technology Developments

The Council developed the following process equipment;

- ☆ Melon Shelling
- ☆ Moringa Oleifera processing equipment
- ☆ Cashew nuts processing plant.
- ☆ Fish smoking plant

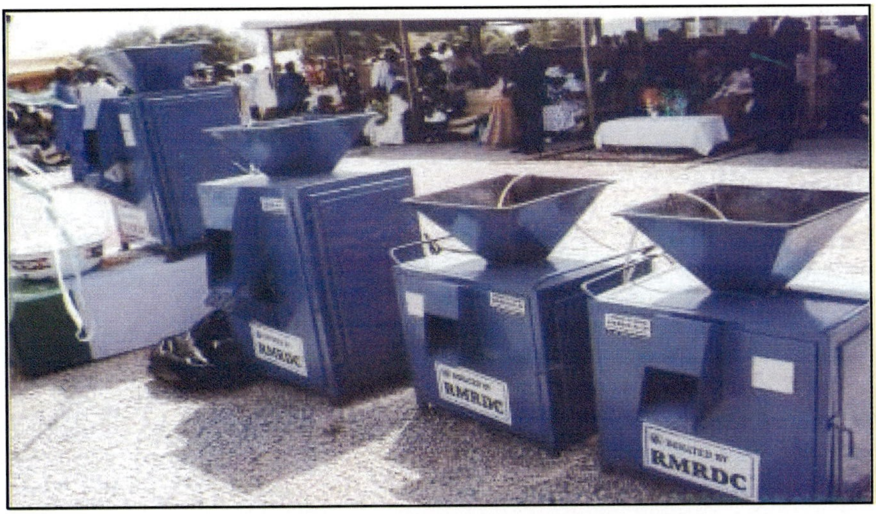

Figure 18.3: Melon Shelling Machines Donated to Women Co-operative Societies in Nassarawa State by RMRDC

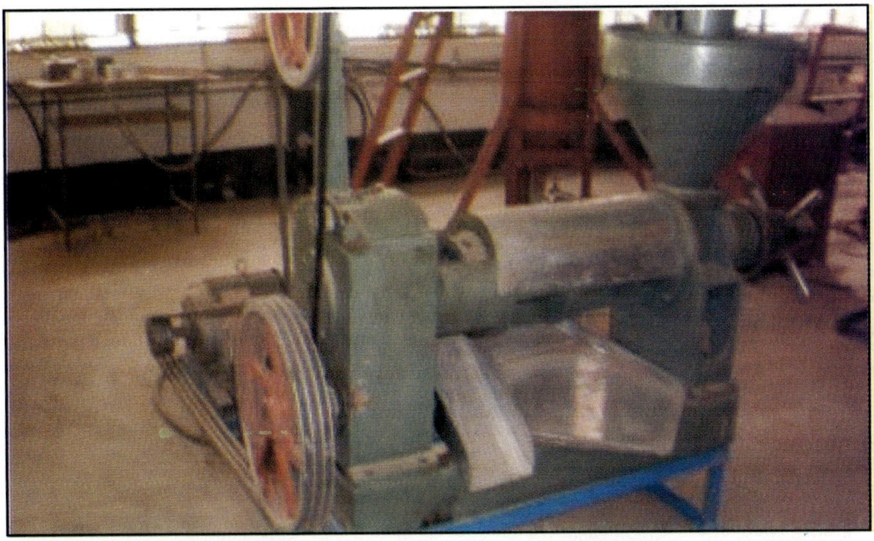

Figure 18.4: Moringa Oil Extractor

- ☆ Castor oil plant
- ☆ Beniseed oil processing plant
- ☆ Essential oil pilot plant
- ☆ Kilishi processing plant
- ☆ Salt Processing
- ☆ Shea butter Production plant
- ☆ Acha dehulling and destoning

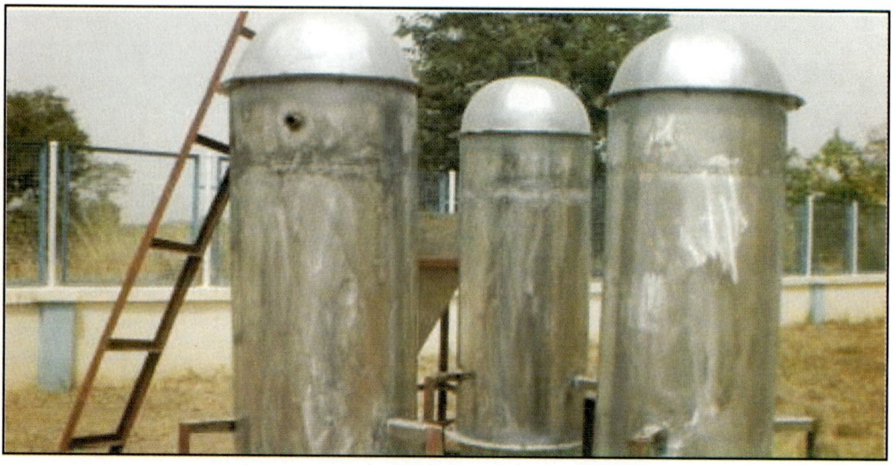

Figure 18.5: Moringa Water Treatment Plant for the Rural Communities

Capacity Building

The Council has organized numerous training/workshops in collaboration with the relevant stakeholders aimed at addressing food security in Nigeria on the following areas:

- Entrepreneurship Development.
- Production of High Quality Cassava Flour (HQCF) and Glucose Syrup from cassava root.
- Production of Dried Mango Chips.

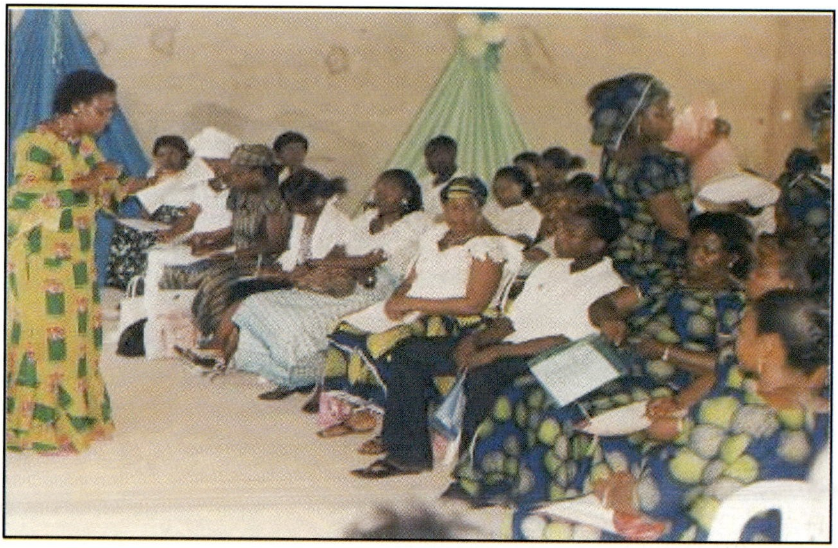

Figure 18.6: Entrepreneurship Development Training

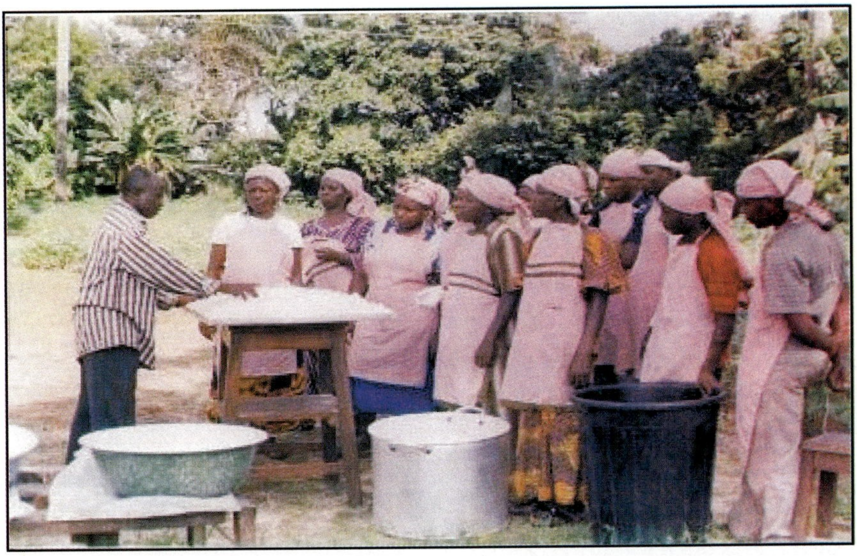

Figure 18.7: Production of Tapioca Flour from Cassava

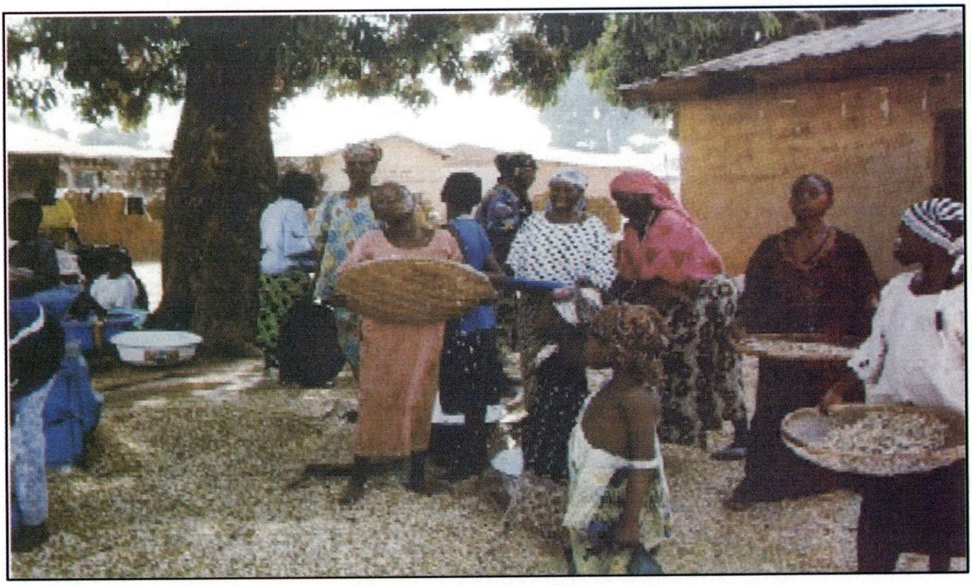

Figure 18.8: Melon Shelling Cluster in Nassarawa State

- ☆ Improved processing technique for shea butter production.
- ☆ Fish smoking.
- ☆ Fulani cattle farmers on appropriate milking process.
- ☆ Cross breeding using exotic breed cattle to achieve enhanced milk production.
- ☆ Establishment of industrial clusters in a rural setting.

- ☆ Aquaculture as a Business
- ☆ Africa Locust Beans (parkia biglobosa)
- ☆ Micro, small and Medium Enterprises
- ☆ Formation of food process clusters

Council's Challenges in the Implementation of Programmes for Food Security and Good Nutrition

- ☆ Poor funding of Research and Development (R&D) activities in the country.
- ☆ Gap between R&D and commercialization
- ☆ Low level of technical expertise/shortage of skilled manpower.
- ☆ Poor infrastructural facilities
- ☆ Political interference

Conclusion

Poverty has been identified as the main cause of ill-health and malnutrition that needs urgent/adequate attention and commitments from global communities to eradicate. Food Processing being the major commercial focus of Nigerian women and its impacts on economic empowerment of Women can not be over-emphasised. The problems and constraints militating against women in embarking on this enterprise needs to be addressed globally because it has direct effect on Women's Health and Nutrition

RMRDC has positioned itself to be a major player in achieving Government initiatives in the areas of food processing by Nigeria Women for good nutrition, and has achieved a lot on strengthening the economic power of Nigerian Women living in the rural areas. We therefore seek for more understanding and unflinching support, including the cooperation and collaboration of International communities to tackle the impediments to women empowerment through food processing and value addition to local raw materials.

Acknowledgement

I am sincerely grateful to the Centre for Science &Technology of the Non-Aligned and other Development Countries (NAMS&T) India which extended the invitation to participate.

International Conference which featured this year on the theme 'Empowering Women in Developing Countries through Better Healthcare and Nutrition'. My appreciation goes to the Director General (RMRDC) Engr. (Prof.) A. P. Onwualu for his nomination moral, encouragement, advice and financial support in putting these documents together. Also my Colleagues Engr. Obasi Ettu, Gimba, Kwaya and others are not left out for their technical assistance in developing, fine-tuning and proof-reading the final draft of the document.

Mostly to the Almighty God whom I trust will enable us have a wonderful Conference that will add meaning to humanity.

Abbreviations

RMRDC: Raw Materials Research and Development Council.
GPZ: Geo-Political Zone.
MDGs: Millennium Development Goals.
NEEDS: National Economic Empowerment Development Strategies.
SEEDS: States Economic Empowerment Development Strategies.
R&D: Research and Development.
MAN: Manufacturers Association of Nigeria.
NACCIMA: National Association 0f Chambers of Commerce Industry Mines and Agriculture.
NASS I: Nigeria Association of Small Scale Industrialists

References

1. Chibuuzor L. Oriuwa KSC: Improving the maternal health and economic status of Women in rural Southeast Nigeria 2009.
2. Oboh Ijeoma P, Fred O. J.Oboh: Sustainable Fish Production through Processing and Product Development: The role of fermented fish products. Paper presented at the TWOWS African Regional Conference in Nigeria 2009.
3. Demographic Data for Development Project "Child Survival: Risk and the Road to Health", Institute for Research Development/Westinghouse 1987.
4. Prof. B. E. B. Nwoke, Prof.P. I. K. Onyeka, Prof. F. O. Nduka: Why Women's Health 2009.
5. Boserup,E. 1970 : Women role in Economic Development, London, George Allen and Unwin.
6. Annon 1974: Nutritional Food and Nutritional Programme Zambia. Nutritional Status Survey. UNDP/FAO, Rome, ESN:DP/ZAN/69/512 Technical report 2.
7. Raw Materials Research and Development Council (RMRDC): Annual reports 2005-2008.

Chapter 19

Nutrition Knowledge, Beliefs and Dietary Habits and their Gender Association amongst Omani Elderly in Nizwa Wilayat: An Input For Policy Implications

Asya Al Riyami[1] and Saleh Al Hadabi[2]*

[1]*Directorate of Research and Studies, Directorate General of Planning, Ministry of Health (HQ), P.O. Box 393, Postal Code 100, Muscat, Sultanate of Oman*

[2] *Director General of Health Services, Ad Dakhaliya Region, Sultanate of Oman*

**E-mail: asyariyami@gmail.com*

ABSTRACT

Nutritional needs of the aging population require special attention. We undertook a cross sectional community based household survey in the Nizwa wilayat, Oman, to understand the nutrition related knowledge and beliefs among the Omani elderly, study their dietary habits and determine their association with gender. The response rate for the household interview was 99.3 per cent from the total sample of 2041 elderly. We found overall poor knowledge of nutrition along with imbalanced nutrition and decreased physical activity. Significant gender difference existed in certain aspects of nutritional knowledge, fluids, milk and sweets consumption, noticing change in appetite and following diet regimen. Also about 45 per cent of our elderly are overweight/obese. This warrants reorientation of the existing health promotion strategy for the elderly.

Keywords: *Nutrition, Knowledge, Beliefs, Dietary habits, Omani, Elderly, Gender.*

Introduction

The WHO acknowledges: Ageing and nutrition- a growing global challenge [1]. Modifying lifestyle factors like diet can prevent, slow or reverse the onset of many of the chronic diseases associated with aging. Identifying dietary patterns and specific dietary components that offer protection against chronic disease is important [2]. Healthy eating perceptions and food group consumption practices of elderly men are largely unexplored [3].

The Food Habits in Later Life project of the International Union of Nutritional Sciences [4] highlights that rapid assessment procedures are valuable to develop food-based dietary guidelines for their aged members. Elderly patients with a compromised nutritional state increase the burden on the existing healthcare infrastructure. Their inpatient burden in Oman is around 10 per cent [5].

This study was undertaken to understand the nutrition related knowledge and beliefs among the elderly, study their dietary habits and determine their association with gender, so as to utilize the findings for health promotion policy.

Methodology

A cross sectional community based household survey of the needs and profiles of non-institutionalized elderly Omanis aged 60 years and above was conducted in the Nizwa wilayat, Ad Dakhaliya region in Oman in 2005.After approval by Research Ethics Committee of the Ministry of Health, Oman, informed consent was obtained. A structured questionnaire based on literature review, expert opinion and as relevant to the elderly in Oman was constructed. It assessed nine different domains (only the nutrition domain is discussed in this paper) and the data was collected by personal interview at home. The interviewers were health educators from the Ministry of Health and volunteers from the community support groups who received 6 days of standardized intensive training. A second questionnaire related to clinical examination and investigations was conducted by a medical doctor in the Nizwa Community Research Center. After the pilot study, the data collection was conducted between June and August 2005.

Our sample frame was the 2003 census data [6]. The total population size of Nizwa wilayat was 68,922 according to census 2003 conducted by Ministry of National Economy. Out of them 4.5 per cent were aged 60 years and above, and this expected to yield 3105 elderly. All of Omani old citizens were recruited in the study except the inhabitants of Jabal Akhdar and remote scattered houses due to logistics' constraints. Nizwa maps of enumeration areas and a list of households consisting of the elderly were provided by Ministry of National Economy, and supervisors were involved on updating the maps and numbering the houses. In the field work, some houses were found empty and some elderly moved out. 1508 houses were visited to yield 2041 elderly citizens. The response rate for the household interview was 99.3 per cent (n=2027) while for the clinical examination and investigation was 80.8 per cent (n=1650).

There is need to prepare uniform food guidelines throughout the Arab region and portion size and food composition tables to suit the Arab food habits and culture[7]. For our analysis we considered the traditional regional [8] and local dietary habits. The portion size information was not collected. Based on this we categorized the dietary (and milk and milk products) intake of frequency equal to/less than 3 times per week as less than adequate while 4 or more times per week as adequate. Milk and milk products were classified as full fat if 2 or more items out of milk, yoghurt and laban were answered as full fat. Regarding fluids consumption per day (water+ milk+ laban + fruit juices + drinks), less than or equal to 1500 ml per day (as measured by number of ORS glasses) was considered inadequate. The physical activity was based on daily chores and walking, with cut off set at 30 minutes per day [9]. BMI [10] was based on WHO criteria.

Data entry was done in the region with Epi data version 3.1 and data management and analysis was done using SPSS 9.0. Descriptive analysis of the nutrition related data was done. Chi square test of significance ($p<0.05$) was used to assess gender difference for the relevant variables.

Results

The respondent sample (Table 19.1) consisted of 51.6 per cent females and 48.4 per cent males with majority residing in the urban area. There were significantly more females between 60-69 years (60 per cent females, males 54 per cent) while less in 70-79 years group (24 per cent females, 31 per cent males).The aged elderly (80+) had equal distribution in both the genders. The illiteracy amongst the females was 95 per cent with 4 per cent studied up to semi primary, the proportions for males being 68 per cent and 26 per cent respectively. Nearly 7 per cent males had primary and above education while less than 1 per cent females had so ($p=0.000$). Amongst males, 91 per cent were married, 5 per cent widowed compared to 45 per cent and 49 per cent respectively in females ($p=0.000$). About 17 per cent males were working while 99 per cent females were housewives. Nearly 72 per cent females and 21 per cent males had no personal income. Overall 21 per cent earned less than 100 Omani Rials (OR) per month while 26 per cent between 100 and 199 OR. The difference in income levels between males and females was significant ($p=0.000$). 97 per cent males were staying with the same family since last 5 years as compared to 94 per cent females ($p=0.000$). Obesity was noted more in females (16 per cent) than males (11 per cent) ($p=0.020$) and 32 per cent of the total sample was overweight with about 8 per cent being underweight. Of the total, 49 per cent were not physically active, amongst the remaining, males were physically more active than females ($p=0.000$).

On assessment of nutrition knowledge and beliefs (Table 19.2), 43 per cent did feel that the quality of nutrition should change with age but only 17 per cent expected the quantity to change with no significant difference between the genders. Only 24 per cent accepted that they should include some specific type of food with advancing age while about 27 per cent were not certain about this. There was a significant gender difference on this above issue with the males having comparatively more affirmative answers. About moderation of consumption of specific food types, significantly less proportion of females gave a negative reply in contrast to males and more females (25 per cent) were not sure about it ($p=0.022$). However marginally increased proportion of females replied positively to reduction in intake of sweets

Table 19.1: Distribution of Background Characteristics According to Gender

		Male (n=982)		*Female (n=1045)*		*Total*	*P*
		n	*Per cent*	*n*	*Per cent*	*Per cent*	
Residence	Urban	877	89.3	935	89.5	89.4	NS
	Rural	105	10.7	110	10.5	10.6	
Age groups	60-69 years	528	53.8	624	59.7	56.8	0.005
	70-79 years	307	31.3	253	24.2	27.6	
	80-89 years	104	10.6	119	11.4	11.0	
	>=90 years	43	4.4	49	4.7	4.5	
Education	Illiterate	662	67.6	996	95.3	81.9	0.0001
	Semi primary	253	25.8	41	3.9	14.5	
	Primary and above	65	6.6	8	0.8	3.6	
Marital status	Never married	14	1.4	13	1.2	1.3	0.0001
	Married	896	91.3	471	45.1	67.5	
	Widowed	52	5.3	509	48.7	27.7	
	Divorced	19	1.9	52	5.0	3.5	
Work status	Working	164	16.7	11	1.1	8.6	NA
	Not working	818	83.3	0	0.0	40.35	
	Housewife	0	0.0	1034	98.9	51.01	
Elderly income/ month	Nil	204	20.8	752	72.0	47.2	0.0001
	<100 OR	205	20.9	221	21.1	21.0	
	100-199 OR	468	47.7	60	5.7	26.0	
	200-299 OR	63	6.4	4	0.4	3.3	
	300-399 OR	15	1.5	3	0.3	0.9	
	400 + OR	27	2.7	5	0.5	1.6	
Staying with the same family since last 5 years	Yes	955	97.3	980	93.8	95.5	0.0001
	No	27	2.7	65	6.2	4.5	
BMI*	Underweight	55	7.8	53	7.4	7.6	0.020
	Normal	358	50.7	325	45.1	47.9	
	Overweight	219	31.0	230	31.9	31.5	
	Obese	74	10.5	113	15.7	13.1	
Physical activity (minutes per day)	no activity	435	44.3	567	54.3	49.4	0.0001
	<30 min/day	335	34.1	329	31.5	32.8	
	=/>30 min/day	212	21.6	149	14.3	17.8	

* Some data missing.

Table 19.2: Dietary Knowledge and Beliefs of the Elderly by Sex

Dietary Knowledge/Belief	Male		Female		Total	P
	n/Total	Per cent	n/Total	Per cent	Per cent	
Quality of nutrition should change with age	424/966	43.9	434/1030	42.1	43.0	NS
Quantity of nutrition should change with age	177/957	18.5	163/1019	16.0	17.2	NS
Eating specific type of food with advancing age						
Yes	248/980	25.3	228/1043	21.9	23.5	0.0001
No	511	52.1	496	47.6	49.8	
Don't know	221	22.6	319	30.6	26.7	
Type of food						
Vegetables	107	10.9	113	10.8	10.9	
Fruits	77	7.9	75	7.2	7.5	
Milk	63	6.5	71	6.8	6.6	
Water	87	8.9	83	7.9	8.4	
Moderation of certain types of food with advancing age						
Yes	387/969	39.9	428/1031	41.5	40.8	0.022
No	375	38.7	343	33.3	35.9	
Don't know	207	21.4	260	25.2	23.4	
Type of food						
Protein	37	3.8	33	3.2	3.5	
Cereals/starch	47	4.9	34	3.3	4.1	
Sweets/sugar	206	21.3	239	23.2	22.3	
Fat	210	21.7	238	23.1	22.4	
Milk	6	0.6	11	1.1	0.9	
Eggs/liver/brain	10	1.0	4	0.4	0.7	
Salt	115	11.9	182	17.7	14.9	
Fruits/vegetables	10	1.0	5	0.5	0.8	
Water	1	0.1	0	0.0	0.	
About use of milk for the elderly	n/980		n/1043			
Rich in calcium	24	2.4	11	1.1	1.7	0.016
Rich in Vitamin D	11	1.1	7	0.7	0.9	NS
Offers protection from osteoporosis	143	14.6	105	10.1	12.3	0.002
Rich in protein	7	0.7	5	0.5	0.6	NS
Helps to prevent constipation	35	3.6	38	3.6	3.6	NS

Contd...

Table 19.2–Contd...

Dietary Knowledge/Belief	*Male*		*Female*		*Total*	*P*
	n/Total	*Per cent*	*n/Total*	*Per cent*	*Per cent*	
Heard about dietary fibers	80/978	8.2	67/1042	6.4	7.3	NS
Use of dietary fibers						
To regulate intestinal movements	36	3.7	28	2.7	3.2	
To relieve constipation	17	1.7	10	0.9	1.3	
Other uses	27	2.8	26	2.5	2.6	
Foods rich in dietary fibers						
Fruits	14	1.4	11	1.0	1.2	
Vegetables	42	4.3	26	2.5	3.3	
Whole cereals	18	1.8	24	2.3	2.1	
Plant proteins	2	0.2	2	0.2	0.2	
Change in dietary habits can protect and control health problems at advancing age						
Yes	309/980	31.5	307/1043	29.4	30.4	0.004
No	355	36.2	328	31.4	33.8	
Don't know	316	32.2	408	39.1	35.8	
Can it control						
Hypertension	194	19.8	218	20.9	20.4	
Diabetes	200	20.4	203	19.5	19.9	
Hyperlipidemia	57	5.8	39	3.7	4.7	
CHD	35	3.6	27	2.6	3.1	
Obesity	36	3.7	23	2.2	2.9	
Anemia	13	1.3	10	0.9	1.1	
Gastric and Duodenal problems	8	0.8	8	0.8	0.8	

and fat (23 per cent) and salt (18 per cent). Overall the detailed knowledge about the value of milk and dietary fibers was quite poor. About 12 per cent were aware of the value of milk in protecting osteoporosis while only 2 per cent knew it as a rich source of Calcium, and there was significant gender difference, with females having less knowledge. 93 per cent of the sample had not heard about dietary fibers and of those who had, less than 3 per cent knew its importance in daily diet. A majority of the elderly could not decide on which foods are rich in dietary fibers. Related to the role of change in dietary habits which would help in protection and control of health problems, a gender difference was noted(p=0.004) with only about 20 per cent of the total being aware that this could be of help in Hypertension and Diabetes, while less than 5 per cent were knowledgeable about the role in other specific illnesses.

The practice of consuming 3 meals per day is seen in 92 per cent of the respondents (Table 19.3). About 34 per cent females compared to 27 per cent males had noticed that there was a change in their appetite (p=0.003), the main reasons overall being, sickness (18 per cent) and having just lost appetite (12.5 per cent) with females attributing these reasons more than males. Ingestion of medicines was attributed as a reason by 2.5 per cent of the elderly. There is no gender difference in consumption of meat related items, cereals, vegetables, fruits, salty food, vitamin/mineral supplements and type of milk products. Nearly 59 per cent consume adequate fish/meat/chicken, 83 per cent adequate cereals, 85 per cent adequate fruits. Vegetable intake is inadequate in 89 per cent of the total. Proportionately more females do not consume any type of sweets (p=0.01) but 58 per cent of the total sample have sweet intake 1 to 3 times a week. About 20 per cent of the sample requires taking additional salt in their diet and 9 per cent take additional vitamins/mineral supplements. Females have significantly less fluid intake per day (p=0.000). There is significant gender difference regards consuming milk and milk products with less females consuming the same (p=0.004). Full fat type appears to be the preference of 39 per cent of the sample. More females follow a diet regimen (p=0.000) with about 15 per cent having fat and cholesterol restriction and 12 per cent salt and sugar restriction.

Table 19.3: Dietary Habits in the Elderly by Gender

		Male		*Female*		*Total*	*P*
		n/982	*Per cent*	*n/1045*	*Per cent*	*Per cent*	
Total number of meals per day	1	15	1.5	11	1.0	1.3	NS
	2	67	6.8	81	7.8	7.3	
	3	900	91.6	953	91.2	91.4	
Noticed change in appetite reasons	Yes	265	27.3	348	33.5	30.5	0.003
Sickness	Yes	147	15.1	209	20.1	17.7	
Taking medicines	Yes	26	2.7	24	2.3	2.5	
Just lost appetite	Yes	116	11.9	135	13.0	12.5	
Lost some loved one	Yes	3	0.3	13	1.3	0.8	
Fish/meat/chicken consumption per week	Adequate	559	58.4	611	59.6	59.0	NS
Cereals consumption per week	Adequate	797	83.0	853	83.7	83.4	NS
Vegetables consumption per week	Adequate	104	10.9	119	11.8	11.4	NS
Fruits consumption per week	Adequate	810	83.7	885	86.2	85.0	NS
Sweets consumption	Nil	315	38.4	393	44.6	41.6	0.01
per week	1-3	506	61.6	489	55.4	58.4	
Consumption of salty food							
Extra salt in diet	Yes	194	19.9	197	19.0	19.4	NS

Contd...

Table 19.3–Contd...

		Male		Female		Total	P
		n/982	Per cent	n/1045	Per cent	Per cent	
Fluid consumption in ml/day							
(water +milk +laban +juices+drinks)	=/<1500 ml	228	23.3	357	34.4	29.0	0.000
	> 1500 ml	749	76.7	680	65.6	71.0	
Milk and milk products consumption per week	=/<3 times	796	81.2	896	85.9	83.6	0.004
	>3 times	184	18.8	147	14.1	16.4	
Milk and milk products type	Low fat/ skimmed	534	59.1	591	63.2	61.2	NS
	Full fat (=/>2 items)	370	40.9	344	36.8	38.8	
Vitamins/minerals supplements	yes	83	8.6	104	10.0	9.3	NS
Follow diet regimen	yes	325	33.3	432	41.6	37.6	0.000
Fat and cholesterol restriction	yes	123	12.6	160	15.4	14.0	
Sugar restriction	yes	94	9.6	125	12.0	10.9	
Salt restriction	yes	84	8.6	130	12.5	10.6	
More iron containing foods	yes	6	0.6	0	0.0	0.3	
More fibers	yes	7	0.7	7	0.7	0.7	

n = Number.

Totals do not add up to sample size due to missing information.

Discussion

This is the first such study conducted in Oman. The respondents were between 25 years and 55(minimum) years of age at the time of the blessed renaissance in 1970, prior to which there were few schools in Oman. Most having by then crossed the age for primary education and very few having the access, explains the high illiteracy. Females in the Arab world had less opportunity for formal education then and this accounts for the significant gender difference. The same is true for work opportunity and hence the elderly income significantly differs across gender.

Changes in lifestyle and socioeconomic status have led to life becoming more sedentary and the pattern of exercising having decreased steeply in most Arab countries [11]. This is true for our overall sample and especially with females who significantly spend less time in physical activity, as perhaps most of them have maids for daily chores and there is less awareness of importance of walking as an exercise. This along with multiparity [11] accounts for the more prevalent obesity amongst females. Similar obesity findings have been noted in rural/semi urban/ urban elderly females in Egypt[8].

Contrary to the general observation, that amongst the elderly, the proportions of females are higher due to the biological component contributing to their survival, in this interior region of Ad Dakhaliya we have less proportion of females in the 70-79 years range while it was nearly similar to males in the 80+ group (Table 19.1). A probable reason could be the unavailability of or wrong birth records in some, leading to misclassification. There are fewer cultural and social barriers for multiple marriages and remarriage by males which accounts for a significant proportion of males being married at the time of this study while a high percentage of females were widowed.

The overall findings suggest that nutrition related knowledge and beliefs need not positively corroborate with daily dietary habits in our elderly.

Elderly in our study, perhaps being accustomed to their dietary habits, resist change. Also they lack knowledge about benefits of nutritional foods resulting in not switching over to their consumption. Majority of our males and females believe that there is no need to change the quantity and quality respectively of nutrition with increasing age. A European study [12] reported 86 per cent of the elderly people believe they don't need to change their eating habits as they already eat healthy. However an Egyptian study reported otherwise [8].

Older persons residing outside of institutions eat reasonably well [13]. There is ample availability of foodstuff from different parts of the world, in Oman. A majority of our elders stay with family and there is a tradition in Arab countries of caring for the elderly. Thus, though there is a significant gender difference on whether the elderly are staying with their families or not, education and income, this is not reflected in their inadequacy of dietary intake of meat related items, cereals, fruits and sweets and also of the frequency of meals per day. Energy intakes fall with advancing age, but average protein intakes remain adequate [13]. High energy intake over decades leads to overweight in both genders [14]. There is a shift in Arab world, from consuming traditional foods to more westernized foods which are characterized by high fat, high cholesterol, low fiber and high sodium [11] The energy intake is by no means falling in our sample as seen from their BMI. The impact of promotional activities of the regional health-care system and of Nizwa Healthy City project of WHO on nutrition domain seems to work positively only for a minimal sample who are aware only of the often canvassed programs like Hypertension and Diabetes.

A high proportion of older adults in England had little basic nutrition knowledge and this presents a barrier to healthier eating [15]. Knowledge of associations between diet and diseases was particularly poor; 90 per cent of subjects being unaware of the benefits of high fruit and vegetable consumption. Men were found to have poorer nutrition knowledge [16]. We found no gender difference but the lack of knowledge related to fruits and vegetables reflects in poor consumption of vegetables but not fruits in our study.

A significant difference across gender was noted for whether, with advancing age, there is need to eat some specific type of food, the need for moderation of certain types of food and whether change in dietary habits can protect and control health problems at advancing age (Table 19.2). Females possessed less knowledge in our sample. In a study[17] related to fat intake from meat, meat products, dairy products and fried foods, females had higher nutrition knowledge scores and more negative views of the fatty foods than did males. More of our females had negative views on specific items like sweets, fat and salt consumption. However, when it came to actual consumption, only sweets were significantly less consumed by females, the other items being consumed equally by both the genders. Nutrition knowledge seems less clearly related to consumption of fatty foods than are more specific beliefs and attitudes [17].

Nutrition knowledge about dairy products is a better predictor of the type of milk consumed (lower fat milk to reduce fat intake) rather than the frequency of milk consumption [18]. We note similar findings. Knowledge about nutritional value of milk was very poor and females were less informed than males. Overall consumption is less than adequate in the total sample and significantly less in females. This shows the poor impact on this age group, of the ongoing Women's Health programme in Oman. Amongst those who consume, 40 per cent take full fat milk and milk products, which again reflects traditional habit.

In the Ageing Nutrition project in Europe [19], comparative analysis of 36 studies showed that the energy intake is too high, especially in some of the 'younger old' and seems not to be adjusted to the energy expenditure whereas it was considerably lower than recommended in some very old seniors in some countries. We cannot comment on the age difference, but energy intake is higher in our sample, which may be inferred from, the number of meals per day, the adequacy of food consumption (meat, cereals, sweets and fruits) and the finding that only 7.5 per cent of the total sample is underweight. Obesity and overweight was also found to be higher than underweight in elderly males and females in Egypt [8]. In UK's ageing population [20], under nutrition in older people is a significant public health issue but our results are contrary to this.

The 'willingness to eat' plays a central role with regard to appetite among elderly [21] and we correlate this with change in appetite noticed. It was decreased mainly due to unexplainable factors and due to illness and medication.

Gender differences were found in food choices and energy and nutrient intakes in older British people, especially those aged 65-79 years [22]. The meal frequency was found to be increased during aging in both genders, especially in men [14]. Women had more regular consumption of fruits and vegetables [23], milk and diary products vitamin supplements [14]. Almost all types of meat, eggs, and vegetables were more preferred by men and their energy intake was also higher. In both genders, fat represented a higher ratio (39 per cent) of energy intake than recommended. In our study the dietary consumption patterns differ significantly only for milk and milk products, sweets and fluids, with females consuming less. However there is no increase in the frequency of consumption or gender difference in the frequency.

Intervention trials[24] demonstrate that there are worthwhile health advantages for older persons in changing risk factors—e.g. weight reduction, sodium restriction, saturated fat reduction—to make later years healthier, more active and less dependent. Effective intervention is required for improving the knowledge among the elderly in our study. Dietary advice should be based on the elderly women's food preferences and habitual foods [25]. It is important to inform about known relations between food and disease. This is vital for our females who have more obesity.

Conclusions

The major limitations of our study were that we did not use a validated questionnaire. Also we could not quantify the food consumption due to non availability of food consumption tables for Oman [26]. Our findings of about 45 per cent of our elderly being overweight/obese and having overall poor knowledge of nutrition along with imbalanced nutrition and decreased physical activity warrants reorientation of the existing health promotion strategy for the elderly. The significant gender difference in nutritional knowledge needs to be addressed. The above findings need to be incorporated in the national strategy for the awareness and education programme for "Active aging and self care" proposed by the Ministry of Health and Ministry of Social Welfare [27]. A further detailed study is necessary in order to prepare a micro nutrient supplementation programme for the vulnerable population which includes the elderly. EMRO has addressed the issue of elderly health for over a decade and the need for appropriate food and nutrition care of the elderly has been identified. But the draft of proposed model national policy for the elderly by EMRO does not mention the nutrition component explicitly [28].The vital recommendations of the Third Arab Conference on Nutrition 2007 resulted in The Abu Dhabi Declaration to promote Healthy Nutrition in Arab countries [7]. But it has not specifically addressed ageing and nutrition-a growing global challenge!

References

1. Nutrition for older persons. World Health Organization http://www.who.int/nutrition/topics/ageing/en/index.html (accessed on 5 Oct, 2008).
2. McKevith B., 2005. Diet and healthy aging. J Br Menopause Soc, 11(4):121-5.
3. Lengyel CO, Tate RB, Bayomi DJ., 2007. Food group consumption and self-rated diets of elderly community-dwelling Canadian men. The Manitoba follow-up study. J Nutr Health Aging, 11(1):8-13.
4. Wahlqvist ML, Wahlqvist ML., 2002. 'Malnutrition' in the aged: the dietary assessment. Public Health Nutr , 5(6A):911-3
5. MOH Hospital Inpatients Morbidity (Table number 9-11) according to age groups and disease category in Annual Health Reports of the Ministry of Health, Oman, 2003 to 2007.
6. Ministry of National Economy, Oman, Census 2003.
7. Abu Dhabi Declaration to Promote Healthy Nutrition in the Arab countries. Recommendations of the Third Arab Conference on Nutrition, Abu Dhabi-UAE, 4-6 December 2007

   http://www.acnut.com/pdf/2ea.pdf (accessed on 10 Oct 2008)
8. Abd El Aty MA., 1990. Health profile of the geriatric group in Assuit governerate, Upper Egypt. Doctoral thesis. Public Health Department, Faculty of Medicine, Assuit University, Egypt.

9. Global Strategy on Diet, Physical Activity and Health. World Health Organization (http://www.who.int/dietphysicalactivity/factsheet_recommendations/en/index.html (accessed on 18 October 2008)

10. WHO Expert Consultation., 2004. Appropriate body-mass index for Asian populations and its implications for policy and intervention strategies. Lancet, 363(9403):157-63.

11. Musaiger AO., 2004. Overweight and obesity in the Eastern Mediterranean Region: can we control it? Eastern Mediterranean Health Journal. Vol 10, No.6, pages 789-793.

12. De Almeida MD,Garça P, Afonso C, Kearney JM, Gibney MJ., 2001. Healthy eating in European elderly: concepts, barriers and benefits. J Nutr Health Ageing, 5(4):217-9.

13. Wahlqvist ML *et al.*, 1995. Food habits in later life—an overview of key findings. Asia Pacific Journal of Clinical Nutrition, 4:1–11.

14. Rurik I., 2006. Nutritional differences between elderly men and women. Primary care evaluation in Hungary. , 50(1):45-50. Epub 2005 Nov 7.

15. Moynihan PJ, Mulvaney CE, Adamson AJ, Seal C, Steen N, Mathers JC, Zohouri FV., 2007. The nutrition knowledge of older adults living in sheltered housing accommodation. J Hum Nutr Diet, 20(5):446-58.

16. Baker AH, Wardle J., 2003. Sex differences in fruit and vegetable intake in older adults. Appetite, 40(3):269-75.

17. Shepherd R, Towler G., 2007. Nutrition knowledge, attitudes and fat intake: application of the theory of reasoned action. J Hum Nutr Diet, 20(3):170.

18. Elbon SM, Johnson MA, Fischer JG., 1996. Developing an instrument to measure the influence of knowledge, behaviours and attitudes on milk consumption patterns in older participants of a community wellness group: a pilot study. J Nutr Elderly, 15(4):21-37.

19. Lesser S, Pauly L, Volkert D, Stehle P and collaborators (Aging nutrition group)., 2008. Nutritional situation of the elderly in Eastern/Baltic and Central/Western Europe-the Ageing Nutrition project. Ann Nutr Metab, 52 suppl 1:62-71. Epub 2008 Mar 7.

20. Holmes S., 2004. What do we know about nutrition and older people? J Fam Healthcare ,14(6):153-5.

21. Wikby K, Fägerskiöld A., 2004. The willingness to eat. An investigation of appetite among elderly people. Scand J Caring Sci,18(2):120-7.

22. Bates CJ, Prentice A, Finch S., 1999. Gender differences in food and nutrient intakes and status indices from the National Diet and Nutrition Survey of people aged 65 years and over. Eur J Clin Nutr ,53(9):694-9.

23. Larrieu S, Letenneur L, Berr C, Dartigues JF, Ritchie K, Alperovitch A, Tavernier B, Barberger-Gateau P., 2004. Sociodemographic differences in dietary habits in

a population-based sample of elderly subjects: the 3C study. J Nutr Health Aging, 8(6):497-502.

24. Horwath CC., 1998. Nutrition and ageing. In: Mann JM, Truswell ST, eds. Essentials of human nutrition. New York, Oxford University Press,499–511.
25. Gustaffson K, Ekblad J, Sidenvall B., 2005. Older women and dietary advice: occurrence, comprehension and compliance. J Hum Nutr Diet, 18(6):421-2.
26. Nutrition Domain in the Seventh Five year plan for Health Development 2006-2010. Ministry of Health, Sultanate of Oman.
27. Dey AB., 2007. Report of the STC, WHO. Old age in healthcare in Primary Healthcare System of Sultanate of Oman.
28. A strategy for active, healthy ageing and old age care in the Eastern Mediterranean Region 2006-2015., 2006. Annex Three. World Health Organization, Cairo,.(WHO-EM/HSG/030/E/01.06/1000)

Chapter 20

A Method for Effectively Employing Graphic Communication Campaigns in the Prevention and Resolution of Health and Nutritional Problems

Yésica A. del Moral Zamudio

Researcher on Graphic Communication,
Dolma House, 1-B, Jogiwara Road, Behind TWA Hostel, P.O. Mcleod Ganj,
Dist. Kangra (H.P.) – 176 219, India
E-mail: ydm@yesicadelmoral.com

ABSTRACT

The main goal of this research paper is to present a practical method for successfully communicating messages – through the use of images – to help prevent and/or alleviate health and nutritional problems. Communication through images preceded writing historically and has been the most effective communication method in humanity's history.

Graphic communication is a process of visual communication with a specific purpose that meets practical requirements. It can be used to help resolve social problems or as a powerful means of manipulation. The effectiveness of any graphic communication process will depend, first of all, on the relevance the message holds for the recipient. For that reason, it is imperative that the sender of the message start with specific knowledge of the culture and the needs of the group being addressed. Such knowledge contributes to finding real solutions to relevant problems that will be applicable within the conditions of the group in question.

In order to build an understandable visual message, we need to get to know the way in which the group in question *understands* graphically. To accomplish that, it is advisable to conduct fieldwork within the community, carrying out different exercises in the reading and production of graphic material, with a focus on the particular problems to be addressed.An analysis of the graphic material compiled will help determine the appropriate syntax of the images to be created. Those images must be tested again within the community to be sure they are correctly putting across the intended message.Over the course of this presentation, I will use the case study of a rural, indigenous community in northern Mexico as an example of the way this method can contribute to the alleviation of specific health problems.

Keywords: *Graphic communication, Images, Visual messages, Method, Graphic campaigns.*

Introduction

Definition of the Problem

The present investigation seeks to demonstrate the value of graphic communication in the development of health and nutrition campaigns, as well as to establish basic parameters that contribute to guaranteeing effective creation of visual employed messages.

"A drawing has always been the easiest means of graphic communication amongst men, even before inventing the alphabet."[1]

To begin, a few brief words on the science of visual communication. A drawing is made up of graphic signs arranged on a surface or format.

Communication through graphic symbols is a language just like any other, with its own syntax or order. The syntactic articulation of the elements and structures of the image translates the principles that govern perceptual organization in formal aspects that are submitted, albeit unconsciously, to complex processes of relation, transformation and interpretation that culminate in the capacity to identify and grasp a meaning.

The job of the graphic communicator is the process of visual creation via methodological instruments applicable to the development of projects that, guided by a clear intention, permit one to reach the obtainment of concrete results.

In that context, graphic design is a process that seeks the resolution of communication problems through the use of images.

These images, when used properly, become powerful tools that can be used as much for manipulation as for social betterment. Within the framework of this conference, we can assert that images can be used to inform and disseminate and to improve the health and nutritional conditions of women and their children, which can result in general results on a societal level.

Justification of the Interest in the Problem

Each year, Mexico spends millions of pesos on the creation of graphic communication campaigns to alleviate health problems. By law, the government must devote part of that budget to indigenous groups.

---

1. German-Fabris. Fundamentos del proyecto gráfico, p. 16

There are fifty-four (54) different indigenous groups living in very diverse geographical zones in Mexico. Each one of them faces specific problems that are not always shared amongst them. Nevertheless, graphic health campaigns meant to apply to all of them equally are organized from the center of the country by the National Health Department. This situation piqued my curiosity as a graphic designer. Thus I decided to work with an indigenous group, in order to study the importance of such graphic health campaigns. The surprising result of what I found not only transformed my outlook on design, but also my understanding of conceptual perception. A significant portion of this research was used in the preparation of my Bachelor's thesis in collaboration with the graphic designer Marco Antonio Sandoval Valle.[2]

The selected health messages were not relevant to the health problems experienced by that group, and the proposed solutions were not applicable within the conditions in which they lived. But in addition, people did not understand the images, and thus they didn't pay them the slightest attention.

With the aid of an interdisciplinary team of experts (anthropologists, medical anthropologists and educators) already working in the region, we very quickly realized that there were essential health problems within the group that could be solved quite simply, using resources that were already available within the communities. So the challenge was to find a way to communicate these ideas using images in a way that people would understand. To that end, it was decided to take a different approach to the problem: Instead of trying to decide the appropriate visual communication approach from the point of view of our mainstream, urban logic, it would be sought from the viewpoint of the community itself and their conceptions.

The next part of the research therefore centered on identifying the way in which the group interpreted and created images, with the goal of utilizing those same graphic elements for the creation of health messages proposed by the experts.

As a result of that work, a functional design object was developed for the group in question. But it has also been my wish to generate a model that can be applied broadly to the creation of graphic communication campaigns that contribute to the resolution of health and nutritional problems and problems of social well-being.

Objectives

To show the value of graphic communication in its application to prevention and relief of women's health and nutritional problems.

To set out a model for the creation of effective graphically communicated messages that promote solutions for health and nutritional problems and to substantiate that model with elements from research conducted in northern Mexico within the Rarámuri indigenous community.

---

2. Del Moral Zamudio Yésica A. and Sandoval Valle Marco Antonio. Promoviendo cuidados para mejorar la salud en la Sierra Tarahumara a través de un objeto de diseño. México. 1997

Hypothesis

It is possible to apply, within a given cultural context, a generally applicable model that can contribute to the construction of effective graphic messages for use in the prevention and relief of women's health and nutritional problems.

Methodology

The approach for this model will be set forth on the basis of a case study with an indigenous community in northern Mexico, known as the Rarámuri or Tarahumara.

It will begin with a general presentation of the group, its environs and several aspects of the community's health that are relevant to the research.

A comparison will be established between the health problems addressed by the previously existing health campaigns and the problems noted by cultural experts, as well as possible solutions to identify messages that target the group's necessities and circumstances.

Some of the results of the fieldwork focused on identifying the way in which the community understands and interprets graphically will also be presented.

Based on fundamental principles established in the field of graphic design by such experts as Germani-Fabris[3], Donis A. Dondis[4] and Wucius Wong,[5] a format for analysis was constructed and then applied both to drawings created in the Tarahumara region and to the existing health-related graphic material. In this document, I will present a drawing exercise as an example of the way in which the analysis of material gathered through fieldwork provides the data needed to understand the group's conceptions of sickness and health that can then be utilized for the creation of effective visual messages.

I will also outline the design solution that was ultimately prescribed to deal with the health problems in the Tarahumara, and finally explain the model for the effective creation of graphic messages.

Main Body

A Case Study as an Example: The Tarahumara, An Indigenous Group in Northern Mexico

The Tarahumara, or Rarámuri, as they prefer to call themselves (*Rarámuri* means "those of light feet"), comprise an indigenous group living in the southern region of the state of Chihuahua, in northern Mexico.

The region inhabited by the Tarahumara is known as the Sierra Tarahumara. It covers an area of approximately 50,000 square kilometers and is made up of a group of mountain ranges that give rise to stark environmental contrasts that impact the inhabitants' way of life. The Tarahumara, in large part, become semi-nomads in

---

3. Germani-Fabris. Fundamentos del proyecto gráfico. Edicionés Don Bosco
4. Dondis, Donis A. Primer of Visual Literacy. MIT Press
5. Wong, Wucius. Fundamentos del diseño bi- y tri-dimensional. Editorial Gustavo Gili

order to adapt to the climatic contrasts created by the mountains (which reach altitudes as high as 3856 meters above sea level) and the valleys (some 500 to 1200 meters above sea level) throughout the various seasons.

The Tarahumara are a people who basically live on agriculture. Their main crops – and thus the staples of their diet – are corn (maize), beans, squash and to a lesser degree potatoes and other legumes. In most cases, they also have some livestock – cattle, goats and sheep – which are for their own consumption or for sale within the community.

Their way of relating to the space around them is a manifestation of their social organization. That is clearly seen in how the Rarámuris organize themselves into *rancherías*, small communities comprising clusters of domestic units, bound together by alliance, family ties or reciprocity.

Each domestic unit possesses its own property, made up of a one- or two-room shack built from stone, wood, adobe or a combination of those materials. Located in the center of their fields, its function is for storage of the family's belongings, for sleeping, and occasionally for cooking. In the area around the shack, one finds: a fire place, which is an important meeting point; a place for storing grain; a chicken coop elevated on four posts in order to keep predators at bay; a livestock pen that can be moved across the fields, to fertilize the earth; and a ceremonial space where rituals and ceremonies are conducted.

The interaction among the clustered domestic units in each ranchería is indispensable for survival in their economic system, which is based on cooperative work.

The obligation of mutual aid goes without saying, and the only payment is *tesgüino*, a thick, milky and nutritious corn beverage that is fermented with the seeds of a local grass. "The *tesgüinada* (a get-together where people drink tesgüino) plays an important role in all aspects of social life, apart from those fulfilled by the group formed by the domestic unit. It is the religious, economic and recreational group, the group at whose heart disputes are settled, where marriages are arranged, and where business deals are made."[6] For a Rarámuri, the most significant group outside his or her family context is the one with whom they drink tesgüino, and that group is made up of guests from different rancherías.

A third form of social organization, introduced by Jesuit missionaries, was the "mission town," which these days servers as the center of civic-religious activity for a given group of rancherías from which people attend meetings there on Sundays to impart justice, celebrate religious rites, and where people go to school. The town is the place where personal, family and matrimonial conflicts are resolved by authorities elected by consensus, and where people go to hear the Tarahumara governor deliver a sermon full of advice that covers most of the necessities of Rarámuri life. These meetings in the town exert a centralizing force. The Rarámuri see their neighbors, find out the latest news, attend hearings and identify with a group that is larger than

---

6. Kennedy, John. Inápuchi, una comunidad tarahumara gentil, p. 119-120.

the domestic unity and the ranchería. Nevertheless, it is important to note the fact that the majority of the Tarahumara do not live in towns, given the fact that it is a place where there is a great *mestizo* (mixed, mainstream culture) influence.

There are strong variations within the Tarahumara population. Depending upon their acceptance of the Catholic or Protestant religions, the contact they have had with mestizos and the area in which they live, there may be linguistic differences or differences in dress.

The Rarámuri conceptions about the world and existence stem from a reinterpretation of elements of the Catholic religion combined with traditional religious concepts.

Health Factors among the Rarámuri

At one of the early stages of this research, Dr. Zuanilda Mendoza González, a medical anthropologist from the Department of History and Philosophy of Medicine at the National Autonomous University of Mexico (UNAM), pointed out a fact which would become a key to the rest of the study: In multicultural countries like Mexico, within the health field, in regard to rural and indigenous communities, we should try to identify first of all what their ideas around health and sickness are. That meant, recognizing that there is more than one way of seeing health and sickness. From that moment onward, identifying those concepts became one of the main purposes of our investigation.

"Addressing sickness would seem to be relatively easy if we do it from the point of view of clinical medicine and the natural sciences, whose focus is made up of nosological entities constructed by a combination of signs and symptoms, with an etiology, a diagnosis, a prognosis and a treatment. As if the disease existed on its own. And for that reason, whenever it was presented before the doctor's eyes, it would be seen in the same way. Yet disease presents a double construction: the one that comes from the doctor and the one expressed by the sick person. Both, in different ways, are conditioned by social, cultural and technical factors."[7]

In the Tarahumara population, one finds endemic diseases such as tuberculosis, chronic vitamin deficiency and malnutrition; seasonal gastrointestinal or respiratory diseases; but psychosomatic illnesses such as bewitchings, contaminations and the loss of a soul also hold an important place.

Amongst the Tarahumara, it is believed that Rarámuri men have three souls, Rarámuri women have four souls and animals and mestizos have two. Life depends upon these souls (which are associated with the breath), and for that reason the Rarámuri believe that death occurs when all of a person's souls have left the body. Nevertheless, souls have a tendency to go for walks at night, which is why dreams occur. And on occasion, those wandering souls can get trapped by some evil force, resulting in serious illnesses.

In the Sierra, there are people with knowledge of medicinal plants (of which there are as many as 600 species in the region); those who suck foreign objects of the

---

7. Mendoza González, Zuanilda. 'Enfermedad para quién' p. 117

body; specialists in plants that have souls (such as peyote); dream wizards who, in their dreams, recover the souls of the sick person that may have gone missing or may have been stolen by following their tracks; and also medical officers at health clinics.

When someone in the Tarahumara falls ill, their family and acquaintances get together to try to discern the causes of the illness. They analyze the relations the person has had with all the beings around them, since some of those, possessors of souls, might have been offended, provoking the person's malaise. In accordance with what social custom indicates for a given cause, they then call for a priest or a native specialist, offer an animal sacrifice or even seek out medicine or official assistance.

A Rarámuri might be in a suboptimal state of health or in fact be chronically ill, but if he or she has enough strength to work and be happy, they are considered healthy. In contrast, if the person is considered to be bewitched, while they may not present a single physical problem, the conviction of their beliefs can even lead them to death.

Different Proposals for the Tarahumara Health Problems

The government's graphic health campaigns at the time of this study were promoted through health centers located in towns which are, as mentioned previously, basically places where people get together once a week, not where the Rarámuri traditionally live. To reach them, the Tarahumara sometimes need to walk several hours. In addition, people generally do not visit those health centers unless they are seriously ill.

During our fieldwork, we had the opportunity to visit several health centers and speak to the doctors and nurses in charge. We also had the good fortune to meet with cultural experts, anthropologists and health educators who were already totally familiar with the problems faced by the Tarahumara. It is based on their comments and observations that I am able to put forth the following ideas:

The main graphic materials distributed in the Tarahumara were posters and leaflets. They emphasized:

- ☆ Construction of latrines.
- ☆ Promoting the boiling of water in order to avoid gastrointestinal illnesses.
- ☆ No-scalpel vasectomy.

But these proposals presented certain problems. For one thing, although towns and schools in the Sierra Tarahumara have made an effort to build latrines, their maintenance has proved very complicated. Some experts in the subject mentioned that a latrine requires at least eight liters of water per day in order to be kept clean. But water is a scarce and much prized resource in the region, given that it must be carried by hand from water sources, rivers or natural springs that may be several kilometers from the home. Simply supplying themselves with enough water to cook each day is a great effort for a family, and for that reason, water would never be used to clean latrines. Thus the latrines become a source of infection.

On the other hand, the cultural experts pointed out that space is not a problem in the Tarahumara, given that the Rarámuri communities hardly have any population density. On the contrary, people live very isolated lives in small rancherías and each house is separated from the others by their fields. Their suggestion, then, was to promote open-air defecation and to teach people to cover their excrement with dirt.

Gastrointestinal ailments play an important role in the Rarámuri communities, but just as water is a scarce resource that is difficult to obtain, wood is, too, and most people cook only with wood. Given a choice between using the wood they have for cooking or for boiling water, the decision is not a difficult one.

In this situation, the anthropologists made an interesting observation: The water in the springs is clean water, accumulated by filtration through tiny natural cavities in the rock, and as such is good to drink. But given that it is found in the open air, it is easily contaminated by organic material, such as leaves, which decompose within the mater. Also, given that these water sources are unprotected, they are open to being transited or consumed by animals. The suggestion, then, was to urge the communities to build a small fence around and roof over the water that would prevent animals from drinking directly from the spring.

While the national government was trying to promote vasectomy among the Tarahumara, the indigenous population in the region was facing infant mortality rates of 50 per cent. Out of every eight children conceived, only four would reach the age of seven. Given the harshness of life in the region, each family needs each of its family members in order to survive. They are not facing problems of overpopulation, but rather the spectre of extinction.

The experts' suggestion once again arose from their deep knowledge of the problem in the context of the community: The majority of Rarámuri women feed their babies nothing but mother's milk for the first two years of life, and that seems to lead to serious problems with malnutrition in the children. Thus the response was to teach mothers to incorporate other foods into the baby's diet beginning at the age of 6 months or when the first tooth emerges.

Through these examples, I would once again like to highlight the vital importance of starting with health messages based on the real needs of the communities, and proposals that present viable options for solving specific, existent problems.

Once the problem and its cause(s) have been identified, it is much easier to find appropriate responses that can be translated into images.

Fieldwork

The fieldwork carried out in the Tarahumara had as its objectives: to identify the way the Tarahumara represent and understand images in general and their graphic approach to the concepts of sickness and health in particular, even in a very basic way, in order to be able to create graphic messages that would communicate to them.

The simplest way to carry out this research was to work in schools that had been set in the Sierra by the National Institute for Indigenous People (Instituto Nacional Indigenista or INI) which were of two types: the first of them being a boarding school where the children live and sleep from Monday through Friday, returning to their homes only on the weekends. The second type is the day (or "unitary") school where children attend from nine in the morning to five at night with the option of going home to sleep at night. The major drawback of that format is the distance, since some children need to walk as much as four hours in each direction in order to attend each day.

The school is not seen as strengthening or incorporating Tarahumara culture. Rather, many Tarahumara people see school as the place where children learn how *not* to be Rarámuri, and they send their children there to reduce the economic pressure of feeding the family or with the idea that their children will learn to read and count in order to be able to defend themselves against the mestizos. Nevertheless, we relied on those schools because they are important meeting places and it would have been practically impossible to achieve our aims in any other way given the vast territory. In addition, children were the group with the most free time available to participate in the project, since adults are busy all day with the activities of their community. Still, the few drawings we were able to collect from adults, along with examples of their weaving which were analyzed, show the use of the same elements that the children used in regard to form, composition and color.

The field research covered three communities: Samachique, Basigochi and Kírare. In the first, work was carried out in three day schools at three different levels: kindergarten, primary school and secondary school. In the second, work was conducted at a day school at the primary-school level and in the third, work was conducted at boarding school covering kindergarten through primary school.

With whatever material they were given – their choice of sheets of paper, poster board, chalk, aniline paints, colored pencils, crayons and acrylic paints – the children created a great number of drawings on a given topic

Some of the topics explored included:

- ✰ The place where you live
- ✰ Draw something hot, something dangerous, a sick person, a form of transportation, something you like, something you don't like
- ✰ Draw your hands
- ✰ Illustrate a given story
- ✰ Let's make masks.

By means of these drawings, we were able to understand the degree to which the children knew their surroundings, how they perceived them and the similarity of their representation to reality. The exercises also contributed relevant data about the cultural concepts associated with the states of health and sickness.

Analysis of the Graphic Material Obtained

A basic analytical format was constructed, underpinned by the principal theories of design, with the purpose of identifying relevant elements in a specific order:

- ✰ Form

- ✩ Representation
- ✩ Size
- ✩ Proportion
- ✩ Depth
- ✩ Composition
- ✩ Equilibrium
- ✩ Color

In regard to form, it was found throughout all the schools that at the beginning, the children utilize absolute forms, inspired by nature, created with lines or abstract surfaces, especially flowers. And as they grow, the children augment the representation of relative forms (those that imitate and reproduce the forms of things that already exist and that describe their surroundings in an exact way), such as the houses around theirs with the exact type of material they are made from or the corrals with the exact type and number of animals they contain. One can observe, even in the work done by kindergarteners, a proportional relation between the size of what is represented and its real size. For example, the relationship between the size of a man and a house, or between a man and a flower, and one can even see a correct proportional relationship between the size of a horse and the size of a burro (a small donkey) or between the size of one house and the other houses around it.

The Rarámuri children's drawings are representations that correspond to their particular cultural environment with great realism and demonstrate a great deal of precision in the details. When the children are very young, they rely upon a minimal number of graphic elements to give the idea of what they're trying to represent, such as a field of flowers made up of horizontal stripes of a single color, indicating the earth, from which vertical stripes of different colors emerge, indicating the flowers. Or they represented elements simply, such as the human figure, passing through a child's natural evolutionary stages, but with a great deal of details based on reality, *i.e.* the father being drawn with his legs uncovered and the mother being drawn with clothing covering her below the knee (exactly like the actual clothing they typically wear).

The technique most often used by the children to give a sense of depth is a gradation of size, on which nearby objects appear bigger, while distant ones appear smaller.

Their way of situating forms in space corresponds to the Germani-Fabris classification of "free" or "dynamic" and "continuous."[8] This is seen in the children who come from the strongest culturally Rarámuri backgrounds. In all the drawings, with the exception of those from Samachique, one can observe a great sense of equilibrium, in the way that Dondis[9] sets out – a constructive horizontal-vertical relation. In fact in Kírare it was common to see that the verticality is subject to the line

8. Germani-Fabris. Fundamentos del proyecto gráfico. pp. 18-21
9. Dondis, Donis A. Primer of Visual Literacy. MIT Press

of the Earth, and therefore they draw curved hills with trees perpendicular to the Earth, even from the position they occupy along the curve of the hill.

It turned out to be complicated to learn the language the Rarámuris attribute to color, though we can deduce a bit from the observations made during the fieldwork, the report from the experts on the culture, and the drawings collected from the Rarámuri. This only marks a beginning, but as a result of analysis of the collected material, it is possible to observe that the Rarámuri adhere completely to reality in their representation of forms, but not in regard to color.

The Rarámuri do not employ any modulation of color – they use only saturated tones without intermediate gradations. Nor do they use achromatic gradations. They handle tonal contrasts, from warm to cold and complementary tones. With respect to the last item, when they place two complementary colors next to each other, they give more surface area to the less luminous color. The children do associate yellow, orange, red and pink with warmth.

It is noteworthy that in places like Kírare, an area with a very strong Rarámuri presence, the children demonstrated a great richness of observation and representation, even in regard to the boarding school they attend. In contrast in Samachique, a town with a large mestizo influence, it is only possible to find that type of drawings among children in kindergarten, because as the children advance through the various classes, the colors lose saturation and their observation and representation of the world is less sharp.

To illustrate the way in which the graphic material compiled during the fieldwork can provide data relevant to the research at hand as well as graphic elements that can be used in graphic messages, I will show one of the exercises carried out.

The children from the Kírare third-grade class (ages seven to nine years) made masks using brown paper bags on which they drew the faces of healthy and sick people using acrylic paints. The purpose was to get to know the concepts culturally associated with those states.

In order to do this, the children put the paper bags on their heads and, assisting one another, drew the area of the eyes. Then they took off the bags and cut out the spaces for the eyes following the outlines they had drawn, thus creating a mask. Then they were instructed to paint sick or healthy people, depending on which group they were in. This principle yielded the result that the children drew the faces life-size, and therefore corresponded with reality. In the masks, it is possible to observe elements that coincide with the general aspects of graphic representation mentioned previously, such as seeking equilibrium based on a horizontal-vertical construction. In this case, the drawings do not indicate depth, but rather are situated on a single plane. With respect to colors, they employed saturated tones without any modulation, but one aspect that made this exercise interesting for the children was that they were only given primary colors that they had to mix in order to obtain secondary ones. That was quite a discovery, and it really amazed them.

The task of analyzing the masks was very simple, and began with the application of primary elements of drawing and a reasoned interpretation of the cultural elements that are identifiable in order to discover elements of the physical manifestation of health and sickness in the children's graphic representations.

Representation of Sickness

It is possible to identify in the masks clear signs indicating sickness through graphic elements. For example, in masks 3 and 4 (below), one can see things coming out of the mouth. In masks 2 and 4, one can observe large bumps covering the face and, in the first case, reaching the hairline, which occurs in diseases such as measles (which is still present in the region). It has already been noted that these children have a great capacity for observation that they demonstrate through their graphic representation, and for that reason it is probable that these faces are examples of real diseases they have observed.

Mask 2 shows the eyes closed, which can refer to a person lying down and therefore definitely sick within the framework of Rarámuri logic. We know this thanks to another exercise in graphic dictation in which the children were asked to draw sick people, not just their faces, but whole people, and the result was that each and every child, without exception, drew people who were lying down.

Mask 3 has large red patches on the cheeks, possibly indicating a high fever.[10]

Upon examining these four masks, it is possible to perceive pain at a glance, but to identify the graphic indicators that represent pain was a bit more complicated task, albeit very interesting.

The basic area where the experience of suffering is expressed is the mouth. Not only in terms of its form or contour but also in terms of the quality of the stroke used, especially as evidenced in its movement. All of them are shown open, and if the faces are transected by a pair of axes to orient horizontal and vertical lines, we find that the four masks that show signs of sickness present the mouth significantly off the vertical axis, which formally generates dynamism and instability, breaking with the equilibrium and symmetry but expressively evoking the experience of pain and discomfort, imitating the gestures one might make in such circumstances.

It is interesting to reflect at this point that the children could not alter the position of the eyes to any great degree, given that they had been outlined and cut out at the beginning of the exercise in order to create the mask. Thus they fell back on the facial element with the next strongest capacity for expression.

Another noteworthy point is the predominance of the color yellow, interpreted here as a sign of sickness due to being an alteration of the natural color of the Rarámuri community (Figure 20.1).

If we trace the horizontal and vertical axes over the features of the face in the masks to observe their form and dynamism, this is what we find shown in Figure 20.2).

---

10. AA.VV. La Medicina Tradicional de los Pueblos Indígenas de México. Tarahumara

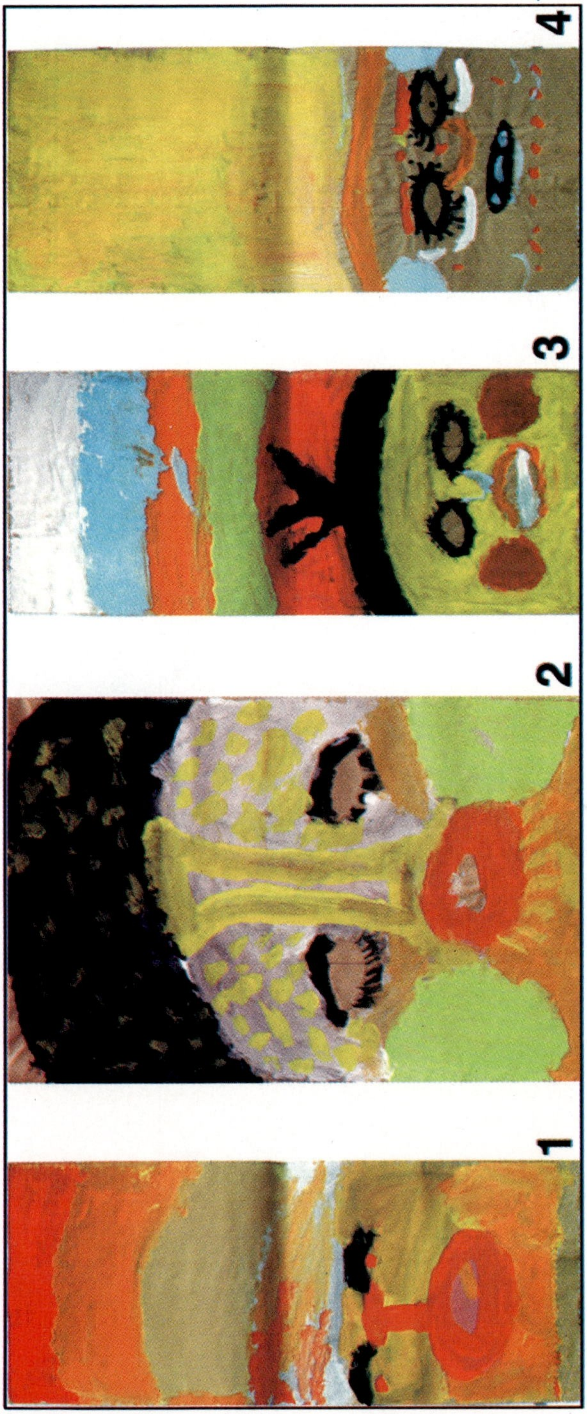

Figure 20.1

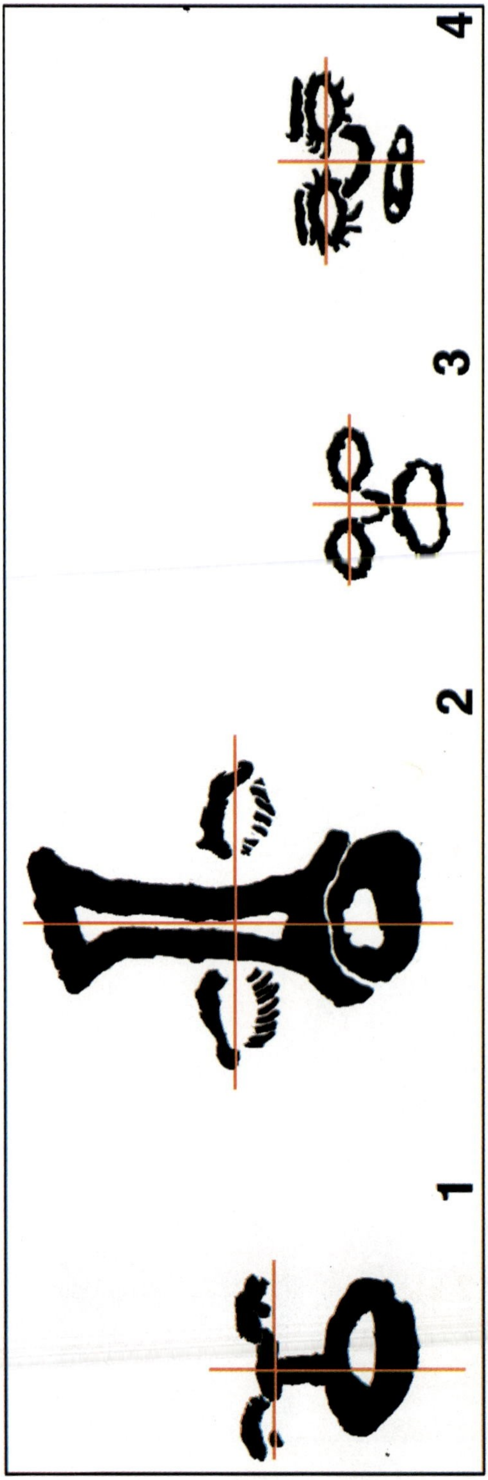

Figure 20.2

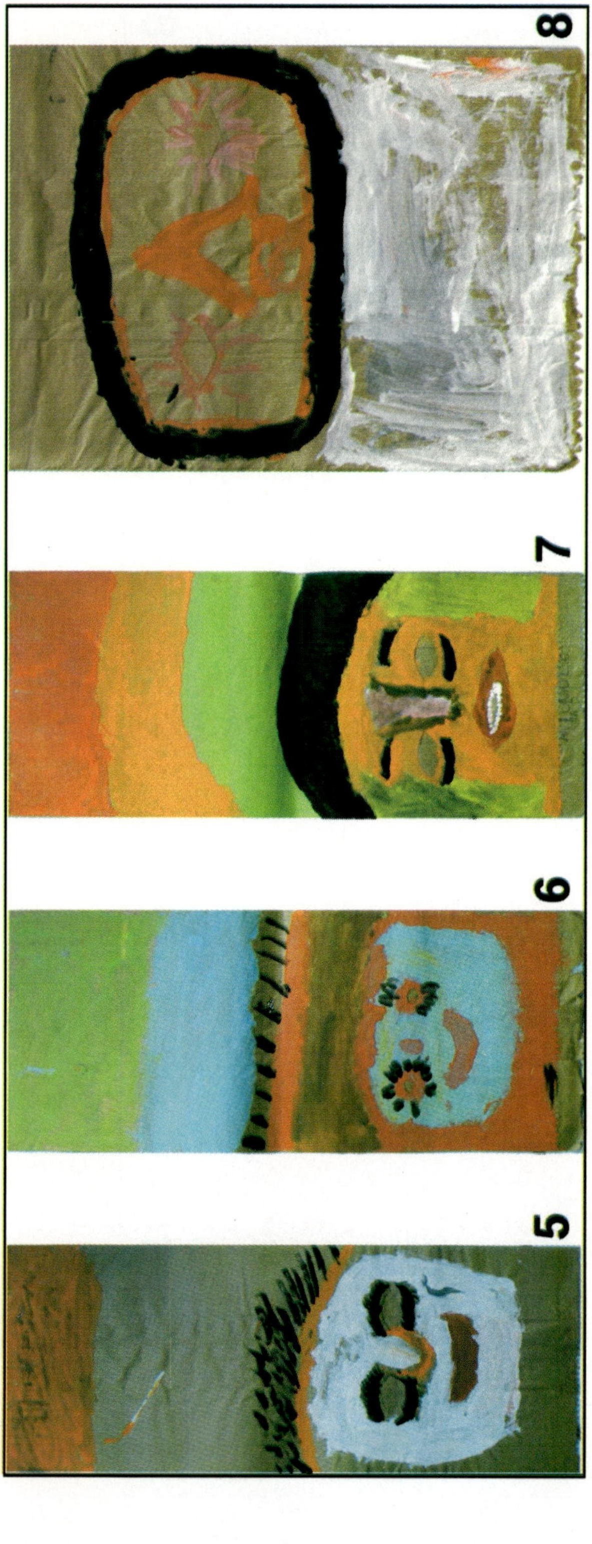

Figure 20.3

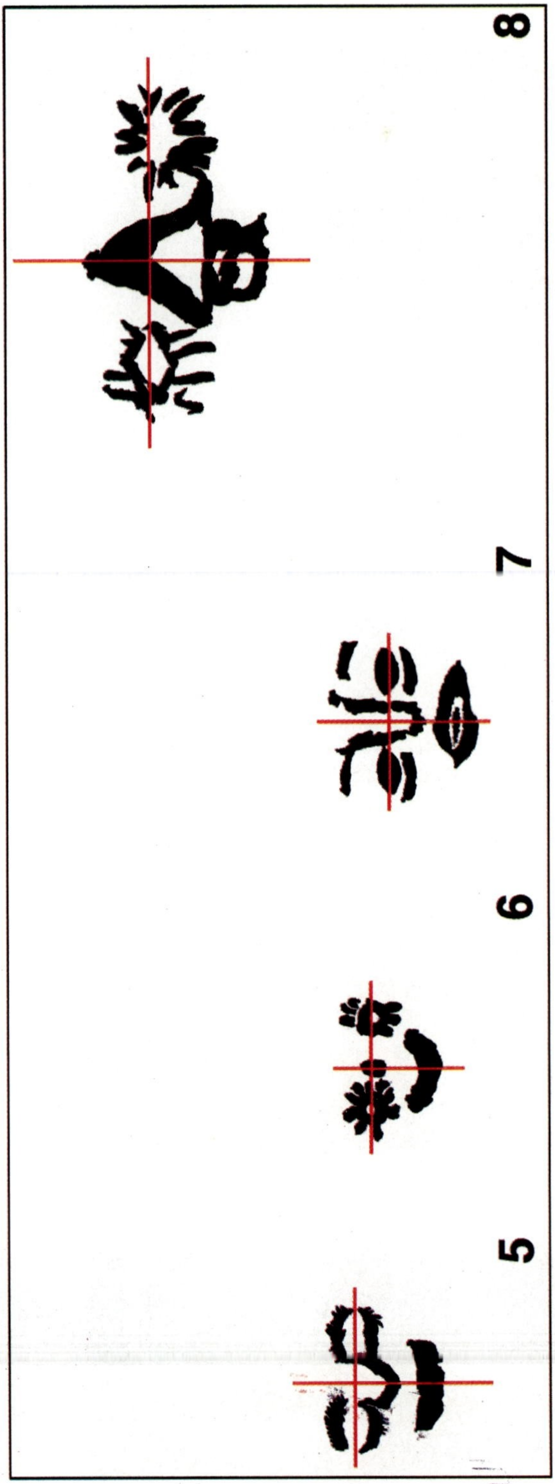

Figure 20.4

Representations of Healthiness

The mouth is once again, in large part, the element indicating the represented experience, happiness, which is manifest basically through the use of a simple curved line (in Figures 20.4 masks 5 and 6), representing a smile. The third mask in the series does not present such a pronounced curve, but it allows the teeth to be seen, which also evokes a smile. The fourth face in the series is shown totally in repose, the area of the mouth being demarcated by two semicircles, which can represent the lips rather simply, in a position parallel to the horizon.

Once again, the children faced the limitation of not being able to play with the position of the eyes due to the aforementioned technique, and curiously they relied upon the same element to communicate what was being asked of them.

Upon applying to these four faces the same lines forming horizontal and vertical axes, we observe greater stability and symmetry than in the faces of the sick people.

These drawings and their analysis show us that the manifestation of the states of healthiness and sickness in the graphic representation of the Tarahumara children is linked to the concepts of happiness and suffering, respectively. That supports the data generated in the documentary research about how the culture defines those states.

The graphic elements employed by the children to communicate those concepts were the form, disposition and movement of the factions of the face, especially the mouth, in relation to the horizontal and vertical axes of the face, breaking or preserving its basic symmetry.

The expression of these states was reinforced by the quality of the strokes and the use of color (yellow in the case of sickness).

Once the analysis of the graphic material obtained in the Tarahumara was completed using formal categories of design, the same analytical scheme was applied to the graphic material distributed by the government health agencies. It was determined that not only that they did not use the same parameters, but in fact that in most cases they relied upon completely opposite elements, which would explain why those graphic messages were not understandable to the Rarámuri population.

Results of the Research in the Tarahumara

As a result of the work carried out with the cultural experts and the observations obtained through the fieldwork, the following health messages, aimed at improving health among the Rarámuri, were agreed upon:

- ☆ Fence in and cover water sources and impede animals' direct access to them.
- ☆ Cover their stools.
- ☆ Enrich children's diets starting with the emergence of their first tooth.
- ☆ Promote the use of water and soap, especially in cleaning children, in order to prevent skin diseases.

These messages were illustrated with drawings that made use of the same special distribution and form of representation used by the Rarámuris, and they were accompanied by short sentences, in the form of advice, as befits Rarámuri discourse. These sentences were interspersed with phrases in Rarámuri.

Given that the Tarahumara cover such a vast space and that their communities live so isolated from one another, it was very important to seek out a design object that was easy to distribute among the Rarámuri population, something that people could have in their homes that would serve as a constant reminder and at the same time fulfill some utilitarian function that would turn it into a valuable object that people would want to preserve. The perfect result of that search was a calendar. Each message would be displayed on a bimonthly page that would include a ritual and agricultural calendar with graphic representations of Rarámuri logic.

At the conclusion of the sketch-drawing stage, members of the interdisciplinary team returned to the community to verify whether or not the messages were clear, and based on that experience, the necessary adjustments were made.

A Generally Applicable Model for the Creation of Effective Graphic Messages that Contribute to the Relief of Social Problems

1. Start with a well-defined group that presents specific problems.
2. Establish familiarity with the group's culture.
3. With the support of specialists in the problem area (for example health, education, etc.), identify the messages to communicate that include concrete options/solutions that can be applied given the conditions and facilities that the people involved in that problem have.
4. Study the way that the group represents and understands graphically. This phase of the process requires fieldwork in the community in question to carry out different types of graphic exercises:

   Studies in visual reading that enable one to get to know how the community understands visually, graphic exercises aimed at understanding how the group represents things graphically, and particularly how the group relates to and thinks about the problem in question.
5. Analyze the graphic material obtained.
6. Identify which type of graphic material is most suitable for that particular community.
7. Sketching stage. Create one or more images using the graphic criteria found in the fieldwork that will clearly communicate the intended message.
8. Test the effectiveness of the image(s) with the group.
9. Make the necessary corrections or adjustments to ensure correct understanding of the message.
10. Print or produce the final graphic material.
11. Distribute the graphic material.

Conclusions

Images are powerful elements that can be utilized in graphic communication campaigns to contribute to social well-being.

In health campaigns, visual messages serve concrete communication functions, spreading information for the betterment of the health and nutrition conditions of specific groups. In the context of this conference, that would be women and their children.

The concepts of healthiness and sickness are determined culturally. In multicultural countries and rural or indigenous communities, it is especially important to identify the attributes linked to those concepts in relation to their context. Once those are identified, it is possible to articulate, through the use of graphic elements, images that are a clear expression of those states, so as to communicate messages that promote prevention and care.

By starting with specific health problems, feasible and complete solutions can be sought, and those can be translated into images for their easily and rapid dissemination. The construction of graphic messages must start with common codes of visual communication that take into account the recipients' way of understanding and representing. To gain that knowledge, a generally applicable model for the development of graphic messages is proposed. It offers the necessary framework for approaching communities which present specific problems and identifying their way of conceptualizing and representing those problems so as to be able to use their own visual language to present viable solutions and alternatives to them

Acknowledgements

This research work was the product of a collective effort of an interdisciplinary group of experts. Without their participation and guidance it would never have been possible to complete it.

I would like to thank my research partner, Marco Antonio Sandoval, and our thesis advisor, Laura Elena Espinosa Aguilar, for their support throughout the research process.

I would also like to especially thank the anthropologists Eduardo Gotés and Nicolás Olivos for opening the doors of the Rarámuri culture for us and guiding us within it.

To Dr. Zuanilda Mendoza and to Laura Prada, who were our guides for aspects of medical anthropology and who made important contributions to this research.

To all the Rarámuri who welcomed us into their homes and in particular to those children who accompanied us on all the paths.

All my gratitude to my professors in my master's and doctoral programs who introduced me to the world of research and showed me all the necessary methodological tools.

To my husband, Peter Aronson, who assisted with the translation of this document and who is a constant source of support, inspiration and motivation in my life.

References

1. AA.VV. 2009. *La Medicina Tradicional de los Pueblos Indígenas de México*. Biblioteca Digital de la Medicina Tradicional Mexicana. México City. http://www.medicinatradicionalmexicana.unam.mx/index.php
2. Anzures y Bolaños, Maria del Carmen, 1978. *Medicina tradicional entre los tarahumaras*. Mexico City.
3. Buenrostro, Manuel, 1994. *Educación y Cultura Tarahumara*. Thesis for Bachelors Degree in Social Anthropology. Escuela Nacional de Antropología e Historia, Mexico City.
4. Dondis, Donis A., 1974. *Primer of Visual Literacy*. Publisher MIT Press. Cambridge, USA.
5. Genest, Serge, 1980. *Introducción a la Etnomedicina*. Revista de medicina tradicional. Volume II No. 8, Mexico City.
6. Germani-Fabris, 1973. *Fundamentos del proyecto gráfico*. Ediciones Don Bosco. Barcelona.
7. Gonzáles Rodríguez, Luis, 1982. *Tarahumara, la Sierra y el hombre*. Editorial Fondo de Cultura Económica, Mexico City.
8. Gotés, Eduardo. Personal interviews. 1994-1996. *La percepción rarámuri*. Director of the Tarahumara language and culture workshop at the Escuela Nacional de Antropología e Historia, Mexico City.
9. Kennedy, John, 1970. *Inápuchi. Una comunidad tarahumara gentil*. Instituto Indigenista Americano, Mexico City.
10. Mendoza González, Zuanilda, 1997. *'Enfermedad para quién' Saber popular entre los triquis*. Artículo académico. http://www.juridicas.unam.mx/publica/librev/rev/nuant/cont/52/cnt/cnt5.pdf
11. Moral Zamudio Yésica A. del and Sandoval Valle Marco Antonio, 1997. *Promoviendo cuidados para mejorar la salud en la Sierra Tarahumara a través de un objeto de diseño*. Thesis for Bachelors Degree in Graphic Design. Universidad Nacional Autónoma de México. ENEP Acatlán. Mexico.
12. Olivos, Nicolás, 1998. *El proceso de incorporación de la Sierra Tarahumara a la Sociedad Nacional*. Thesis for Bachelors Degree in Social Anthropology. Escuela Nacional de Antropología e Historia, Mexico City.
13. Wucius, Wong, 1992. *Fundamentos del diseño bi- y tri-dimensional*. Editorial Gustavo Gili. Mexico City.

Chapter 21

Narratives Around Dietary and Exercise Practices of Young Urban Females

M.H. Sedibe[1] and Shane Norris[2]

[1]Faculty of Health Sciences, University of the Witwatersrand
111 Quintus van der Walt Street Norkem Park
[2]WITS University, Birth to Twenty Research Programme
Faculty of Health Sciences, University of the Witwatersrand
7 York Road Medical School, Parktown
E-mail: [1]sedibemh@gmail.com, [1]modiehi.sedibe@wits.ac.za,
[2]san@global.co.za

ABSTRACT

In many low- and middle-income countries exists a scenario of a "double burden" of disease (childhood malnutrition and adult obesity) that threatens to overwhelm the health services of many resource-poor countries. The paper reports dietary and lifestyle practices of 16-19 year old females living in Soweto, South Africa. The purpose of the study was to describe young females' narratives around lifestyle practices across various areas of influence - community, home, school, peers, and self. Fifteen pairs of friends were interviewed with the use of semi-structured, open ended questions. Participants expressed that people in Soweto respect each other and the elderly. There are not many recreational activities that young women engage in within the community; some site concerns for safety and limited availability. Families have favourite dishes/recipes and scheduled cooking, some family food taboos exist. Families share meals, especially supper, while watching television. At school the girls share money and food with their peers. The girls often eat the filling "kota" for lunch. The participants wish there was more variety of food, but some say they would still buy the "kota". The "kota" is also eaten as a snack after school or on weekends as a lunch option by individuals and some families. As friends, Sowetan young women mostly listen to music, watch TV, eat together, go to shopping malls, chat at street corners, and study together. The participants mentioned personal food likes and dislikes, with most vegetables being unpopular due to taste, smell, and cooking methods. Some of the young women say they have tried to diet, but stopped before seeing any results, as it was very hard. In conclusion, this study highlights barriers to healthy eating and exercising. Future research should focus on the multidimensionality of influence around lifestyle to understand the critical factors and possible areas of intervention.

Keywords: *Narratives, Dietary practices, Lifestyle practices, Community, Home, School, Peers, Self.*

Introduction

The World Health Organization (WHO) finds itself needing to deal with the new pandemic of obesity and its accompanying non-communicable diseases (NCDs), while the challenge of childhood malnutrition has far from disappeared, TB and malaria rates are escalating, and the scourge of AIDS has emerged (Prentice AM, 2006)· The diet and lifestyles of children adolescents are of public health concern due to evidence relating poor nutrition in childhood to subsequent obesity and elevated risks for type II diabetes, the metabolic syndrome and CVD (Cañete R *et al.*, 2007), all of which are increasing in prevalence (WHO, 2004). Identifying dietary and lifestyle practices among adolescents and the factors that influence them, may assist in targeting at-risk groups and developing strategies to improve lifestyle and dietary practices. WHO warns that the greater future burden of obesity and diabetes will affect low- or middle-income countries. South Africa is no exception, with the greatest prevalence in African females. Further research is needed to understand the lifestyle precursors to obesity risk.

Materials and Methods

Study Sample

Setting

The study was undertaken in Soweto, the largest black township in Gauteng, South Africa. It has been estimated that 65 per cent of Johannesburg's residents live in Soweto. The Nov 10, 2009 official estimate of its population was 1, 3000,000 (www.*shopsoweto.com/population/*)

Study Design

To describe young adults' narratives around lifestyle practices across various areas of influence, we conducted in-depth, semi-structured, pair interviews with young females and their best friend. The best friend was defined as "someone of your own age, you know very well, with whom you meet regularly (*i.e.* couple of times a week), you are engaged with in activities, hang out and/or chill out with and you share emotional moments. This can be someone from the same neighborhood and may not be from the same school". Study participants were interviewed as pairs, so as to facilitate greater information sharing about activities in and outside schools, eating and physical activities with friends and in the community. We defined the selection criteria as within the age range of 16 and 18 years of age and still attending high school within the Soweto area. This study was approved by the Human Research Ethics Committee (Medical) at Witswatersrand University.

Selection and Recruiting

Recruiting was done by submitting an invitation and study information letter to the Gauteng Soweto Education district office. After permission was granted to visit six longest existing high schools in different areas of Soweto, the study was explained to the principals and teachers to assist in recruiting Grade 12 female students, who represented the 16-18 years age group. Three schools agreed to participate in the study; the reason for non-participation was exam preparations. Of the three schools, one was a private school, and two were public government schools. Sessions were organized by the study researchers to explain and encourage students to participate in the study. Only the students who showed interest were issued with information sheets and consent forms to give to their caregivers/parents to read and contact numbers to call in case of inquiries. Interested students were encouraged to recruit a best friend into the study. Information sheets and consent forms were also given to the best friend. A day was arranged to collect the signed consent and assent forms from the students at their respective schools. Parents of the participants who returned the consent and assent forms were contacted telephonically to confirm consent, and interview dates were scheduled with the participants. Recruitment for the study took place over a period of six weeks.

Only participants whose caregiver/parent/guardian, best friend, and friend's caregiver/parent/guardian could be contacted for confirmation were included in the study. A sample of 29 female adolescents and their best friends was selected. This number allowed saturation of concepts to be achieved across the different domains of the study.

Development of Instrument

A semi structured, open ended interview schedule was formulated with the expertise of a panel of qualitative and nutrition researchers. The questions were based on domains identified in the theory of Triadic Influence (Flay, 1993). This theory presumes that intentions to certain behavior derive from three streams of influence, namely the cultural environment, the social environment and biological and personality factors. For the purpose of this study we focused mainly on the social stream of influence. The aim of this study was to describe young adults' narratives around lifestyle practices across various areas of influence, namely: community, home (household), school, peers, and self (personal).

Conceptual Research Model

Our conceptual research model was based on the model of the Theory of Triadic Influence (Figure 21.1) (Flay 1993; Flay, Petraitis *et al.*, 1995; Flay 1999). This theoretical approach of predicting health-related behaviours presumes that there is an intention to engage in certain behaviours, *e.g.* food sharing behaviour, derive from three streams of influence; namely the cultural environment, the social environment and biological

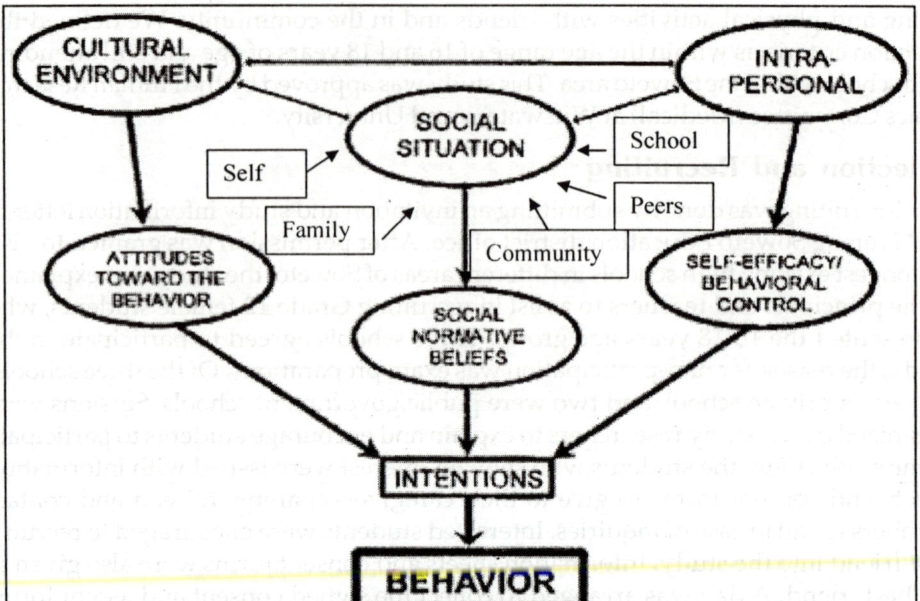

Figure 21.1: The Conceptual Framework

and personality factors. Factors on a proximal and distal level are most likely to predict certain behaviour, unlike ultimate influences which are beyond easy control of adolescents and less changeable. This model has been successfully used in previous nutrition research (de Bruijn, Kremers *et al.*, 2005; Wiefferink, Peters *et al.*, 2006). The present study mainly focused on the middle, social environment, stream of this model to explore the distal (*i.e.* social normative beliefs) and proximal factors of influence that potentially affect the behaviour of food sharing in the context of food choices and dietary patterns. Like Flay (1993), we expect these beliefs of adolescents are rooted in the attitudes and behaviours of the ones with the closest bond to them like family members, peers and other immediate surroundings. Relative influences of these immediate surroundings in the home and school environment as well as other situations were taken as the basic concepts for coding and analysis. Although both of the other streams, namely the cultural environment and biological and personality factors, were taken into account in this research, they were not the main focus of this research.

Interview Procedure

The questions were piloted on a total of four pairs of friends who were not part of the study population, and adjustments were made to the interview schedule accordingly. Changes made to the schedule included rephrasing of questions for better understanding, changing questions to accommodate local languages and understanding. A question about birthdays was deleted as most girls in the population seemed not to have birthday parties or celebrations. A question on funerals of families or friends was deleted due to some of the girls having lost biological parents, and were therefore uneasy talking and attending funerals.

All interviews were conducted and digitally recorded in a quiet room with the two participants, the interviewer and an observer. Each interview lasted for an average of 90 minutes. The interviews were conducted in languages that the participants were most comfortable with. In most cases, interviews were conducted in three different local languages, as the friend would be *e.g.* Zulu, and the main participant would be Southern Sotho, and there would be some usage of English. Data collection took place during the 2009 winter school holidays (29 June – 17 July) at Chris Hani Baragwath Hospital site, Soweto.

Participants were asked about their definition of a best friend, activities they engage in together and with other peers, daily dietary practices with emphasis on breakfast, eating at school, eating after school and supper, eating and activities with family, cultural foods, community activities and foods, money saving management (shown in Box 21.1).

At the end of data collection, the schools were presented with appreciation certificates for participation in the study.

Data Analysis

The transcripts were analyzed for emerging themes around dietary and exercise practices. The data of the participants was analyzed individually and the connectivity between the friends was not part of the analysis. The expected connectivity was not identified in the pairs. Based on data, the friendships were mostly based on emotional support, mutual respect, and honesty, than on time spent together, activities done together, foods shared, and things in common. Most of the friends were found to actually be very different, and to be spending time with other friends. The recorded interviews were transcribed and translated by private local transcribers who understand English and the different local languages. The quality of the transcripts was checked by the study researcher and feedback given to transcribers.

Five transcripts were read, coded and discussed in detail by two researchers (M.H.S and C.V) based on the themes emerging from the interviews. Themes were developed based on the Triadic Model framework areas of influence and based on the narratives of the participants. Preliminary analysis occurred concurrently with the continued administration of interviews to identify emergent sub-themes to pursue in subsequent interviews (Guest *et al.*, 2006). The remaining transcripts were read repeatedly and coded manually for emerging themes and their repetitions and variations by the researcher (M.H.S) with the help of the principal advisor (Strauss and Corbin 1990, Ryan and Bernard 2003).

Results

Personal/Self

Participants were asked about personal dietary and lifestyle practices. Questions were asked about breakfast practices, and amongst those that do not eat breakfast during schools days, some of the reasons cited were that breakfast is not a priority, it

Tell me about your day today, from when you got up this morning. (probe for breakfast, why she or does or doesn't eat, probe for composition)

Do you usually eat anything before going to school (probe for reasons for behavior)?

Probe for who prepares breakfast

What is your opinion about breakfast?

What do you believe breakfast should consist of?

Do you eat anything on your way to school, or before school starts, besides what you eat at home? Do you usually eat something just before school?

School - Eating and activities at school (during break(s)) – tell me about your eating and activities during lunch and other breaks at school (probe for who she eats with, what she eats, how eating happens amongst peers, how they decide on what to eat, what is available at schools, lunch boxes and attitudes towards lunch boxes)

After school – Tell me about what happens after school (probe for activities, foods, family chores, etc.)

Family – who cooks at home (probe for cooking schedules, favorite meals, favorite family dish, family activities, and chores) Food taboos (probe for reasons and detail of the taboos)?

Peers – Activities with peers (probe about activities and foods when hanging out, and when just chilling with peers)

Personal – Favorite fruits and vegetables, favorite cultural food/dish; Your least favorite food (probe for reasons and food allergies/sicknesses); favorite thing to eat at home, and away from home, favorite thing to do; health beliefs and experiences in relation to dieting, health beliefs about high blood pressure, heart diseases, junk foods, exercise, healthy foods?

Community - Soweto foods and activities, probe about their personal opinion of Soweto foods, probe about Soweto culture

Box 21.1: Main Interview Schedule

makes them fall asleep or feel tired in class, when they eat breakfast, they feel hungry quicker at school, and therefore cannot concentrate in class when they feel hungry. Some said they don't have enough time before going to school. Some quotes from those who don't eat breakfast were "What I would like to have for breakfast is not available at home", "I don't make time to eat breakfast", "I am very slow when I prepare for school, so I don't get time to eat breakfast", "I eat if there's bread, I don't like soft porridge", "If my mom gets up and cooks oats, I will eat, otherwise I don't eat".

Reasons given for eating breakfast included energy; some are just used to eating breakfast, and others were brought up with that practice. Participants said breakfast is the most important meal of the day. One participant said she eats soft porridge because her mother doesn't want them to waste food.

The participants mentioned personal likes and dislikes, with most vegetables being unpopular due to the taste, smell, and methods of cooking. A few who don't like mashed potatoes will eat fries, some will eat potato salad, since it has mayonnaise added, this could show the role that taste plays, as they say "I don't like mashed potatoes, they have no taste", or "they smell bad". Some of the young women say they have tried to diet, but stopped before seeing any results, as it was very hard. Dieting was defined as food deprivation, eating a balanced diet, and eating less. Some of the methods included drinking lemon water, only eating snacks, not eating supper, not eating starch. Participants said exercise is important, with some having engaged therein, but concern for community safety, and the need to study now that they were in grade 12 at school, were some of the reasons for ceasing to exercise.

Eating supper depends on what is on the menu. Some said "Sometimes I don't eat because of the smell of the food". At time some eat "kota" after school when they are hungry, and would at times not eat supper as they would still be full. Majority of the young women like simple sugars, they add a lot of table sugar to their tea or coffee, (between 4-10 teaspoons in a tea cup). They say "I like sugar, I like sweets". The few who don't add sugar at all or who add less, do so because "My grandmother has diabetes, and she says we should not add sugar", "My mom has sugar disease (diabetes), and she says we should not eat much sugar, it will make us sick". The ones, who eat less sugar, do so because of some kind of family influence.

Participants save money to buy sanitary essentials, to help the family with bread money if the caregiver doesn't have money, to help with lunch money in case the caregiver doesn't have money to give to participant for lunch the next day, to go to the movies, to buy stationary and school essentials like uniforms. Some say "I just save money, without a specific reason", "to buy snacks" "I save money, and I go to Pick n' Pay and buy chips, Ultramel (custard), and snacks, and I shut myself in my room, and indulge, some of the food I eat when I cross- night". The sources of the savings money is amongst others: plaiting people's hair (hair dressing), lunch money, and money from family members.

Home/Household

Families have favorite dishes/recipes and scheduled cooking. Some family food taboos emerged such as, "my mom says I should not eat lots of eggs, as they will increase my libido", "eggs will cause me to menstruate more", "chicken livers are not for girls", but some adolescents don't adhere to them, as they claim not to see any physical difference in their lives. A few of the participants feel that whatever the elderly say about cultural food taboos must be respected because the elderly know what they are talking about. Families share meals, in particular supper, while watching television.

On weekends, some adolescents eat the "kota" when there is no cooked meal at home. The "kota" is sometimes eaten by the whole family, as a fast food alternative (it is cheaper, quicker, easily accessible, and filling) – see picture below. Majority of the

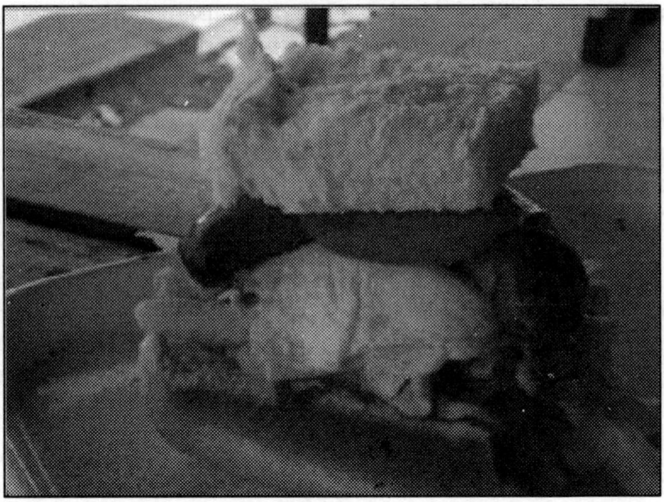

Figure 21.2

adolescents can cook, especially their "favorite home meal to eat". Some don't cook, but help with food preparation, and household chores. Those who don't cook have different reason for not doing so:" I don't like to cook"; "I get home late, I only cook my favorite meal. The participants who don't eat supper with the family for the following reasons: "I don't like the way they cook"; "I am on a diet"; "I don't like what they eat"; "I would rather eat something else". Caregivers mainly influence what the family eats.

Peers/Friends

As friends, the Sowetan young women mostly listen to music, watch TV, eat together, go to the shopping mall, attend parties, eat "kotas", relax at street corners, and study together.

School

During the interviews the participants were asked to say something about what they do and eat during breaks at school. Questions probed for what they eat, whether they eat together with friends, share their meals, their own lunch from home or buy their lunch and why they adopt this behaviour. Lunch breaks at school were extensively discussed in most of the interviews. The girls share money and food with their peers. "If one of my friends doesn't have lunch money, as a group, we combine our money, buy food, and share with her". The girls eat "kotas" at school because the "kota" is energy dense/filling. The participants wish there was more variety of food, but some say they would still buy the "kota", as they like it. The "kota" is also eaten as a snack after school or on weekends as a lunch option by individuals and by some families. As friends, the Sowetan young women mostly listen to music, watch TV, eat together, go to the shopping mall, relax at street corners, and study together.

Community

Participants expressed that people in Soweto love each other, as a young person in Soweto you are expected to greet your elders when you meet them in the street, Sowetans like to have fun, and they take interest in each other's business. There are not many recreational activities that young women engage in within the community; some site concerns for safety and limited availability.

The most popular cultural dishes are boiled tripe, samp with beans, fat cakes, "kota", boiled and fried chicken feet, street roasted chicken, maize meal pap. Community activities within Soweto include: Poetry, local museums, community parks, local restaurants serving cultural food, Braais (barbecues) at street corners, hanging out at street corners, car racing, and street bashes/parties.

Discussion

The most popular breakfast food on weekends for families and individual adolescents is fat cakes. The "kota", samp and beans dish are common lunch options for individuals and families. Some families cook meals for Saturday lunch, but if there's no meals cooked, families will eat "kotas". The Sunday meal is still common, with different vegetables, some of the participants said "the Sunday meal has all seven colors". Participants eat this meal as families, even those who are on some "diet" during the week. Some participants don't eat breakfast because they are just lazy to prepare it. They will eat if something has already been prepared by a sister or elder in the house; some don't always have bread to eat, which may reflect inconsistency in availability or limited choices. Some just don't prioritize breakfast, giving reasons such as, having no time, being too slow, just not thinking about breakfast before going to school. Some don't eat at home, but will buy fat cakes at school, or even ask someone to buy them something before school starts.

Most participants dislike lunch boxes, but will take a lunch box to school on Mondays, as they bring Sunday left-over food to school, this meal consists mainly of rice, salads, chicken or other protein source. This could suggest that adolescents want to take tasty, colorful food to school. Some say it's because they have more time on Sundays evening to prepare lunch boxes, as opposed to during the week, but this is food that is already prepared/cooked. The few who take lunch boxes to school on other days take mostly processed meats (polony and cheese).

Two of the interviewees reported that they were smoking and this could affect their taste and choice of foods. Alcohol drinking came up as a social activity that peers participate in (especially at parties, or when chilling with friends on weekend), some seemed to be shy to mention or talk about it. Some interviewees view alcohol drinking as bad for health, and therefore they don't participate in it.

Conclusions

This study highlights real barriers to healthy eating and exercising and it is important for future research to focus on the multidimensionality of influence around lifestyle in order to understand the critical factors and possible areas of intervention.

The study stresses the need for future research to focus on the still elusive but important role the immediate social surrounding (*i.e.* friends, caregivers and environmental factors) have in determining the food consumption of an individual. Interventions to reduce obesity rates are needed in which these social factors should be addressed. This study and the established literature stresses the importance of intervening broadly, on different levels and on multi facets with a tailor made evidence based approach specific for the particular community.

There may also be a need to focus on ways to help provide nutritious and more affordable food options at schools. There is need to investigate what items are being consumed in urban communities, and to increase recreational activities for young females.

References

References from Journals:

1. Cañete R, Gil-Campos M, Aguilera C and Gil A (2007) Development of insulin resistance and its relation to diet in the obese child. Eur J Nutr 46, 181-187.
2. de Bruijn, G. J., S. P. Kremers, *et al.* (2005). "Determinants of adolescent bicycle use for transportation and snacking behavior." Prev Med 40(6): 658-667.
3. Flay, B. R. (1993). Youth tabacco use: Risk patterns, and control. Nicotine addiction: Principles and management. C. T. O. J. Slade. New York, Oxford: 653-661.
4. Flay, B. R. (1999). "Understanding environmental, situational and intrapersonal risk and protective factors for youth tobacco use: the Theory of Triadic Influence." Nicotine Tob Res 1 Suppl 2: S111-114; discussion 569-170.
5. Guest G., Bunce A. and Johnson L. (2006) How many interview are enough? An experiment in data saturation and variability Field Methods 18, 59-82.
6. Prentice AM. The emerging epidemic of obesity in developing countries. Int.J.Epidemiol. 2006 Feb;35(1):93-99.
7. Ryan G.W. and Bernard H.R. (2003). Techniques to identify themes. Field Methods 15, 85-109.
8. Strauss A.L. and Corbin J.M. (1990) Basics of qualitative Research: Grounded Theory Procedures and Techniques. Sage Publications, California.
9. Wiefferink, C. H., L. Peters, *et al.* (2006). "Clustering of health-related behaviors and their determinants: possible consequences for school health interventions." Prev Sci 7(2): 127-149.

References from other Literature

10. World Health Organization (2004) Global strategy on Diet, Physical Activity and Health. Geneva: WHO

References from Books

11. Flay, B., J. Petraitis, *et al.* (1995). Chapter 3: The Theory of Triadic Influence: Preliminary evidence related to alcohol and tobacco use. Alcohol and tobacco: From basic science to clinical practice. J.

12. Fertig and J. Allen. Washington DC, National Institutes of Health, U.S. Government Printing Office: pages 37-58.

References from Websites

13. http://www.*shopsoweto.com/population/* (accessed 15 february 2010)

Definition of Terms

"kota" – quarter sized bread cut from a full loaf, filled with fried chips, atchaar, cheese, fried egg, vienna, etc varying in price from R5 up to R15

Chapter 22

Prevalence of Under-nutrition and Associated Factors Among Females Aged 13–16 Years in Plantation Sector Medical Officer of Health (MOH) Area in Sri Lanka

*A.M.S. Niranjala[1] and N. Gunawardena[2]**

[1]Assistant Medical Officer of Health, Thihagoda, Sri Lanka
[2]Senior Lecturer in Community Medicine, Faculty of Medicine, University of Colombo, Sri Lanka
**E-mail- nalikaguna@hotmail.com*

ABSTRACT

Under-nutrition among female adolescents is associated with adverse consequences that span generations. Nearly 9 per cent of the population of Sri Lanka lives in estates. There is evidence that health indicators in this sector are lower compared to other sectors. Research data on prevalence of under-nutrition among adolescents in estates are lacking. This study aimed to estimate the prevalence of under-nutrition and socio-demographic factors associated with it among the female adolescents aged 13-16 years in estate sector in Haliela Medical Officer of Health (MOH) area.

A community based descriptive study was carried out in out in all 12 estates in Haliela MOH area. A sample of 524 females aged 13-16 years was selected based on probability proportionate to size of the population living in each estate and were interviewed using a structured questionnaire. Anthropometric indicators were measured using standard techniques and prevalence of under-nutrition was estimated based on age and sex specific Body Mass Index (BMI) charts by National Centre for Health Statistics and cut off values recommended by World Health Organization.

Prevalence of under-nutrition (categorized as 'thinness' with BMI <5th percentile) was 39.1 per cent. A proportion of 58.2 per cent were categorized as 'normal' (with BMI 5th-85th percentile) and 2.7 per cent were categorized as at 'risk of over weight' (with BMI >85th percentile). Prevalence of under-nutrition showed a decreasing trend with increasing age. Under-nutrition was more among low socio-economic strata ($p<0.001$). Adolescent not schooling ($p=0.79$), mother being literate ($p=0.18$), mothers having received school education ($p=0.08$), mother being employed ($p=0.49$), family size >6 ($p=0.15$), presence of a sibling within one year of age ($p=0.30$) were not significantly associated with under-nutrition.

The study highlighted that under-nutrition among female adolescents in estates is a public health problem and nutritional intervention programmes need to target the adolescents in the poorer families in the estates.

Keywords: *Estates, Under nutrition, Adolescents, BMI, Prévalence, Females.*

Introduction

Under-nutrition

Nutritional status is one of the important indicators that reflects a populations' overall health status (World Health Organization, 1995b). Human suffering caused by malnutrition remains a challenge now as ever in the past. Malnutrition exists in some form in every country. Commonest form of malnutrition in many developing countries is still under-nutrition while overnutrition is an emerging problem (Gopalan, 1992). Under-nutrition is defined as inadequacy of food supply or inability to use the nutrients in food.

Socioeconomic, health and environmental factors that directly or indirectly linked to poverty can be considered as contributing to under-nutrition status. Difficulty in reducing prevalence of under-nutrition has been attributed to this complex nature of interaction between various factors related to poverty.

Poor nutrition starts before birth, and generally continues into adolescence and adult life and can span generations giving rise to intergenerational under-nutrition. Chronically malnourished girl children are more likely to remain undernourished during adolescence and adulthood, and when pregnant, are more likely to have morbidity and mortality associated with pregnancy and delivery, and increase risk of delivering low birth-weight babies (World Health Organization, 2006). Low Birth Weight (LBW) is said to be the best indicator and the predictor of this persistent effect of under nutrition through the life cycle. LBW indicates that the mother was malnourished during her own infancy, childhood, adolescence and pregnancy. One third to two thirds of all babies born in south Asia are born with low birth weight (United Nations Children's Fund, 1996).

The period of adolescence is from 10 to 19 years. This period is referred to as second window of growth because of the growth spurt that occurs during this stage

(World Health Organization, 1995a). According to World Health Organization (WHO) adolescent population constitutes 18 per cent to 25 per cent of total population in the South-East-Asia region and males outnumber females in all the countries in the region (WHO, 2006). Adolescence is characterized by the onset of major maturational events, principally the spurt in somatic growth and accompanying appearance of secondary sexual characteristics. This rapid growth and increase in physical activity create special nutritional needs with nutritional requirements being higher during adolescence than at any other time in life. Failure to consume adequate diet at this time can potentially retard physical growth and intellectual capacity, and delay sexual maturation (Aneja and Patwari, 2006). Improving nutrition during adolescence is the last opportunity a child has, to improve his/her linear growth.

Prevalence of Under-nutrition

Malnutrition, particularly under-nutrition is a global problem. It was estimated that 200 million children under five years of age were undernourished in the year 1995 (WHO, 1995b). Approximately half of child deaths (56 per cent) in the developing country have been attributed to effects of under-nutrition, while 83 per cent of the deaths are attributable to mild to moderate forms of under-nutrition (Pelletiro, 1995).

A large percentage of adolescents in the South East Asian region are thought to suffer from under-nutrition (WHO, 2006). However, very few studies provide data on nutritional status of adolescents. Prevalence of under-nutrition (less than 5th percentile of National Centre for Health Statistics standards) in 1992-93 among Mumbai school children in 10 to 19 years was 53 per cent (Kurz, 1996). In rural Bangladesh it was 67 per cent (Shahabuddin, 2000). Approximately one third (36 per cent) of rural Nepal children suffer from under-nutrition (Kurz, 1996).

Since gaining independence in 1948, though Sri Lanka has achieved dramatic improvements in selected social, health and educational indicators in the country, indicators pertaining to nutritional welfare of the population and poverty indicators do not show much improvement. Much of this available evidence is in relation to under-nutrition among children. Evidence of under-nutrition among adolescents is scarce in the country.

Nationally representative survey in Sri Lanka (n=6264) conducted among 10 to 15 year old school going adolescents showed that prevalence of thinness was 47.2 per cent. This prevalence was more among boys than among girls (57.9 per cent vs 36.1 per cent; $p<0.05$) (Jayatissa and Ranbanda, 2006). Another study done in Kalutara MOH area among grade 11 students (n=639) showed that prevalence of thinness among girls was 28.7 per cent (De Silva, 2008). A school based study (n=1224) done in Colombo revealed that prevalence of thinness, stunting and underweight among girls were 23.1 per cent, 5.2 per cent and6.8 per cent respectively (Wickramasinghe *et al.*, 2004).

Justification

The population of Sri Lanka lives in three distinct sectors the urban, rural and the estate sector with nearly 9 per cent living in estate sector. There is evidence that health indicators in the estate sector are lower compared to other sectors of the country

(Department of Census and Statistics and Ministry of Healthcare and Nutrition, 2009). However, above studies on adolescents nutritional status have not indicated the nutritional status of estate adolescents. In anaemia survey done in 2001 by department of the Nutrition of Medical Research Institute (MRI) through out the country except North and East, anthropometric indices were assessed among 3052 adolescents provided the sectoral differentiation. This study found an overall prevalence of thinness of 33.3 per cent. Prevalence of thinness was 27.5 per cent, 33.6 per cent and 36.1 per cent in urban, rural and estate sectors respectively (Piyasena and Mahamithawa, 2003).

Poor nutritional indicators of estate residents are evident from surveys on childhood nutrition.

The Demographic and Health Surveys are conducted every ten years in Sri Lanka (SLDHS) in a nationally representative sample of households. These surveys have revealed that under-nutrition among children under five years of age is a persistent problem in the country. The demographic and health surveys have found a wide variation of prevalence of under-nutrition in sectoral analysis with the estate sector having worst indicators (Department of Census and Statistics and Ministry of Healthcare and Nutrition, 2009).

In the SLDHS 2006-07, conducted by Department of Census and Statistics and Ministry of Healthcare and Nutrition (DCS and MoH) the overall prevalence of stunting (height for age below -2 SD or chronic under-nutrition), wasting (weight for height below -2 SD or acute under-nutrition) and underweight (weight for age is lower than two standard deviations or both acute and chronic under-nutrition) in age under five were 17.3 per cent, 14.7 per cent and 21.1 per cent respectively. The corresponding figures for estate sector were 40.2 per cent 13.5 per cent and 30.1 per cent respectively (DCS and MoH, 2009).

Low birth weight rates (percentage of children of children with a reported birth weight less than 2.5kg), which is considered as a predictor of the persistent effect of under nutrition through the life cycle in Sri Lanka is 16.6 per cent in the year 2006-07. In sectoral analysis highest LBW prevalence (31 per cent) was recorded from the estate sector.

With this back ground, the present study was planned to estimate the prevalence of under-nutrition and to describe socio-demographic factors associated it, among females aged 13 to 16 years in plantation sector in Haliela Medical Officer of Health (MOH) area. Haliela MOH area, is situated in Badulla district in Uva province. Haliela consists of twelve estates and rural areas. According to 2001 census, population of Haliela divisional secretariat was87, 476 with estate population of 28,761 living in the twelve estates. The ethnic distribution was, 63.5 per cent Sinhalese with 32.4 per cent, 3.6 per cent and 0.5 per cent Tamils, Sri Lankan Moors and others respectively (DCS, 2004). Most of the adults living in estates, work as labourers while the main occupations in rural areas are paddy farming and vegetable cultivation. In Haliela the total population in 13-16 year age group was 7523 according to census 2001 (DCS, 2004).

Methodology

Study Design and Study Population

We conducted a community based descriptive cross sectional study during the period of August to December 2009. Females aged 13 to 16 years who have been residing in the same estate for a period of at least six months comprised study population. Those who were pregnant at the time of survey and those who were diagnosed to be suffering from long term illnesses which affect the nutritional status were excluded.

Sample Size and Sampling Technique

The sample size was calculated to determine prevalence of under-nutrition using 36 per cent as the estimated prevalence of under-nutrition among adolescents in estate as found in a previous study (MRI, 2003). We added a design effect 1.4 as the study employed cluster sampling technique and after allowing for a non response rate of 6 per cent the final sample size was 526.

We conducted the study in all 12 estates in Haliela MOH area. Estates are divided in to divisions according geographical areas. There are 48 divisions in twelve estates in this MOH area. A division within an estate was considered as a cluster in this study. A total 20 adolescents were included from each cluster hence study included 27 clusters. The number of clusters included in the study from each estate was based on the probability proportionate to size of the population living in each estate and the required number of clusters from each estate, was through a random sampling technique.

A random procedure was used for selection of the starting point of the cluster. This was done by dropping a pin on the map of the cluster. After selecting the starting point randomly, houses were visited in a pre determined direction. Only one eligible adolescent was included in the study from a household. If there were more than one eligible adolescent in a house, the adolescent to be included was selected randomly. If a house was closed or if the eligible individual was not available at the time of data collection visit, the house was revisited later in the same day or next day to include eligible adolescents.

Collection of Data

A pre testing structured interviewer administered questionnaire was used to gather information on socio-demographic characteristics of the adolescents. Age, state of schooling, number and type of household members, details of parents, family income, household assets were the variables included in this section. The socio economic status was objectively assessed using a validated approach (Thalagala, 2004). An asset index for each household was calculated using a set of standardized asset item weights corresponding to different asset items and by summing them up.

Two Public Health Midwives (PHM) who had sound knowledge on Tamil and Sinhala were trained to administer the questionnaire.During the training a description of the study design and its objectives were given. Selection of eligible persons, obtaining informed consent, ensuring confidentiality and minimizing non-response were highlighted during these sessions. Administration of each section of the questionnaire was explained in detail. Training included a practice data collection session in the field in an estate in Ella MOH area, following which actual practical problems were discussed.

Data were collected during the school vacation, so that finding the children in the community was easy. Households were visited between 8a.m to 6.p.m during week days and week ends. During house hold visits the eligibility criteria was checked and the verbal informed consent and permission was obtained from the parents/ guardian and from subjects prior to the data collection to conduct the interview and to perform measurements by a prior trained PHM and Public Health Inspector in the afternoon of the previous day. The participants and parents were informed about the purpose and importance of the study, methods of data collection, voluntary nature and the confidentiality that will be maintained during the data collection.

The interviewer administered questionnaire was administered by the data collectors after selecting the study units within the household. Privacy was ensured by conducting the interviews within the house but in a place where there were minimum disturbances from household activities.

Following administering the questionnaire, an identification card was given to the respondent to be used as identification for the purpose of anthropometric measurements. The participants were then requested to come to the nearest crèche or dispensary for measurements on the same day. Height and weight measurements were taken to estimate BMI which was the measure of under-nutrition. Height and the weight of the adolescents were marked at the end of each questionnaire in relevant cage. The principal investigator performed the anthropometric measurements with assistance of a Public Health Nursing Sister.

Measurements were taken at a common place to ensure ground facilities to make accurate measurements and to ensure that PI perform all the measurements to ensure accuracy. Privacy of the subjects was protected by taking measurements in a room with a female chaperon. It was ensured that the filled questionnaire relevant to the study units in whom the measurements were made were available to the PI at the time of anthropometry and the PI entered the figures in the questionnaire after verifying the identification number.

Weight and height of all the subjects were measured according to the standard procedures using standard equipments by the principal investigator (WHO, 1995a).

For measuring height, a stadiometer was used and measurements were made to the nearest 0.1 cm. Weight was measured by electronic digital weighing scale to the nearest 0.1kg. Weighing scale was calibrated with a known weight before each day prior to a weighing session and batteries were replaced as required. All weight measurements were done when participants were in light indoor clothing, without foot wear or heavy items in pockets.

Many measures were adopted at the stage of designing the questionnaire, during selection of sample, at the time of data collection and data entry to ensure validity of data.

At the stage of designing the questionnaire, literature related to measuring of relevant variables were perused and relevant scales validated for Sri Lanka were used. Experts in the field of public health and nutrition were consulted regarding content included, wordings used etc. Questionnaire consists of simple self explanatory questions that were easily understood. Open ended questions minimized to avoid interviewer bias.

Non response rate was minimized by conducting the interviews at a time convenient for the respondents, explaining the purpose of the study participants and confidentiality of all the information provided. Non availability was minimized as it was conducted during school vacations. Participants and their parents were made aware about the study and at the same time. PI was available in the field throughout the data collection period and the measurements were taken at a specified place on the same day of administering the questionnaire which also contributed to reduce the non response rate. Those who were not available at the time of visit were visited again and included in the study.

Only females were used for data collection to ensure better response and accuracy of data collected. Use of interviewer administered questionnaires in both Sinhala and Tamil languages and utilizing Sinhala and Tamil speaking data collector's ensured inclusion of respondents of all levels of educational background and all ethnic groups ensuring validity.

In assigning the PHM for data collection, care was taken not to assign the PHMM to her own area of duty to maintain similar familiarity among data collectors and respondents from all areas. The interview was conducted as far as possible in a location away from the usual to avoid disturbance of others in the household and to ensure the accuracy of the information.

Principal investigator (PI) was available in the field during the whole period of data collection to clarify any doubts of the data collectors. All the anthropometry measurements were done by the PI. Weighing scale was an automated device so that it did not influenced by observer. All instruments were calibrated before use. All the measurements were taken according to the standard procedure. Standard protocols for anthropometry were followed to minimize errors in measurements. Duplicate measurements were taken in a 10 per cent of the sample to ensure validity. All the measurements were recorded immediately in the questionnaire.

Analysis of Data

Statistical analysis was performed by PI using statistical package for social sciences (SPSS) version 12.0.

Prevalence of under nutrition of 13 to 16 years old females was based on the Body Mass Index. Body Mass Index was calculated for each adolescent from the measured weight and height using the formula BMI = weight (kg)/height^2 (m^2).

The study units were categorized in to three groups of nutritional status using sex specific BMI for age percentile charts developed by the National Centre for Health Statistics (NCHS). Those who were below 5th percentile for age of the reference population were taken as suffering from under-nutrition. Those with BMI 5th-85th

percentile were categorized as 'normal' and those with BMI >85th percentile was categorized as at 'risk of over weight' (WHO, 1995a).

In calculating the prevalence of under-nutrition, number of study units with thinness constituted the numerator while the number of 13 to 16 years old females who were included in the study constituted the denominator.

The socio-economic and demographic characteristics were presented using frequency distributions and were cross analyzed with nutritional status. Chi-squared test was used wherever appropriate to assess whether the factors were associated with under-nutrition. A p value of 0.05 was used to determine significance.

A standardized asset item weights corresponding to different asset items were summed up to generate an asset index for each household. The Asset Index was then categorized in to Quintiles using cut off points (Thalagala, 2004)

Ethical Considerations

Informed verbal consent was taken from the parents of the study units and study units were inquired into willingness to participate in the study to ensure autonomy.

Ethics clearance was obtained from the Ethics Review Committee of Faculty of Medicine, University of Kelaniya.

Results

Study included 524 females in 13 to 16year age group with a response rate of 99.6 per cent (524/526).

Socio-Demographic Characteristics of the Study Population

Mean age of study population was 14.5 years (SD± 1.1years). Proportions of study units included from each of the four years of age were more or less equal.

All the study units were in the schooling age. Of the 524 of study units, 43 (8.2 per cent) were not attending school at the time of survey. Those of who were not attending school were inquired into the highest grade of schooling. A majority 12 (27.9 per cent) of those who were not attending school had studied up to grade 6.

A household was defined as a group of individuals who live in a residential unit and purchase and prepare food together. The number of members living in the household and their relationship to the study unit were inquired into. A majority 379 (72.3 per cent) of population had five or less than five members living in the household. Mean house hold size is 4.9 (SD±1) in the study population.

Among the participants 476 (90.8 per cent) had their mothers living with them and 480 (91.6 per cent) had their fathers living with them. Nearly 356 (68 per cent) of them had an either grandparent living in the household. Of those whose mothers were not living in the same household (48), a majority, 26 (54.2 per cent) were abroad for employment. Mothers were not living in 15 study units.

Among mothers 125 (24.9 per cent) had never been to school and 257 (51.2 per cent) had been educated only up to grade five while among fathers corresponding numbers were 70 (14.6 per cent) and 266 (55.4 per cent) respectively. However, 375

(74.7 per cent) mothers were able to write at least in one language and 393 (78.3 per cent) were able to read at least in one language. Among fathers 86 per cent were able to write and 88.3 per cent were able to read at least in one language. Among the mothers, a majority 256 (51.6 per cent) were tea pluckers, 105 (20.9 per cent) were tea factory workers and 115 (22.9 per cent) were housewives and among fathers, 315 (65.6 per cent) were working in tea estate/factory.

Of total study population only 188 (35.9 per cent) had a sibling with a one year age gap.

The study units were inquired regarding the monthly income of their family and 39 (7.4 per cent) study units did not know to respond to this. Most, 280 (53.4 per cent) reported that monthly family income was less than 5000 Sri Lankan rupees (<USD 44), 160 (30.5 per cent) reported an income of 5000-10,000 Sri Lankan rupees (USD 44-88) with only 45 (8.7 per cent) of the study units reported an income more than 10,000 Sri Lankan rupees (>USD 88).

An asset index was calculated for each house hold by adding a set of standardized asset item weights as described in the methodology. By adopting validated quintile cut off points the study units were separated into different socio-economic strata and the results are shown in Table 22.1.

Table 22.1: Frequency Distribution of Socio Economic Strata of Study Population

Socio-Economic Quintile	*Frequency*	*Percentage*
Poorest	193	36.8
Second	231	44.1
Middle	47	9.0
Fourth	37	7.1
Richest	16	3.0
Total	524	100.0

A majority of the study population 231 (44.1 per cent) belonged to second quintile of socio-economic stratum which was followed by the proportions in the poorest (36.8 per cent) quintile of socio-economic stratum.

Regarding presence of selected individual household assets, a great majority (479, 91.4 per cent) were having electricity in their houses. Equally high number of households had a radio and a television set which were 424 (80.9 per cent) and 423 (80.7 per cent) respectively. A small number of households (80, 15.3 per cent) possessed a refrigerator.

Prevalence of Under Nutrition Among the Study Population

The mean weight of the study population was 39.54kg (SD ±7.48kg) with 22.1kg being the minimum and 61.3kg being the maximum.

The mean height of the study population was 1.493m (SD ± 0.069m). Minimum height was 1.22m and the maximum was 1.71m.

Frequency distribution of BMI of the study population by age is shown in Table 22.2.

Table 22.2: Frequency Distribution of BMI of the Study Population by Age

Age in Years	*Mean BMI (kg/m²)*	*SD*	*Median*	*Minimum Value*	*Maximum Value*
13-	16.53	2.1	15.27	13.55	23.34
14-	17.49	2.4	17.40	13.60	24.32
15-	18.29	2.3	18.48	13.57	25.78
16	18.92	2.4	19.40	14.73	25.96
Total	17.61	2.5	17.67	13.55	25.96

The mean BMI of the study population was 17.61 kg/m^2 (SD ± 2.5 kg/m^2). A slightly increasing trend in mean BMI with increasing age was observed.

Table 22.3 shows the frequency distribution of the study population by nutritional status categorisation and age.

Table 22.3: Frequency Distribution of the Study Population by Nutritional Status Categorisation and Age

Age in Years	*Thinness**		*Normal***		*At Risk of Over Weight****		*Total*	
	No	*Per cent*	*No*	*Per cent*	*No*	*Per cent*	*No*	*Per cent*
13-	61	47.6	65	50.8	02	1.6	128	100.0
14-	52	39.6	79	57.5	03	3.0	134	100.0
15-	53	37.9	82	58.6	05	3.5	140	100.0
16	39	31.9	79	64.8	04	3.3	122	100.0
Total	205	39.1	305	58.2	14	2.7	524	100.0

*: Thinness- <5th percentile; **: Normal-5th to less than 85th percentile;
***; At risk of overweight-≥85th percentile.

Among the study group the prevalence of under nutrition was 39.1 per cent while 58.2 per cent were normal and 2.7 per cent were at risk of over weight. Highest prevalence of under nutrition (47.6 per cent) was seen among 13 year olds with nearly half of them suffering from under nutrition. Prevalence of under nutrition decreased with increasing age.

Socio-Demographic Characteristics Associated with Nutritional Status

The state of schooling of the study population, characteristics of the family and mother were cross analysed to with their nutritional status to assess the associations and the results are shown in Table 22.4.

Table 22.4: Frequency Distribution of Study Population by Nutritional Status and Selected Socio-Demographic Characteristics

Socio-Demographic Factors	*Thinness*		*Normal/ At Risk of Over Weight*		*Test of Significance*
Pattern of schooling at the time of survey					
Schooling	189	39.3	292	60.7	$\chi^2 = 0.072$
Not schooling	16	37.2	27	62.8	df = 1
					p = 0.788
Family size					
5 or less	141	37.2	238	62.8	$\chi^2 = 2.11$
≥6	64	44.1	81	55.9	df = 1
					p = 0.146
Presence of a sibling within one year of age					
Present	68	36.2	120	63.8	$\chi^2 = 1.073$
Absent	137	40.8	199	59.2	df = 1
					p = 0.300
Mothers receiving school education or not (n=502*)					
Not been to school (n=125)	58	46.4	67	53.6	$\chi^2 = 2.988$
Gone to school (n=377)	142	37.7	235	62.3	df = 1
					p = 0.084
Ability to read at least one language (n=502*)					
Not able to read (n=127)	57	44.9	70	55.1	$\chi^2 = 1.803$
Able to read (n=375)	143	38.1	232	61.9	df = 1
					p = 0.179
Ability to write at least one language (n=502*)					
Not able to write (n=109)	47	43.1	62	56.9	$\chi^2 = 0.624$
Able to write (n=393)	153	38.9	240	61.1	df = 1
					p = 0.429
Employed or not (n=502*)					
House wife (n=115)	49	42.6	66	57.4	$\chi^2 = 0.477$
Employed (n=387)	151	39.0	236	61.0	df = 1
					p = 0.490

* Study units whose mothers were separated and passed away were not included.

Proportions of study units suffering from under-nutrition was similar among schooling (39.3 per cent) and non schooling (37.2 per cent) study units (p =0.788). Under-nutrition was seen more among study units living in a family of six or more members (44.1 per cent) compared to those living in families with five or less (37.2 per cent) The association was not statistically significant (p=0.146). Prevalence of under-nutrition among those having siblings within one year of age (36.2 per cent) and those not having siblings within one year of age (40.8 per cent) were similar (p=0.30).

Though a higher proportion of study units whose mothers have not received school education (46.4 per cent) were undernourished compared to those whose mothers had received school education (37.7 per cent) this difference was not statistically significant (p=0.084). A higher proportion of study units whose mothers were housewives (42.6 per cent) had under-nutrition compared to those whose mothers were employed (39.0 per cent) but this difference was not also statistically significant (p=0.49).

Table 22.5 shows the frequency distribution of study population by nutritional status and amalgamated socio economic strata based on the Asset Index.

Table 22.5: Frequency Distribution of Study Population by Nutritional Status and Amalgamated Socio Economic Strata

Socio Economic Strata	*Thinness*		*Normal/At Risk of Over Weight*		*Total*		$\div^2 = 136.97$ df = 1 p <0.001
	No	*Per cent*	*No*	*Per cent*	*No.*	*Per cent*	
Poorest/second/middle	200	56.3	155	43.7	355	100.0	
Fourth/Richest	05	3.0	164	97.0	169	100.0	
Total	205	39.1	319	60.9	524	100.0	

Under-nutrition was seen more among amalgamated quintiles of poorest, second and third quintiles(56.3 per cent) than among fourth and richest quintiles (3.0 per cent). And this difference was statistically highly significant (p<0.001).

Discussion

The implications of poor nutritional status on adolescents, especially its life long continuing effects for female adolescents is clearly described in scientific literature. Adolescents comprise 17.5 per cent of the population of Sri Lanka (DCS and MoH, 2009). Evidence on nutrition status of children in estates have indicated that problem of under-nutrition among children is worse in estates compare to other sectors in the country. This highlights the importance of generating research evidence on adolescent under-nutrition in the estate sector in Sri Lanka.

A cross sectional descriptive study design was used to assess the under-nutrition and its associated socio-demographic factors among females aged 13- 16 years in Haliela MOH area. A community based study as opposed to a school based or a clinic based study ensured that non school going adolescents and adolescents who do not have access to health services were also included in the sample improving the validity of the results. The sampling technique adopted, which is the cluster sampling with probability proportionate to size to population living in each estate, helped in identifying a representative sample of from all estates, making the results generalizable to estates in Haliela MOH area.

Use of an interviewer administered questionnaire as the data collection tool, all the team of survey members being females and the fact that study was conducted in their homes during school vacation would have contributed to the minimum non response rate. This ensured validity of the results in relation to the target group of the study. Study utilised a validated process using an assets index to categorise the study population into socio-economic strata.

Principal investigator performed all the anthropometric measurements to ensure the accuracy. Body weight was measured to the nearest 0.1 kg with electronic digital weighing scale and height was measured using a stadiometer to nearest 0.1cm. Weighing scale was an automated device therefore the measurement was not influenced by the observer. Weighing scale was calibrated with a known weight before each day prior to a weighing session and batteries were replaced as required. All the measurements were taken according to the standard procedure. Standard protocols for anthropometry were followed to minimize errors in measurements. Duplicate measurements were taken by the PI in a 10 per cent of the sample to ensure validity. All the measurements were recorded immediately in the questionnaire.

A majority (53.4 per cent) of the units reported monthly family income was less than ₹ 5000. Similarly a majority of the study population (80.9 per cent) belonged to poorest and second quintile of socio-economic strata. In SLDHS 2006-07 the proportion of poorest and second quintile was 90.4 per cent in estate sector.

Availability of household assets indicated that availability of main items such as electricity and items to obtain information such as radio and television are high in estates. Among the study population 91.4 per cent were having electricity in their houses while 80.9 per cent households had a radio and 80.7 per cent had a television set. In DHSSL 2006-07, the corresponding figures for estate sector was lower with only 65.1 per cent having a radio and 63.7 per cent having a television.

Prevalence of Under-nutrition among Adolescents

Body Mass Index-for-age cut off values recommended by the WHO using NCHS reference data was used to asses under-nutrition as used by other national and international researchers, making the results comparable.

The mean BMI of the study population was 17.61 kg/m^2 (SD ± 2.5 kg/m^2). A slightly increasing trend in mean BMI with increasing age was observed indicating that BMI can be expected to improve by the time the adolescents reach their reproductive age.

Among the study group the prevalence of under-nutrition was 39.1 per cent, indicating that under-nutrition among estate adolescent females is a public health problem in the country. Highest prevalence of under-nutrition (47.6 per cent) was seen among 13 year olds. This observation was in agreement with a national study done in 2002 among school going adolescents of 10-15 years, where the overall prevalence of under-nutrition for the whole country was 36.1 per cent in females (Jayatissa and Ranbanda, 2006). However, this study included only school going adolescents and did not take the sectoral differences into account.

In the present study, the prevalence of under-nutrition between 13 to 16 years decreased with increasing age. In the study by Jayatissa and Ranbanda (2006) showed similar results.

De Silva (2008) showed that prevalence of thinness among grade eleven female students was 28.7 per cent in the study conducted in Kalutara which is done among only urban and rural settings. The relatively low prevalence can be attributed to sector difference and the latter study constituted students more than half from upper social classes (De Silve, 2008).

In another study carried out among 8 to 12 age group (n=1224) in urban schools the prevalence of thinness among girls was 23.1 per cent (Wickramasinghe *et al.*, 2004). The relatively low rates observed in this study may be due to differences in age, and the study setting was urban schools.

Socio-economic and Demographic Factors Associated with Nutritional Status

In assessing association between under-nutrition and socioeconomic status, it was shown that under-nutrition was seen significantly more among poorest, second and third quintiles (56.3 per cent) than among fourth and richest quintiles (3.0 per cent) ($p<0.001$). This is in conformity with established association of poverty and under-nutrition.

Almost all researches on factors associated with adolescent nutritional status in Sri Lanka, irrespective of their study setting have found similar results (Jayatissa and Ranbanda, 2006; Wickramasinghe *et al.*, 2004; Rathnayake and Weerasinghe, 1990; De Silva, 2008).

The present study found that under-nutrition was more among study units living in a family of more than six members (44.1 per cent) compared to those living in families with five or less (37.2 per cent) but the association was not significant ($p=0.146$). in keeping with this, the study in rural areas in India among 12,124 adolescents too revealed that stunting was not significantly associated with family size (ventaiah *et al.*, 1998). However, the study in urban areas of Pakistan among infants between six to eighteen months found that family size more than six members was associated with stunting indicating the association of overcrowding with under-nutrition (OR=1.7,CI1.2 to 3.8) (Baig Ansari *et al.*, 2006).

The difference of this finding between adolescents and infants may be highlighting that though overcrowding is a known factor associated with childhood under-nutrition it may not be a factor associated with under-nutrition of adolescents.

Present study found that those whose mothers have not received school education (46.4 per cent) showed higher prevalence of under-nutrition compared to those whose mothers had received school education (37.7 per cent). However, this difference was not statistically significant ($p=0.084$).The national study done by Jayatissa and Ranbanda in 2006 in Sri Lanka among adolescents, parental education has not been studied. The study done in grade eleven students (n=639) in Kalutara MOH area showed that higher proportion of thinness was observed where mother's education was less than G.C.E O/L and even in this study the difference was not statistically significant (De Silva, 2008).

In a household survey done among pre-schoolers (n=4450) in Sri Lanka in all districts except North and East revealed that children's nutrition had a clear relationship with mothers' education level with lower education being associated with higher prevalence of stunting ($p<0.05$) and underweight ($p<0.05$), (Rathnayake and Weerasinghe, 1990). Similar finding is shown in the study in Pakistan among

399 infants between six to eighteen months in year 2000, where mother's non-education was associated with stunting (OR 3.2, CI 1.6-4.9) (Baig Ansari *et al.*, 2006).

The observed difference between preschoolers and adolescents may be due to the reason that adolescents are more independent than preschoolers regarding their dietary practices. Preschoolers diet depend more on maternal education which is associated with, practice of child care feeding, sanitation, food preparation and healthcare.

Limitations

Conventionally nutritional status was assessed using anthropometric indices but these indices were known to be influenced by sexual maturity, and ideally needs to be adjusted for it. These adjustments were not done in the present study due to lack of information required. The international and local studies among adolescents have also not used adjusted indices thus it allowed the present study to be readily compared with other studies.

World Health Organization currently recommends using BMI for age compared to reference standard (NCHS) (WHO, 1995a). However, it does not distinguish acute from chronic under-nutrition (Aneja and Patwari, 2006.) Furthermore, when compared to the NCHS population BMI curves of affluent Sri Lankan children were far below the NCHS curves (Wikramanayake and Amarasinghe, 1990). Still the above standards were used in the present study due to non-availability of other Asian standards.

Conclusions

The overall prevalence of under-nutrition among the females in13 to16 age group in Estates in Haliela MOH area was 39.1 per cent indicating that it is a public health problem. Therefore, it is necessary to plan and implement nutritional intervention programmes to improve the nutritional status of this population.

In exploration of the demographic factors associated with under-nutrition, though not statistically significant, a higher proportion of under-nutrition was found among adolescents whose mothers who were not being to school, not able to read or write at least one language and who were unemployed at the time of the study. It gives us an indication of the importance of the female education in prevention of under-nutrition among future generation. However, this factor has to be further studied and tested in a larger scale study.

Low socio economic status was associated with under-nutrition indicating that nutritional intervention programmes need to target the adolescents in the poorer families in the estates. This study provides evidence that Asset Index is a valid measure of socio economic status even in estates.

Abbreviations

BMI: Body Mass Index

DCS and MoH: Department of Census and Statistics and Ministry of Healthcare and Nutrition

LBW: Low Birth Weight

MOH: Medical Officer of Health area
MRI: Medical Research Institute
NCHS: National Centre for Health Statistics
PHM: Public Health Midwives
PI: Principal investigator
SLDHS: Demographic and Health Survey Sri Lanka
WHO: World Health Organization

References

1. Aneja, S., Patwari,A. K., 2006. Malnutrition in adolescence,in: Bhave, S. Y., Bhave's Textbook of Adolescent Medicine. New Delhi: Jaypee Brothers Medical publishers.
2. Beig-Ansari, N., Rahbar, M.H., Bhutta, Z.A., Badruddin. 2006. Food and Nutrition Bulletin, 27(2).
3. Department of Census and statistics, 2004. Census of Population and Housing Sri Lanka -2001, Colombo: Department of Census and statistics.
4. Department of census and statistics and Ministry of Healthcare and Nutrition, 2009. Sri Lanka demographic and health survey 2006-07.Colombo: Department of census and statistics.
5. De Silva, S., 2008. The nutritional Status of Grade Eleven Students in the MOH area Kalutara. Journal of the College of Community Physicians of Sri Lanka,13(2), pp. 34-8.
6. Gopalan, C., 1992.Nutririon in Developmental Transmission in South East Asia. New Delhi: World Health Organization.
7. Jayatissa, R and Ranbanda, R.M., 2006. Prevalence of challenging nutritional problems among adolescents in Sri Lanka, Food and nutrition bulletin, 27(2).
8. Kurz,K.M., 1996. Adolescent nutritional status in developing countries. Proceeding of the Nutrition Society, 55(1B), pp. 321-31.
9. Pelletire, D.L.,1995. The effects of malnutrition on child mortality in developing countries. Bulletin of WHO, 73(4), pp. 443-8.
10. Piyasena, C., Mahamithawa, A.M.A.S.B., 2003. Assessment of Anaemia Status in Sri Lanka. A Summery Report. Colombo: Medical Research Institute of the Department of health services, Ministry of Health, Nutrition and Welfare, Sri Lanka.
11. Ratnayake, R.M.K., Weerasinghe, S., 1990. Sri Lanka Nutrition status survey 1988/89. Ceylon Journal of Medical sciences, 32; (2), pp. 31-45.
12. Shahabuddin, A.K., Talukder, K., Talukder, M.K., Hassan, M., Seal, A., Rahman, Q., Mannan, A., Tomkins, A., Costello, A., 2000. Adolescent nutrition in a rural community in Bangladesh. Indian Journal of Paediatrics, 67(2), pp. 93-8.

13. Thalagala, N.I., 2004. An index to Measure Socio Economic Status: Asset Approach. Journal of the College of Community Physicians of Sri Lanka, 9, pp. 32-40.

14. United Nations Children's Fund, 1996. Atlas of South Asian Children and Women. Kathmandu, Nepal: United Nation's Children's Fund, Regional Office for South Asia.

15. Wickramasinghe, V.P., Lamabadusuriya, S.P., Atapattu, N., Sathyadas, G., Karuparanantha, S., Karunarathna, P., 2004. Nutrition status of school children in urban areas in Sri Lanka. Ceylon Medical Journal, 49(4), pp.114-8.

16. World Health Organization, 1995a. Physical status: The use and interpretation of anthropometry. Report of WHO Expert Committee. Technical report series, No 854. Geneva: World Health Organization.

17. World Health Organization, 1995b. Nutrition Highlights of recent activities in the context of the world declaration and plan of action for nutrition. Geneva: World Health Organization.

18. World Health Organization, 2006. Adolescent Nutrition : A Review of the Situation in Selected South Asian Countries. New Delhi: World Health Organization.

Chapter 23

Role of Elected Women in Panchayati Raj and their Knowledge Level in Reproductive and Child Healthcare

Geeta Malhotra[1] and Kailash Kumar Mishra[2]

[1]Country Director, READ INDIA
707, HEWO Towers, Sector 56, Plot 42, Gurgaon – 122 001, India
[2]Managing Trustee and Chief Executive, Bahudha Utkarsh Foundation
"Ramnandan-Dulari", B2/333, Tara Nagar (Duggal Farm), Kakrola, Dwarka Sector 15, New Delhi – 110 078, India
E-mail: [1]geeta.malhotra16@gmail.com, [1]geeta@read-india.org
[2]kailashkmishra@gmail.com, [2]kailashkumarmishra@ymail.com

ABSTRACT

In this article an attempt is made to evaluate the role of elected women in Panchyati Raj and their knowledge level in reproductive and child healthcare. The authors on the basis of their direct experience from the field and interaction with the people as NGO professionals and scholars in various geographical pockets of India with special reference to Haryana and Western Uttar Pradesh have evaluated the impact of the 73rd and 74th Amendment Acts of the Indian Constitution. The women were well respected and always treated as the equal half in the Vedic and Puranic periods. The texts of the Rig-Veda, Athrva-Veda and Manusmriti confirm such facts. However, because of over dominance of male ego geniture, and patriarchy the women were subjugated and lost their individual and gender freedom in the changing phases of the Indian history. Gandhi as pioneer of Indian politics and architect of new India talked about the participation of women in every sphere of life and he also advocated for the decentralization of power from centre to the Panchayat and village levels. His concept of gramswarajya is a major contribution in this respect. Post 1993 the Indian villages and also the women and dalits of India tasted the new form of democracy and started sharing the decision making process in all possible affairs. Health of the child as well as the mother is one of major concerns where women representatives were supposed to respond with their positive concern and attachment. The economic and other issues are also very important. The proxy voting, dominance of males and the representatives from higher caste and class are, however, very clearly observed in the entire process of Gram Panchayat. The initiatives of the government agencies and Planning Commission in this specific area are also discussed on the basis of the ground reality. The author suggests some meaningful suggestions as well.

Keywords: *Panchayti raj, Gram sabha, PRI, NGO, 73rd and 74th amendment acts, Gramswarajaya, Dalit.*

Introduction

Reflections

Panchayats in India are an age old institution for governance at village level. It is a peculiar country where the people of 3000-plus of castes, all major religions and more than 427 odd Tribal communities have been living together maintaining an exemplary communal harmony from thousands of years. It is rooted in its traditions. The Indian history confirms that we had civil society right from the Vedic period. Vedic hymns describe about egalitarian and democratic norms of their society. Some people's assemblies like *vidath, sabha* and *samiti* have been mentioned. *Vidath* was a general meeting of the *Jana* (whole community), which had redistributive functions. Vedic seers also described about *kilvis samprat i.e.,* general consensus. In all the Vedic assemblies' decisions were taken on the basis of consensus only.

Sabha was a body of village elders and it assisted the *janasya gopah.* The etymological meaning of *janasya gopah* is the protector of the people or fellowmen as well as their cattle wealth. But in practice it was used for the *rajanya i.e.,* ruler. *Samiti* was a general assembly in which all the members of the community participated. Its main function was to elect the ruler. The most remarkable fact about all these assemblies was that women also participated in it. *Sabha* and *samiti* had been depicted as the two daughters of Prajapati and especially *samiti* has been termed as *narista* that means a place where intellectual discourses or discussions can be made. *Sardh, vrat* and *gana* are the three other assemblies about them also we have a number of references. Mention can be made of *gosthi* that was like a modern days *Chaupal* in which discussions regarding day today socio-economic problems of village life were discussed. The Vedic seers used a fascinating term, *madhyamsiriv i.e.,* in case of indecision or altercation in the assembly the elders should opt the middle path to maintain the harmony and solve the problems. So Vedic period assures a balanced and ordered civil society. Later also all rulers, political thinkers and seers tried hard to honor the individual as well as the group liberty.

Manu has talked very high about the women. He says: Prosperity reigns supreme where women are held in high esteem. All their actions fail to bring wellbeing, where women are held in disrespect.

But, sadly the later phase of India created a male dominance (rather over dominance) and women were subjugated in all directions and dimensions. Slowly and gradually the urbanization sidelined the needs and requirements of the Indian villages, untouchables, Tribals and women. This concern was very much realized by Mahatma Gandhi (1869-1948). As early as 1936 he remarked, "I would say that if villages perish India would perish too. I believe and repeat times without number that India is to be found not in few cities but in its 7,00,000 villages." His role was crucial in awakening the most dormant and stagnant sector of Indian society, *i.e.*, villages of India.

Gandhi's Gramsvaraj was not the resurrection of the old village but the formation of fresh independent units of villages having a self-sufficient economy. Self-suffiency in basic needs was one of the fundamental conditions of Gandhian village reconstruction. Food, clothing and other basic necessities should be produced at the village itself, which would lead to full employment of almost each able-bodied person and would prevent the rural – urban migration in search of employment and better opportunities.

Illustrating the idea of Gramswaraj Gandhi speaks: "My idea of village swaraj is that it is a complete republic, independent of its neighbors for its vital wants, and yet interdependent for many others in which dependence is a necessity. Thus the village's first concern will be to grow its own food crops and cotton for its cloth. It should have a reserve for its cattle, recreation and playground for adults and children. Then if there is more land available, it will grow useful money crops, thus excluding ganja, tobacco, opium and the like. The village will maintain a village theatre, school and public hall. It will have its own water works ensuring a clean water supply. This can be done through controlled wells or tanks. Education will be compulsory upto the final basic course. As far as possible, every activity will be conducted on cooperative basis. There will be no caste, such as we have today with their graded untouchability. Nonviolence with its technique of *satygraha* and non-cooperation will be the sanction of the village community. There will be a compulsory service of village guards who will be selected by rotation from the register maintained by the village. The government of the village will be conducted by the Panchayat of five persons annually elected by the adult villagers, male and female, possessing minimum prescribed qualifications. They will have all the authority and jurisdiction required. Since there will be no system of punishment in the accepted sense, this Panchayat will be the legislature, judiciary and executive combined to operate for its year of office. Any village can become such republic without much interference, even from the present Government whose sole effective connection with the villages is the exaction of village revenue. I have not examined here the question of relations with the neighbouring villages of the centre, if any. My purpose is to present an outline of village government. Here there is perfect democracy based upon individual freedom. The individual is the architect of his own government. The law of non-violence rules him and the government."

Mahatma Gandhi's imagination of "Self Government" came to reality in 1992 when the Indian Parliaments gave rights, power and duties to the Gram Panchayats through 73rd amendment in the Constitution. Here the Panchayats are defined as "institutions of self- government." The Act provides for a three-tier Panchayati Raj system at the village, block and district level with a fixed tenure of five years. Seats have been reserved in favor of SC/ST and women so as to enhance their participation. The Act also provides for setting up a Finance Commission and an Election Commission.

What we Did?

For the first time in India through the initiative of the Governments and also with the interventions of likeminded NGOs, social thinkers, social workers, women representatives etc., countless numbers of measures were initiated to decentralize the administrative as well as financial power (including the decision making process) from top to bottom through a three-tier structure (district-block-village).

It was firmly and universally decided and accordingly it became a law to carry out the development programmes at all levels through these bodies.

With the involvement of people, community, planners and decision makers, strategists, politicians and political thinkers, parliamentary affairs and judiciary, several steps were taken in various phases of Indian history, mainly after the Independence and a special provision was made to assure that the women and underprivileged groups of India whether living in rural and urban India should be given equal opportunity through proportionate reservation in the every affairs, post, and functions of Panchayati Raj.

These bodies are now given real powers of implementation with sufficient financial resources so that they can carry out their responsibilities. 73rd and 74th Amendment Acts of the Indian Constitution are certainly the mile stones which changed the fate of women, underprivileged groups and brought them in the mainstream.

73rd and 74th Amendment Acts

The new Panchayati Raj Institutions (PRIs) in India acquired a constitutional status in 1993, with the 73rd constitutional amendment – a landmark in the history of decentralized planning and governance. The Panchayati Raj Act became applicable all over the country. It gave the vision of village level democratic governance and paved the way for rural development to be both, participatory and community based.

The passage of the 73rd Constitution Amendment Act, 1992 marks a new era in the federal democratic set up of India and provides Constitutional status to the Panchyati Raj Institutions. The salient features of the Act are: (i) constitution of panchayats at village, intermediate (block) and district level; however, panchayats at the intermediate level may not be constituted in a State having a population not exceeding twenty lakh; (ii) regular elections to Panchayats; (iii) reservation of seats for Scheduled Castes/Scheduled Tribes and Women (33 per cent); (iv) setting up of an independent State Finance Commission for strengthening finances of local bodies at all levels; (v) constitution of an independent State Election Commission to hold PRIs elections on a regular basis; (vi) legal status to Gram Sabhas; and (vii) addition of Eleventh Schedule to the Constitution listing 29 Subjects within the jurisdiction of PRIs. Further, the 73rd Constitutional Amendment Act contains provisions for devolution of powers and responsibilities upon panchayats at the appropriate level with reference to (a) the preparation of plans for economic development and social justice; and (b) the implementation of such schemes for economic development and social justice, as may be entrusted to them. The Provision of the Panchayat (Extension to Scheduled Areas) Act 1996 (PESA) extends panchayats to tribal areas in nine States. It enables the tribal society to shape their own development and preserve and conserve their traditional rights over natural resources.

The application of decentralization in PRIs has meant administrative and financial devolution of powers from top to bottom through a three-tier structure with bodies at each level, linked to one another. The development programmes at all levels are to be carried out through these bodies. These bodies are to be given real powers of implementation with sufficient financial resources so that they can carry out their responsibilities. The PRI Act has provisions, which enforce community participation, especially of the women, poor, and the marginalized sections of the region. The Gram Sabha (GS) is the backbone of the PRI. The term 'Gram Sabha' literally means village assembly/council and it includes all the adults in the village whose names are registered as voters. It is mandatory to have at least 4 GS Meetings in a year. The planning and development of resources is to be done through the Gram Sabhas. The 73rd Amendment provides for periodic elections to be conducted by an autonomous body and reservation of seats for women/SC/ST at all the levels.

The 11th schedule comprising 29 items of work provides a clearly defined role to Panchayats. Article 243 (G) of 73rd Amendment Act assigns Panchayats the responsibilities of preparation and implementation of plans for economic development and social justice. The items under the 29 responsibilities are:

- ☆ Primary Education
- ☆ Public works and construction
- ☆ Education and literacy
- ☆ Social and gender justice
- ☆ Health and disease
- ☆ Reproductive and Child Health
- ☆ Environment and Health
- ☆ Health and Nutrition
- ☆ Water
- ☆ Family welfare
- ☆ Agricultural development
- ☆ Land development
- ☆ Food grain supply and distribution
- ☆ Village development
- ☆ Animal husbandry

The above responsibilities are directly linked with the women and hence their intervention and active participation are very essential to make these responsibilities successfully undertaken.

In addition, the 74th amendment for Urban Local Government called Municipalities Act, there is provision for District Planning Commission (DPCS). These are combined Planning Committees for Panchayats and Municipal areas. Not less than 4-5 of the total number of members of such committees are required to be elected from amongst the elected members of Panchayats and municipalities in the district by the members themselves. This is to be in proportion to the ratio between the population of the rural and the urban areas in the district.

The constitutional amendment brought through 73rd and 74th Acts meant for community development at the grassroots level with one third reservation for women. Post-1993, all the Indian states have formulated their legislations accordingly, completed their elections and brought new Panchayats into existence. For the first time in India, nearly eight lakh women became members/chairpersons at the three levels of Panchayati Raj. It included, as per the new Act, the election of SC/ST women of not less than one-third of total SC/ST members/chairpersons. This is a unique experiment in the world of democracy, wherein women at grassroots level, irrespective of their education and socio-economic-political background have occupied local governing bodies. (Kaushik, Susheela, 2002[1]).

Now the change in the status of women, both in rural and urban India, is clearly visible. The women now in many cases are active in governance. This can easily be understood with the help of quantifiable data given below:

- ✰ Rural population of India: 744 Million-plus
- ✰ 537 District Panchayats elect15694. Out of this 5779 are women
- ✰ Total No. of Elected reps: 2828779: Out of this : 1038989 are women
- ✰ 198 Dist. Panchayat are headed by women.
- ✰ 232913 village Panchyats elect 2656476. Out of this 975116 are women.
- ✰ 1970 Block Panchayats are headed by women.
- ✰ 77,210 Village Panchayats are headed by women
- ✰ Total Urban population: 391 Million plus
- ✰ 112 City Corporations. Out of this 34 City Corporations are headed by women
- ✰ 1430 Town Municipalities. Out of this 476 Town Municipalities are headed by women.
- ✰ 2009 Nagar Panchyats. Out of this 670 Nagar Panchayats are headed by women
- ✰ Women Elected Representatives in Panchayats at all levels: Bihar 54.1 per cent and Karnataka 42.9 per cent.

Had there been no provisions for reservation, they would never have got such a chance.

---

1. Kaushik, Sushila, 2002, "Women and Panchayati Raj Institutions", in *Towards Comprehensive Women's Health Programmes and Policy* (ed.), Renu Khanna, Mira Shiva, Sarala Gopalan. pp. 515-516.

Status of Women vis-a-vis Improved Health and Nutrition

The 73rd Constitutional Amendment Act has given a new dimension to the process of women's empowerment in India. Apart from one-third reservation of women in Panchayati Raj Institutions (PRIs), the act has given constitutional powers and responsibilities for a range of issues including resource management, family planning, education and health. With the participation of women in PRIs, inter- personal relations within their families have changed for the better and this political process has heightened women's perceptions of their own capabilities. Even much-marginalized women have taken participation further to become activists despite constraints like illiteracy, lack of experience, family responsibilities, restrictive social norms, lack of enabling environment and violence (Singh, D.P., 2008)[2].

PRI's have been assigned several development activities including health and population stabilization. The Gram Sabha acts as a community level accountability mechanism to ensure that the functions of the PRI respond to people's needs.

Progress in engaging PRI has been uneven across states. While fiscal devolution is a significant issue, lack of institutional modalities and clear guidelines on PRI participation and variable capacity among PRI are key lacunae.

Articulation of PRI Engagement in Policy Documents

- The National Population Policy 2000 and the National Health Policy, 2001, include decentralization and convergence of service delivery at village levels and recognize the PRI as the agency responsible to ensure this. In 2001, the Planning Commission's Task Force reviewed PRI involvement and found that: Currently *the PRI are not equipped to take on such planning and monitoring functions, nor is there a cognizance in the health system of the role of PRI.* The Tenth Plan document also emphasizes the critical role and function of PRI in development.
- In August 2003, the Central Council of Ministers of Health and Family Welfare, resolved "that the States would involve PRI in the implementation of HFW programmes by progressive transfer of funds, functions and functionaries, by training, equipping and empowering them suitably to manage and supervise the functioning of healthcare infrastructure and manpower and further to coordinate the activities of the works of different departments such as: Health and Family Welfare, Social Welfare, and Education which are functioning at the Village and Block Levels".
- Despite geographic disparity, social inequity, poor status of women, illiteracy and the caste system, Panchayat elections do take place in most states every five years. I*n the context of health and family welfare, perhaps the most significant impact of the amendments is the ability of women to get elected to local bodies.* In some areas, women PRI members take an active role in polio eradication, health camps, mobilize women for services and monitor attendance of staff.

---

2. Singh, D.P., 2008, "Impact of 73rd Amendment Act on Women's Leadership in the Punjab". International Journal of Rural Studies, p.1, Vol. 15, No.1.

☆ Initiatives by MOHFW and donors in various states have focused on engaging PRIs in health programmes. MOHFW has supported the development of a training module for community and women's health, which deals with Panchayat engagement. MOHFW has also implemented the community needs assessment, the National Maternity Benefit Scheme and the Referral Transport scheme through PRI in various states. *Most experiences have been positive, but recognized that the enabling environment for panchayats to function needs strengthening.*

☆ The Kerala experience in strengthening PRIs, while not immediately and completely replicable, offers useful insights and lessons. Several factors influence the progress of decentralized planning and implementation, not the least being political will, and people's readiness to engage with decentralization.

Issues and Recommendations: Critical Role of Panchayati Raj Institutions in the Success of the National Rural Health Mission

☆ The National Rural Health Mission (NRHM) is seen as a vehicle to ensure that preventive and promotive interventions reach the vulnerable and marginalized through expanding outreach and linking with local governance institutions. *PRIs are seen as critical to the planning, implementation, and monitoring of the NRHM.* Implementation of the NRHM in achieving its outcomes is significantly dependent on well functioning gram, block and district level panchayats. At the District level a District Health Mission will coordinate NRHM functions. *Key to NRHM success are: intersectoral convergence, community ownership steered through village level health committees at the level of the Gram Panchayat, and a well functioning public sector health system with support from the private sector.*

☆ ASHA, (Accredited Social Health Activist), the mechanism to strengthen village level service delivery, will be a local resident and selected by the Gram Panchayat or the Village Health Committee. She will be supported in her work by the AWW, school teacher, community based organizations, such as SHGs, and the VHC. Her role would be to facilitate care seeking and serve as a depot holder for a package of basic medicines. She will be reimbursed by the panchayat on a performance based remuneration plan. The Village Health Committee (VHC) will form the link between the Gram Panchayat and the community, and will ensure that the health plan is in harmony with the overall local plan.

Empowerment of Panchayats through and the Assured Availability of Adequate Funds, Clear Articulation of Functions, and Transfer of Requisite Functionaries to Carryout such Functions

☆ State legislatures have been behindhand in framing laws that endow Panchayats with power and authority to enable their functioning. It has largely been a matter of political will in each state and is governed by different legislations, despite the central mandate. While PRI are mandated to carry out health activities, they are not backed by the necessary policy/ legal framework, authority or fiscal commitments. Many centrally sponsored schemes and others are implemented outside the purview of the panchayats, thus keeping them out of the loop and undermining their credibility. Issues of political patronage hamper functioning.

☆ Funds transfer to PRI for effective functioning of health services. Transfer of funds to PRI is a critical must before they could be expected to play a meaningful role in HFW activities. While several states have taken steps to complete financial devolution commensurate with functions still has a long way to go. With financial devolution other processes such as fiscal management, systems training and appropriate checks and balances need to be introduced.

☆ Clear articulation of functions of PRI at various levels: In areas where little devolution of power or funds has taken place, PRI representatives and particularly women lack clarity on their roles in development functions, including health. Line department staffs have to recognize that PRI carry the mandate of the people.

☆ Transfer of functionaries with commensurate authority and accountability guidelines. PRIs are expected to undertake monitoring of functionaries, particularly of line departments such as health and family welfare for increased accountability and improved functioning, without any authority over them. Transfer of functionaries is critical to ensure adequate functioning, monitoring, and accountability. Safeguards must be in place to protect against intimidation, wrongful harassment, and corruption.

Enlisting NGO Support in Building Capacity among PRI Members to Effectively Handle Development Related Functions

☆ Capacity building of PRI is required in thematic areas and leadership skills, negotiating, monitoring, ability to withstand patronage and political interference. Capacity building processes need to be tailored to literacy levels, sex and circumstances of PRI members.

☆ Joint orientation and sensitization meetings between PRI and health and medical professionals could help to bridge the gap in education and social strata. Developing Citizen Charter of Rights and Codes of conduct also lay down guidelines for boundaries of operation and accountability.

☆ NGOs could be involved in PRI strengthening in a variety of ways, including: consciousness raising, provision of technical advice, support in participatory planning, capacity building and facilitating monitoring processes, such as community and social audits to improve accountability.

Repealing Penalties and Disincentives such as the Two Child Norm, which Violate Individual Rights and Discriminate against Women's Participation in Panchayats

- ✩ Several states include disincentives in their population policies. The *most draconian is that which bars people who have more than two children from holding office.* Such policies are anti- women, threaten to undo the good of a decade's work in enabling women to participate in political processes and violate women's freedom and individual rights. They feed son preference actions such as sex selective abortions, pushing down an already unfavorable sex ratio. There are cases of women being abandoned, the third child given away or disowned, and consequent denial of the child's rights.
- ✩ Policies and laws such as this need to be repealed or they might have serious negative consequences for women and society at large. Population stabilization is a function of women's empowerment, access to high quality RH services and equal participation of men. PRIs should be encouraged to support these interventions to further promote improved health.

There are enough portents to suggest that PRI engagement in improving key health indicators will become a reality. However in order to expedite the process and to make it more effective, consideration of key issues related to empowerment of panchayats through funds, human resources and capacity are critical. PRI engagement is perhaps the only existing mechanism to achieve large-scale community participation and reach the marginalized and vulnerable, particularly women, children, and the poor. Locating NRHM functions within the gram panchayat and implementing it through a village health committee/gram Sabha will facilitate the process and make health for all an achievable reality.

Role of Panchayati Raj Institutions (PRIs) as Defined by Planning Commission

The Planning Commission has constituted a Task Force to formulate operational guidelines for the involvement of the Panchyati Raj Institutions in schemes of selected Central Ministries and Departments. Such Task Force is necessarily required to examine the PRIs-NGOs interface which is another area of concern and suggest norms for their harmonious relationship consistent with the spirit and provisions of 73rd Constitutional Amendment Act.

The Task Force of the Planning Commission has reviewed the status of the PRIs in the country, transfer of administrative powers and provision of financial resources to the PRIs, the conceptual dimensions of PRIs - NGOs interface, in the matrix of autonomy and accountability for effective functioning of the PRIs. The Report has considered in detail the role of PRIs in the implementation of specific centrally sponsored and central sector schemes of a few Ministries such those of Rural Development, Health and Family Welfare, Social Justice and Empowerment, Women and Child Development, Environment and Forests, Agriculture, Irrigation and Education and made specific recommendations on the manner in which involvement of different tiers of PRIs in their implementation and monitoring can be effected.

Similarly, dovetailing of PRIs in existing management structures for Externally Aided Projects has also been dealt with. The other relevant Ministries not specifically covered through schematic references in the report are also expected to formulate appropriate guidelines concerning their centrally sponsored / central sector schemes in the light of the recommendations of the report of the Planning Commission of India.

If the recommendations are followed seriously it will ensure following points:

- ✰ Gram Sabha to be involved in the identification of key target groups
- ✰ Gram Panchayat to designate a fixed day service for service provision to ensure regularity
- ✰ Panchayats will ensure ANM visits through a roster and facilitate the visits by ensuring mobility
- ✰ Panchayats will facilitate referral of community members as required to the PHC/CHC.
- ✰ Gram and block Panchayat will undertake periodic review of programme implementation
- ✰ Block Panchayats will ensure attendance of doctors, and other staff and identify bottlenecks to services at PHC/CHC

The structuring can easily be shown through a Table 23.1

Table 23.1: Planning Commission: Task Force Report Recommendations on PRI Involvement in HFW

Key Programmes	*Specific Interventions*	*Role of PRI–Various Levels*
Family Welfare (RCH) schemes	✰ Identification of pregnant women and children 0-12 months ✰ Ensuring antenatal and postnatal coverage of target group in the ANM's allotted villages. ✰ Arranging for immunization ✰ Referral of cases to PHC/ CHC ✰ Delivery of contraceptive services	✰ Gram Sabha to be involved in the identification of key target groups ✰ Gram Panchayat to designate a fixed day service for service provision to ensure regularity ✰ Panchayats will ensure AM visits through a roster and facilitate the visits by ensuring mobility ✰ Panchayats will facilitate referral of community members as required to the PHC/CHC. ✰ Gram and block Panchayat will undertake periodic review of programme implemen-tation ✰ Block Panchayats will ensure attendance of doctors, and other staff and identify bottlenecks to services at PHC/CHC

But there are many grey areas where the government, the NGOs, social workers, planners and thinkers have to think, plan and act to assure autonomy, respectful position to the women so that the RCH and other issues can very well be taken. This situation may bring the equal justice for women and all deprived sections of the society.

Observations

We, as grass root NGO professionals, have been working with the rural and urban communities of India across geographical and cultural boundary. However, in order to focus our attention in some prioritized geographical pockets, we have decided to share our observations from Haryana and western Uttar Pradesh.

During pre-evaluation of their knowledge and experience level, they did not share anything about RCH, Immunization, Nutrition and Health, Institutional deliveries and their role in addressing these issues in Panchayat meetings.

After interventions with them, discussions, providing them the platform to share, they expressed the present status of Health, home deliveries, functioning of the PHC and other related issues.

If the platform is provided with freedom of expression, they know how to express not in an articulated manner, but they are capable of putting their ideas, suggestions and recommendations.

There is a need for regular exposure to such platforms, regular interactions on issues and platform to perform.

Limitations of `The Success` Stories

- ✰ Women still face considerable handicaps to their involvement in politics; for example, inadequate exposure, the burden of reproductive and productive roles, a lack of self-confidence and the opposition of entrenched cultural and religious views.
- ✰ Need to provide women with specific kinds of support which go beyond technical training. They need support to build solidarity amongst women, through strengthening links between women's organizations and elected bodies.
- ✰ Need information about innovative organizations and NGOs which enhance women's lives. It is also necessary to strengthen women's sense of common identity by articulating the elements of a feminist consciousness and presenting it as the special quality of women's leadership.
- ✰ There has been insufficient elaboration of what that leadership has to offer which distinguishes it from men's leadership and which commends it as something special. Such an elaboration through feminist discourse and action is essential for this revolution to deliver the promise it holds.
- ✰ The lesson of PRI is clear: if the wisdom of grassroots organizations, especially the courage and clarity of women, is to become policy, it will not be through the art of intellectual persuasion but by the arrangements made within a political system for their voice to have power.

- ☆ Women's entry into local government in such large numbers, often more than the required 33.3 percent, and their success in campaigning, including the defeat of male candidates, has shattered the myth that women are not interested in politics, and have no time to go to meetings or to undertake all the other work that is required in political party processes. Though there is a need for devolution of project design and monitoring powers from central government to the elected bodies, so that the latter can play their requisite role, developing their own policies, reflecting the views of their own representatives rather than those of central government, and be held accountable for them.
- ☆ There is a need to build global coalitions. This includes bringing women into political structures and supporting the backward and forward linkages of women's presence in politics, linking household and family priorities with macro-planning processes. Campaigns and training programmes to prepare the women both as electors and elected.
- ☆ In the case of Haryana, a formal stocktaking is yet to be undertaken in this regard at the level of the government. Some efforts in terms of training etc., though, have been there at an informal level during the recent years, particularly in the area of orienting elected women panchayat representatives for making their personal participation possible in the first place. However, even such half-hearted efforts have been found lacking in case of those coming from dalit background in general and dalit women in particular as a distinct category.
- ☆ At the outset it is to be recalled that vested interests had never taken kindly to the provision of reservation in the new Act. A clause, 175(1) (q), was therefore incorporated in Haryana Panchayati Raj Act 1994 at the time of its ratification by the state assembly. Under this clause, a dubious condition was imposed that a person having more than two children cannot stand for election. Any elected representative is further liable to be unseated if a third issue is born to him or her. This retrograde provision has adversely affected not only the persons coming from poorer background in general but the Dalits and women in particular. Ironically, these were the very sections for whose supposed benefit the reservation was provided.
- ☆ Secondly, in the given social milieu it is the rural rich who continue to hold the levers of socio-economic power. They get their womenfolk elected on seats reserved for women while they themselves continue to function as *de-facto* representatives with impunity. Sarcastically called as *Sarpanch Pati or Panch Pati*, these proxy men are being unhesitantly entertained at all administrative levels as elected representatives. The government has never issued instructions to discourage this open fraud and clear cut offense of impersonation.
- ☆ Thirdly, most of the Dalit sapanches are sought to be remote controlled by influential people upon whom they have to remain dependent due to various compulsions. In the event of defiance or self assertion by a Dalit sarpanch, the panchayat is virtually made defunct by unique methods.

Panches belonging to upper caste would tactically stay away from the officially convened meetings which then cannot take place for want of required quorum. Instances of public humiliation and even physical intimidation of dalit sapanches, including of women, have often been reported in the media.

- ☆ Most of the elected panchayat members in Haryana are still working within the traditional mode as far as the functions and areas of activities are concerned. These are mainly confined to digging of ponds, construction of roads, auctioning of village common lands for cultivation etc. while key aspects of village life in the social domain like health, education, sports, food security, managing potable water, sanitation (including drainage), housing, environment (including forestry), social justice and cultural affairs remain still untouched by the panchayats.
- ☆ Absence of toilet facilities for women continues to be the most haunting problem. There is also the issue of giving residential plots for the landless. Until these problems are addressed within and even outside the panchayat system from the angle of Dalits, women and the youth, neither the panchayats become participatory nor these ignored sections could be empowered in any significant way.

Suggestions and Conclusions

On the basis of our experience and interaction with the women, change agents, social thinkers, etc., we may suggest the following points:

- ☆ Devolution of 29 subjects according to XIth schedule must be compulsory.
- ☆ There should be effective and continuous training programmes for PRI leaders and officials. (This has already been initiated but we want it in focused manner with the help of seasoned professionals and successful achievers.
- ☆ Training arrangement should be made at block level and at the district level too.
- ☆ Gram Sabha should be effectively empowered.
- ☆ Presence of women should be made a compulsory and to check the proxy of women role the punitive measures must be introduced.
- ☆ Government must effectively empower PRIs. Reservation of seats for Sarpanch, chairman of Panchayat Samiti and President of Zila Parishad should not be rotational.
- ☆ Political interference must be abolished in the elections, structure and functioning of PRIs.
- ☆ There should be separate cadre of Panchayati Raj services, with one third women officials.

Abbreviations

DPC: District Planning Commission
HFW: Health and Family Welfare
MOHFW: Ministry of Health and family Welfare
NGO: Non Governmental Organization
NRHM: National Rural Health Mission
PESA: Panchyat Extension to Scheduled Areas (Act 1996)
PRI: Panchayati Raj Institution
RCH: Reproductive Child Health
VHC: Village Health Committee

References

1. *Athrava-Veda* (5.17.1)
2. *Athrava-Veda* (5-17-13)
3. *Atharva-Veda* (5-17-16)
4. *Atharva-Veda* (5-17-18)
5. Kaushik, Sushila, 2002, "Women and Panchayati Raj Institutions", in *Towards Comprehensive Women's Health Programmes And Policy* (ed.), Renu Khanna, Mira Shiva, Sarala Gopalan, pp. 515-516.
6. Malhotra Geeta, 2010, *Role of Women Members of Panchyati Raj Institutions in Effective Utilisation of RCH Services*, Doctoral Thesis ready for the Submission of PhD award from the Anna Malai University.
7. Mishra, Kailash Kumar, 1994, "Role of Factionalism in a Panchayat Election: Study of an Ahir Village of Haryana", *Indian Anthropologist*.
8. Mishra, Kailash Kumar, 1994, "The Unhealthy State of the National Health Policy." *Indian Anthropologist* (Vol. 24).
9. Mishra, Kailash Kumar, 2004, "Chaupal as Multidimensional Public Space", in M. D. Muthukumaraswamy and Molly Kaushal edited, *Folklore, Public Sphere and Civil Society*, pp. 123-137; Delhi and Chennai; IGNCA and NFSC, 2004.
10. Singh Inderji, 2005, "Looking Beyond Elections: State of Panchyati Raj in Haryana", *People's Democracy*, Vol. XXIX, No. 20
11. *Rig-Veda* (10.109.1)
12. Singh, D. P., 2008, "Impact of 73rd Amendment Act on Women's Leadership in the Punjab", *International Journal of Rural Studies*, p.1, Vol. 15, No.1.
13. Singh, Surat, 2004, "Working of Gram Sabha: The Haryana Experience" in Surat Singh (Ed), *Decentralized Governance in India: Myth and Reality*, Deep and Deep Publications, New Delhi.

Chapter 24

Traditional Leafy Vegetables as a Source of Pro-Vitamin A Carotenoids for Under Five Year Olds in Uganda

A. Atero Angella, Agnes Namutebi and Margaret Kabahenda*

Science and Technology Communications Officer, Uganda National Council for Science and Technology (UNCST), Uganda

E-mail: *atero_angella@yahoo.com, a.atero@uncst.go.ug

ABSTRACT

Vitamin A Deficiency (VAD) status in Uganda is still alarming, despite the fact that the Government of Uganda has put programs in place to try and alleviate the problem. It is estimated that child deaths that occur annually in Uganda due to Vitamin A deficiency are 29,000, while the percentage of children less than 6 years of age in Uganda with sub-clinical Vitamin A deficiency is 66 (UNICEF, 2005). In 2006 it was noted that, 20 per cent of children (6-59 months) in Uganda are categorized as having Vitamin A Deficiency (<0.835 micromoles/liter of Retinol Binding Protein (RPB)), levels those are always considered to have functional consequences in terms of morbidity and mortality. Children in East Central Uganda, where Iganga District is located, were noted as having the highest (32 per cent) VAD levels in the whole country compared to the national average of 20 per cent (UBOS, 2006). Iganga District where the study took place is located in the Lake Victoria Basin which is rich in plant biodiversity including traditional leafy vegetables[1]. These traditional leafy vegetables are rich in pro-vitamin A carotenoids and thus can be used to reduce the high prevalence of VAD

---

1. Traditional Leafy Vegetables are those plants whose leaves or aerial parts have been integrated in a community's culture for use as food over a long span of time.

in that region and the whole country at large. Leafy vegetables are relatively easy to produce; inexpensive and accessible/available almost all year round (Rodriguez-Amaya, 1997; Maundu *et al.*, 1999). Data was collected from 363 children in Iganga District in the month of July 2008 during the wet season. Data collection was done using Gibson's 24 Hour Dietary recall method and a qualitative food frequency questionnaire (FFQ). Information was provided by mothers and female caretakers with children between 6 - 59 months. Analysis of date was done using Statistical Package for Social Sciences (SPSS) and Nutri-survey and the level of significance used was $p<0.05$. A total of 21 species of traditional leafy vegetables and 1 non-traditional leafy vegetable were consumed at least once a week by children aged between 6-59 months in Iganga district. Of all these leafy vegetables, only five were mostly consumed and these included; *Amaranthus lividus* (booga) (93.7 per cent), *Cucurbita maxima* Lam (eisun*sa(83.2 per cent)), Colocasia esculenta* (timpa*) (72.5 per cent), Cleome gynandra* (eiyobyo)(66.3 per cent), and *Brassica Oeracea Var.capitata* (non-traditional)(85 per cent). For the rest of the vegetables, less than 50 per cent of the respondents consumed them at least once a week. However, results from the 24 Hour Dietary Recall showed that of all the leafy vegetables mentioned above, only 5 had been consumed by the children 24 hours preceding the survey. They included *Amaranthus lividus* (18.75 per cent), *Cucurbita maxima Lam* (6.25 per cent., *Colocasia esculenta* (2.08 per cent), *Vigna unguiculata* (0.60 per cent) and *Brassica Oeracea Var.capitata* (8.93 per cent) (Non-traditional). Compared to other food groups it was discovered that TLVs were the second least consumed (27 per cent). It was also discovered that 94 per cent of mothers and caretakers had no knowledge of the nutritional value of TLVs and only 20.1 per cent of households cultivated TLVS. There is generally a low consumption of traditional leafy vegetables in the region by children aged between 6-59 months. The low consumption could be attributed to the fact that there is limited knowledge on the nutritional value of traditional leafy vegetables among the mothers/caretakers. Similar results were reported by Kikafunda *et al.* (2006). Another reason could be that there is limited cultivation of these traditional leafy vegetables, Rubaihayo, (1997) in his study also reported similar results. Most households depended on volunteer plants[2] during the rainy seasons. This therefore means that those traditional leafy vegetables whose seeds have short dormancy periods are disappearing. Peasant farmers prefer to cultivate the introduced exotic vegetables like *Brassica Oeracea Var.capitata* for urban markets. Food groups like meat and meat products and dairy products that are rich sources of Vitamin A were also among the least consumed. 28.72 per cent and 23.3 per cent of the respondents indicated that they consumed meat and its products and dairy products at least once a week. Therefore there is low consumption of other foods rich in vitamin A. All the reasons above explain why there is a high prevalence of VAD in East Central Region (30 per cent) compared to the national figure which is 20 per cent.

Keywords: Traditional leafy vegetables, Vitamins.

Introduction

Vitamin A Deficiency (VAD) status in Uganda is still alarming, despite the fact that the Government of Uganda has put programs in place to try and alleviate the problem. It is estimated that child deaths that occur annually in Uganda due to Vitamin A deficiency (VAD) are 29,000, while the percentage of children less than 6

---

2. Volunteer plants are those that have resulted from natural propagation as opposed to having been deliberately planted by humans seed.

years of age in Uganda with sub-clinical Vitamin A deficiency is 66 (UNICEF, 2005). In 2006 it was noted that, 20 per cent of children (6-59 months) in Uganda are categorized as having Vitamin A Deficiency (<0.835 micromoles/liter of Retinol Binding Protein (RPB)), levels that are always considered to have functional consequences in terms of morbidity and mortality. Children (6-59 months) in East Central Uganda (where Iganga District is located) were noted as having the highest (32 per cent) VAD levels in the whole country compared to the national figure which is 20 per cent (UBOS, 2006). Iganga district where the study took place is located in the Lake Victoria Basin which is rich in plant biodiversity including traditional leafy vegetables. These [3]traditional leafy vegetables are rich in pro-vitamin A carotenoids and thus can be used to reduce the high prevalence of VAD in that region (east central Uganda) and the whole country at large. Leafy vegetables are relatively easy to produce; inexpensive and accessible/available almost all year round (Rodriguez-Amaya, 1997; Maundu *et al.*, 1999)

Methodology

Data was collected from 363 children in Iganga District in the month of July 2008 during the wet season. Data collection was done using Gibson's 24 Hour Dietary recall method and a qualitative food frequency questionnaire (FFQ). Analysis was done using Statistical Package for Social Sciences (SPSS) and Nutri-survey and the level of significance used was $p<0.05$.

Results

Consumption of Leafy Vegetables

A total of 21 species of traditional leafy vegetables and 1 non-traditional leafy vegetable were consumed at least once a week by children aged between 6-59 months in Iganga district. Of all these leafy vegetables, only five are mostly consumed and these include; *Amaranthus lividus* (booga) (93.7 per cent), *Cucurbita maxima* Lam [eisunsa (83.2 per cent)], *Colocasia esculenta* (timpa) (72.5 per cent), *Cleome gynandra* (eiyobyo) (66.3 per cent), and *Brassica Oeracea* var. *capitata* (non-traditional)(85 per cent).

For the rest of the vegetables, less than 50 per cent of the respondents consumed them at least once a week. However, results from the 24 Hour Dietary Recall showed that of all the leafy vegetables mentioned above, only 5 had been consumed by the children 24 hours preceding the survey. They included *Amaranthus lividus* (18.75 per cent), *Cucurbita maxima Lam* (6.25 per cent), *Colocasia esculenta* (2.08 per cent), *Vigna unguiculata* (0.60 per cent) and *Brassica Oeracea Var.capitata* (8.93 per cent) (non-traditional).

Compared to other food groups it was discovered that TLVs were the second least consumed (27 per cent).

---

3. Traditional Leafy Vegetables are those plants whose leaves or aerial parts have been integrated in a community's culture for use as food over a long span of time.

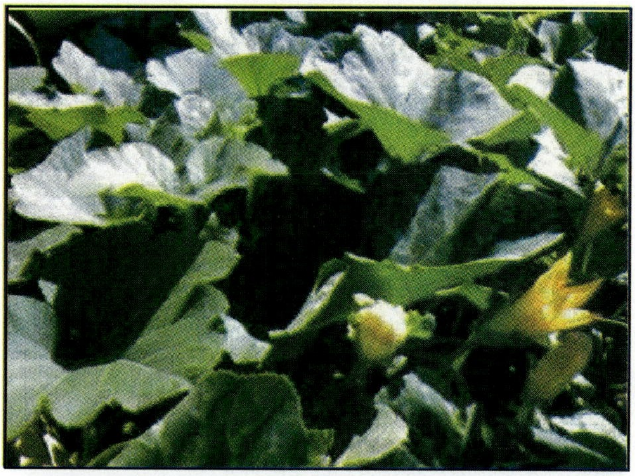

Cucurbita maxima **Lam (Eisunsa) (83.2 per cent)**

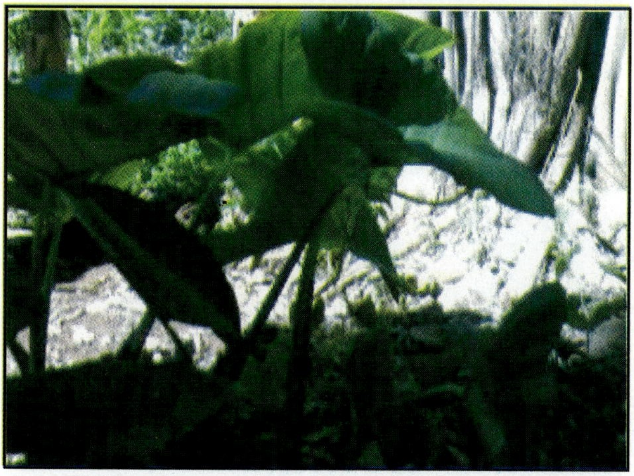

Colocasia esculenta **(Timpa) (72.5 per cent)**

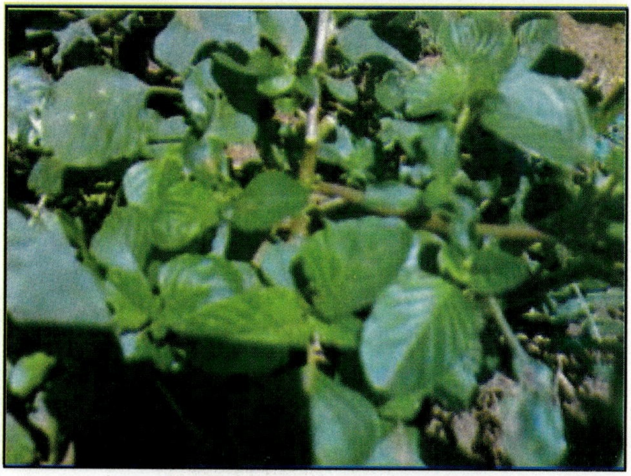

Amaranthus lividus **(Booga) (93.7 per cent)**

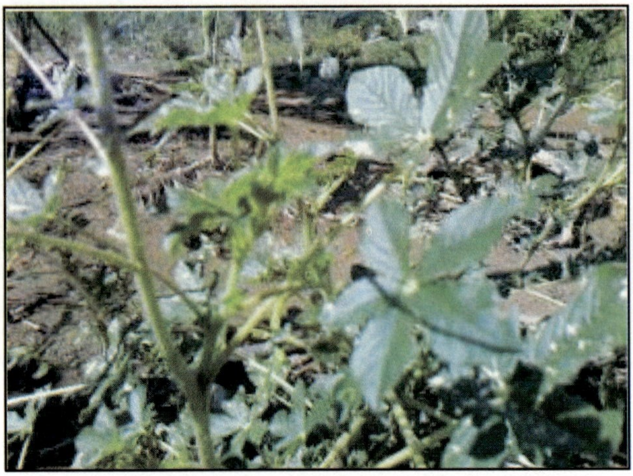

Cleome gynandra **(Eiyobyo) (66.3 per cent)**

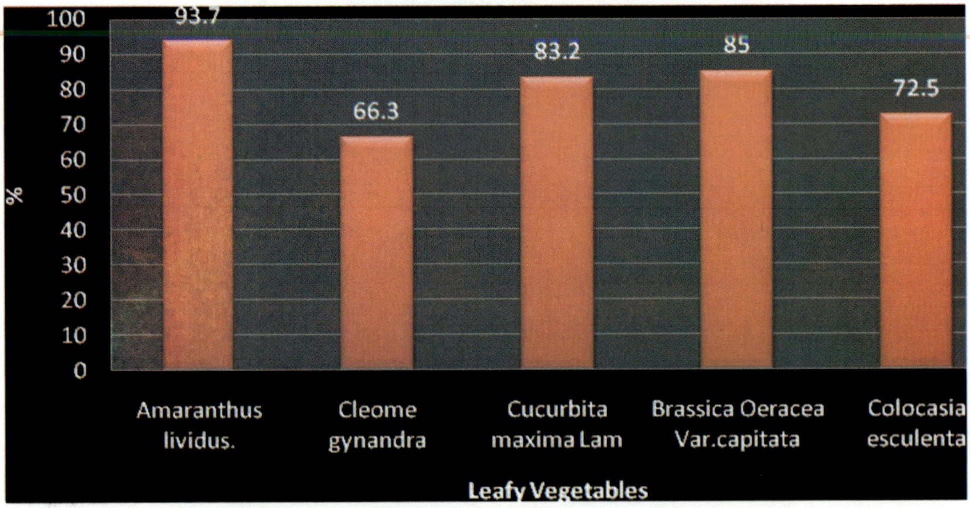

Figure 24.1: Per cent Consumption of Different Varieties of Leafy Vegetables

Knowledge of the Nutritional Value of TLVs

It was also discovered that 94 per cent of mothers and caretakers have no knowledge of the nutritional value of TLVs

Cultivation of TLVs

About 20.1 per cent of households cultivate TLVS.

Discussion

There is generally a low consumption of traditional leafy vegetables in the region by children aged between 6-59 months. The low consumption could be attributed to

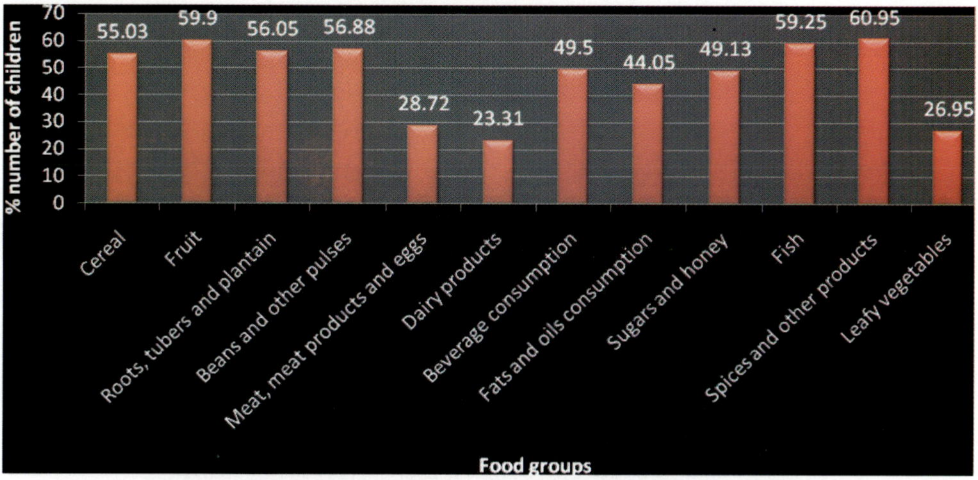

Figure 24.2: Consumption of Different Food Groups

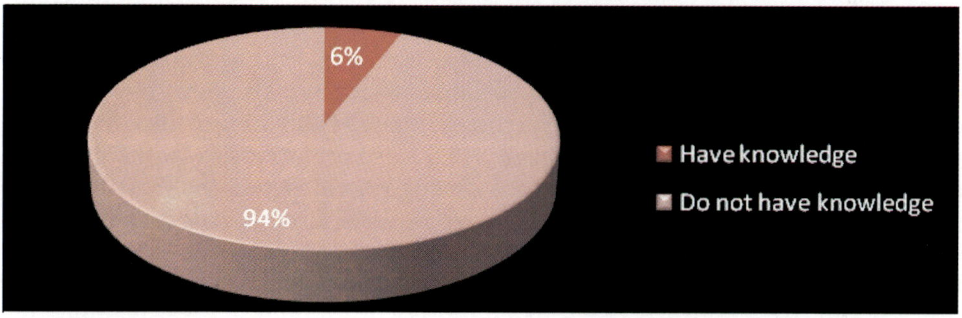

Figure 24.3: Mothers/Caretakers Knowledge of the Nutritional Value of TLV

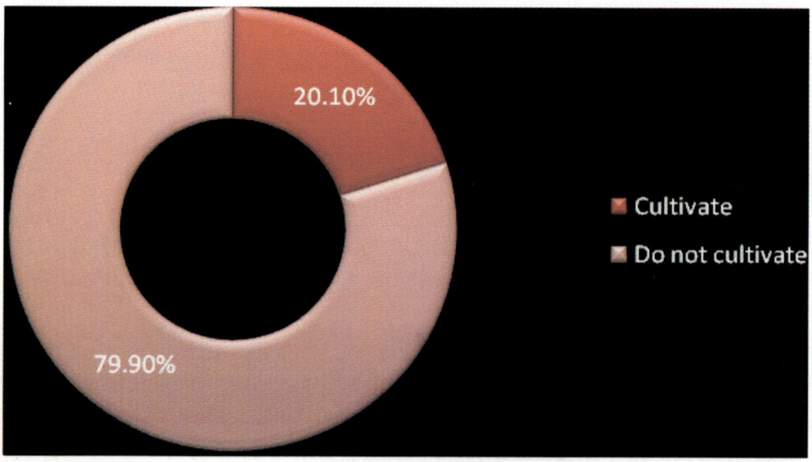

Figure 24.4: Cultivation

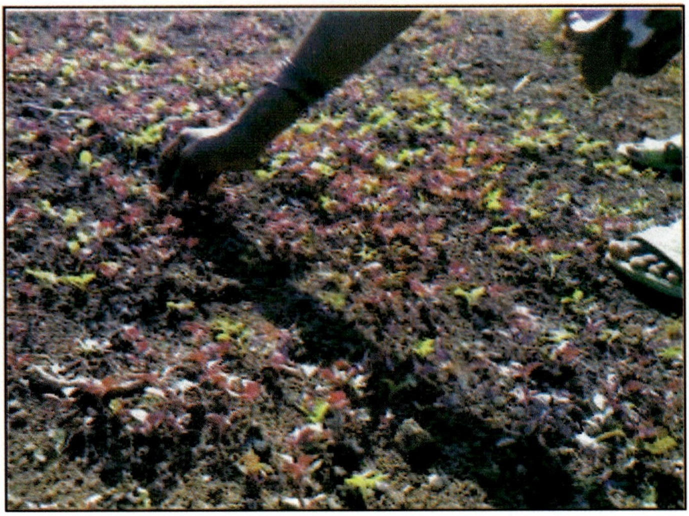

Figure 24.5: A Woman Weeds her Vegetable Garden in Iganga District

the fact that there is limited knowledge on the nutritional value of traditional leafy vegetables among the mothers/caretakers. Similar results were reported by Kikafunda *et al.* (2006). Another reason could be that there is limited cultivation of these traditional leafy vegetables, in his study Rubaihayo, (1997) also reported similar results. Most households depend on [4]volunteer plants during the rainy seasons. This therefore means that those traditional leafy vegetables whose seeds have short dormancy periods are disappearing. Peasant farmers prefer to cultivate the introduced exotic vegetables like *Brassica Oeracea Var.capitata* for urban markets. Food groups like meat and meat products and dairy products that are rich sources of Vitamin A are also among the least consumed. 28.72 per cent and 23.3 per cent of the respondents indicated that they consumed meat and its products and dairy products at least once a week. This shows a low consumption of other foods rich in vitamin A.

These reasons are an explanation as to why there is a high prevalence of VAD in East Central Region (30 per cent) compared to the national figure which is 20 per cent.

Recommendations

- ✰ The traditional leafy vegetables with high levels of pro-vitamin A carotenoids, need to be identified such that diversification of diets through increased utilization and consumption would help in alleviating hidden hunger and malnutrition.
- ✰ Improving the consumption of these TLVs through sensitization of the public of their nutritional value would go a long way in improving their cultivation. This will intern reduce infant mortality due to VAD in the region.

---

4. Volunteer plants are those that have resulted from natural propagation as opposed to having been deliberately planted by humans seed.

Conclusion

Traditional Leafy Vegetables can be used as a cheaper source of Pro-Vitamin A carotenoids if there utilization and cultivation is improved. Low consumption of traditional leafy vegetables combined with low consumption of other foods rich in Vitamin A have continued to cause high levels of VAD among children aged 6-59 months in Iganga district as reported in the Uganda Demographic Health Survey report of 2006 (UBOS, 2006). Therefore increasing mothers and caretakers knowledge on the nutritional value of traditional leafy vegetables would lead to their increased consumption and thus cultivation. This would in turn lower levels of VAD and therefore mortality among the children.

References

1. Kikafunda J and Kiremire B.T. (2006). Utilization of Indigenous Food Plants in Uganda, A case study of south western Uganda www.bioline.org.br
2. Maundu P., Njiro E., Chweya J., Imungi J., and Seme E. (1999). The biodiversity of traditional leafy vegetable- Kenya chapter- IPGRI www.bioversityinternational.org/publications
3. Rubaihayo E.B. (1997). Conservation and use of traditional vegetables in Uganda: Traditional African Vegetables. Proceedings of the IPGRI International Workshop on Genetic Resources of Traditional Vegetables in Africa: Conservation and Use 29-31 August 1995, ICRAF-HQ, Nairobi, Kenya. http://www.bioversityinternational.org/publications
4. Rodriguez-Amaya. (1997). Carotenoids and Food Preparation: The Retention of Provitamin A Carotenoids in Prepared, Processed, and Stored Foods. John Snow, Inc/OMNI Project. http://www.mostproject.org/PDF/carrots2.pdf
5. Uganda Bureau of Statistics (UBOS) and Macro International Inc. (2007). Uganda Demographic and Health Survey 2006- Calverton, Maryland, USA: UBOS
6. UNICEF (2005). A partnership drive to end hidden hunger in Sub Saharan Africa. http://www.micronutrient.org/vmd/countryfiles/subsaharan

Chapter 25
Maternal and Child Health

Doomun Aryamah Kumaree

Principal Nutritionist, Ministry of Health and Quality of Life/Nutrition Unit
153, Jasmin Street, Morcellement Montreal, Phase 2, Coromandel, Mauritius
E-mail: angel_timeline@yahoo.com

ABSTRACT

Malnourished pregnant women do not receive nutritional supplements from government programs. However, all pregnant women receive Iron, Calcium and Multivitamin tablets during their antenatal treatment in their local health centers or at hospital level. However, according to the Quarterly Bulletin of the Nutritional Surveillance System, for Percentage of infants having a low (<2.5 kg) birth weight is 16.7 per cent (Health Statistics, 2008). Percentage of exclusively breastfed infants under 6 months – No clear cut data is available. The months of July – September 2009, absolute breastfeeding practices for infants at 14 weeks are 48.9 per cent. Exclusive breastfeeding for six months is officially promoted. A national system for giving nutritional supplements to malnourished children does not exist. However, children in the 'ZEP'(Zone d'Education Prioritaire) Schools do benefit from the Food Supplementary Programme where they receive a supplementary meal representing a balanced diet with all the seven essential food elements (carbohydrates, fats, proteins, vitamins, minerals, roughage and water) present in adequate amounts).

Keywords: *Maternal health, Child health, Family planning, Abortion, HIV/AIDS, Disease, Breast cancer.*

Introduction

Population

The estimated resident population of the Island of Mauritius at the end of 2008 was 1,234,042 (609,261 males and 624,781 females) as compared to 1,227,075 in 2007, growing at a rate of 0.57 per cent.

Health Delivery System

In the Island of Mauritius, as at the end of 2008, there were five regional hospitals with a total of 2,410 beds and two district hospitals namely Souillac Hospital with 30 beds and Mahebourg Hospital with 63 beds. There were also a psychiatric hospital with a bed complement of 751, and other hospitals for chest diseases (61 beds), eye diseases (57 beds), ear, nose and throat (ENT) diseases (65 beds) and heart diseases (63 beds). This brought the total number of beds in government institutions to 3,500 as compared to 3, 819 in 2000.

In the public sector, primary healthcare, curative and high-tech medical care are provided free of any user cost at the point of use to the entire population.

In the private sector there were, as at the end of 2008, seventeen nursing homes (private clinics) with a total of 582 beds.

While the private health institutions cater for around 15 per cent of the total healthcare requirements, the public sector provides services to the remaining 85 per cent of the population.

The total number of beds in the public and private sectors as at the end of 2008 was thus 4,082, that is, 3.3 beds for 1000 inhabitants. In 1997, the corresponding ratio was 3.0 beds.

All regional and district hospitals as well as the Psychiatric, Eye, ENT and Cardiac hospitals have an out-patient department. Out-patient services are also delivered in two community hospitals, two medi-clinics, 21 Area Health Centers (AHC) and 113 Community Health Centers (CHC).

The basic services delivered at the Health Centers include the treatment of common diseases and injuries, maternal and child care, and family planning. In addition to these services, AHC also provide dental care. This service is also delivered in a few CHCs.

Out-patient care is also provided in the private sector, including several clinics and dispensaries on sugar estates. There were also 13 health offices, a chest clinic, a social hygiene clinic, and a National Centre for the Immuno-suppressed in operation as at the end of 2008.

The number of contacts with government preventive and curative health services, which includes attendances for the treatment of diseases and injuries at outpatient departments of hospitals, mediclinics, area health centers, community health centers and ayurvedic clinics, together with admissions and attendances at hospitals for other services such as haemodialysis, diet clinis and physiotherapy which decreased from 8.4 million in 2006 to 8.2 million in 2007, was 8.4 million in 2008 with a daily average of around 23,000.

There is at least one service point which is easily accessible to the community within 2 to 3 km of their place of residence.

Maternal Health

Situation Analysis

The number of maternal deaths registered in 2008 was 6. The maternal mortality rate (MMR) per 1000 live births was then 0.38 (38 maternal deaths per 100,000 live births) as compared to 0.9 in 1984. This represents a decrease of 57.8 per cent. The lowest rate with only one death due to complication following childbirth was 0.05 in 2002.

The prevalence of anemia among pregnant women is 9 per cent (2004 NCD/ Nutrition Survey).

As at the end of 2008, a total of 678 females were detected with HIV/AIDS.

Maternal Health Services

The following services form part of the Maternal Health Programme of the Ministry of Health and Quality of Life:

Antenatal Clinics

Ante-natal care is easily accessible at primary healthcare centers [21 Area and 113 Community Health Centers].

In the antenatal clinics, the following services are offered:

- ✰ Regular follow up by skilled health personnel for the duration of the pregnancy.
- ✰ Check up for blood pressure, growth of foetus, oedema and other medical conditions.
- ✰ Voluntary blood testing and counseling for Sexually Transmitted Diseases (STIs) and HIV/AIDS.
- ✰ Early detection of problems complicating pregnancy *e.g.*, anemia, hypertensive disorders, bleeding, malpresentations, multiple pregnancy.
- ✰ Routine echography.
- ✰ Routine counseling of all pregnant women by trained healthcare staff on self care at home, nutrition, safe sex, preparation for breastfeeding, family planning, healthy lifestyle and management of diarrhea and other childhood illness.
- ✰ Weekly session by Gynecologists at all Area Health Centers.

Functional referral systems exist from the primary care to hospital level.

Care of Mothers during Labour and Postpartum

Trained personnel attend all deliveries, and monitor all mothers before, during and after delivery.

Care during Labour and Delivery includes

- ✰ Diagnosis of labour

- ☆ Monitoring progress of labour, maternal and fetal well-being with partograph
- ☆ Providing supportive care and pain relief
- ☆ Detection of problems and complications (*e.g.* malpresentations prolonged and/or obstructed labour, hypertension, bleeding, and infection)
- ☆ Delivery and immediate care of the newborn baby, initiation of breastfeeding
- ☆ Newborn resuscitation
- ☆ Active management of third stage of labour.

Immediate Postpartum Care of Mother

- ☆ Monitoring and assessment of maternal well being, prevention and detection of complications (*e.g.* hypertension, infections, bleeding, anemia)
- ☆ Treatment of moderate posthaemorrhagic anemia
- ☆ Information and counseling on home self care, nutrition, safe sex, breast care and family planning.

Health Promotion

Education of women and their family members is carried out during antenatal clinics, post partum clinics and in the well baby clinics.

A handbook for parents providing information on how to deal with common childhood medical problems is distributed for information of parents, carers and other members of the community.

Family Planning

Reproductive health services are accessible to all individuals through the primary healthcare system. There are 160 service points that provide family planning services and information throughout the island. These service points include 1 Community Hospital, 2 Medi-Clinics, 23 Area Health Centers, 114 Community Health Centers, 4 Family Health Clinics, 2 Family Planning Clinics, 1 Family Planning Supply Centre and 13 Industrial Family Planning Supply Centers. Moreover, about 2,125 women in the reproductive age group were served per point in 2008. In the same year, 9 family planning clinics provided services after working hours, on Sundays and on public holidays.

The FP programme has formulated its objectives in line with the Plan of Action adopted at the 1994 Cairo International Conference on Population and Development, and the major part of the ICPD goals have been achieved.

A National Action Plan on Sexual and Reproductive Health is under preparation.

Abortion

This is a serious health problem because it can leads to many complications, especially in those cases where it is performed in improper settings. Abortion is illegal in Mauritius, but many women procure abortion for an unwanted pregnancy. Legalization of abortion remains a very sensitive issue.

A draft Pregnancy Control Bill is under consideration, and will be prepared in consultation with other stakeholders in order to address issues concerning abortion, especially in cases of sexual assault. Government may consider legalizing abortion in certain well defined cases.

Teenage Pregnancy

Talks are held by qualified staff from Ministry of Health, MFPWA and Action Familiale in secondary schools on reproductive health, and information leaflets on reproductive health and prevention of HIV/AIDS are distributed to pupils.

Two Youth Friendly Service Centers are fully functional. One is situated on the campus of the University of Mauritius and the other one in the City Centre. Staffs at these centers provide counseling to the youth on reproductive health issues. It is planned to set up more such centers in other parts of the island, including one in Rodrigues.

HIV/AIDS

Until now Mauritius can be considered as a low prevalence HIV/AIDS country. The first case of AIDS was notified in October 1987. As at the end of 2008, a total of 3,844 cases of HIV/AIDS were detected, of whom 3,671 (2,993 males, 678 females) were Mauritians; 243 of these Mauritians were known to have passed away. 76 per cent of the 3,671 HIV infected Mauritians were in the age group 25 to 49 years and 17.9 per cent in the age group 15 to 24 years. At the beginning of the epidemic, the mode of transmission of the HIV virus was predominantly heterosexual. The rising incidence as from year 2000 was driven by Injecting Drug Users (IDUs) acting as the main mode of transmission. The gradual shift in mode of transmission from heterosexual to IDUs became evident in 2003. The distribution of the 3,671 infected Mauritians by mode of transmission is as follows: 74.9 per cent Intravenous Drug Users; 16.9 per cent heterosexuals; 5.5 per cent heterosexual IV Drug Users; 0.7 per cent Homosexual/Bisexual; 0.6 per cent Mother to Child transmission and 1.4 per cent other and undetermined cases.

Sexually Transmitted Diseases

The main STIs (Gonorrhoea and Syphilis) as reported by Health Statistics Annual are showing a decreasing trend in the last decade. For 2008, 47 cases of Gonorrhoea (45 male, 2 female) and 13 cases of Syphilis (7 male, 6 female) have been reported.

Cervical and Breast Cancers

Married and sexually active women in the age group 35-60 are screened for cervical and breast cancers. Pap smears are done – there is visual examination of the cervix, using a speculum and specimens are taken for cytology. Suspicious smears are reviewed. As far as breast cancer is concerned, there is clinical examination of the breasts. The family history of premenopausal breast cancer in a first-degree relative is one among the key elements of the programme. Suspected cases are sent for mammography and onwards treatment and follow-up.

Non-Communicable Diseases

Mauritius has registered a shift in the burden of diseases since the early nineteen eighties. Whilst at one time communicable diseases were the main problem, over the past decades, the major health concern has become the high prevalence of NCDs, namely Type-2 diabetes, hypertension/ischaemic heart disease and cancer. Communicable diseases have to a large extent been successfully been controlled, with some diseases such as Malaria having been eradicated.

The high prevalence of diabetes increased from 14.3 per cent in 1987 to 19.5 per cent in 1998 and then slightly to 19.3 per cent in 2004 (age ≥ 30 years); that is, one in every five adult in this age group had Type-2 diabetes. The age-standardized prevalence of diabetes in the Mauritian population aged 20-74 years was 15 per cent (15 per cent in males, 15.1 per cent in females).

The age-standardized prevalence of hypertension in adults aged 20-74 years was 23.1 per cent (24.2 per cent in males, 22.8 per cent in females). In adults aged 30 years and over the prevalence has remained at around 30 per cent during the period 1987-2004.

A total of 10 per cent of the Mauritian population aged 20-74 years are obese (BMI>30) and another 25 per cent are overweight (25<BMI ≤ 30). The prevalence of overweight and obesity in both sexes taken together show an increase from 31 per cent in 1987 to 41 per cent in 1998 and a subsequent decrease to 36 per cent in 2004.

Child health

Situation Analysis

There have been significant improvements in the survival of infants over the past four decades.

During the year 2008, 15,590 live births were registered, giving a crude birth rate of 12.7 per thousand mid-year resident populations. In 1997, the crude birth rate was 17.4.

Life Expectancy at birth, 66.4 for males and 74.3 for females in 1997, was estimated to be 69.1 and 76.1 respectively in 2008.

The number of deaths registered in 2008 was 8, 798, corresponding to a crude death rate of 7.1 per thousand mid-year resident population as compared to 7.3 in 2006 and 6.8 in 2007.

The number of infant deaths, that is deaths among children aged under one year, registered in 2008 was 223, corresponding to an infant mortality rate (IMR) of 14.3 per thousand live births as compared to 15.3 in 2007. The IMR which was 19.6 in 1995 increased to 22.2 in 1996, the highest rate in the last decade. Following the opening of the Neonatal Intensive Care Service at one of the regional hospital in May 1999, the IMR drastically fell from 19.2 in 1999 to 15.8 in 2000. The lowest IMR (12.4) was recorded in 2003.

Low Birth Weight

The percentage of low birth weight babies (less than 2,500 grammes) among live births in the public sector, which increased from 14.3 per cent in 2000 to 17.2 per cent in 2005, was 16.7 per cent in 2008.

Under-five Mortality Rate

Considerable improvement was observed in <5MR from 17.9 in 2000 to 15.9 per 1000 live births in 2006. However there has been an increase in 2008 to 16.4 per 1000 live births.

Breast Feeding

The mean duration of exclusive breastfeeding is 2.0 months and the mean duration of any breastfeeding is 13.6 months.

NCD/Nutrition Survey 2004

In children 5-11 years:

The prevalence of overweight is 7.9 per cent among boys and 7.5 per cent among girls.

8.5 per cent of boys and 7.8 per cent of girls are obese

Prevalence of underweight is 24.3 per cent.

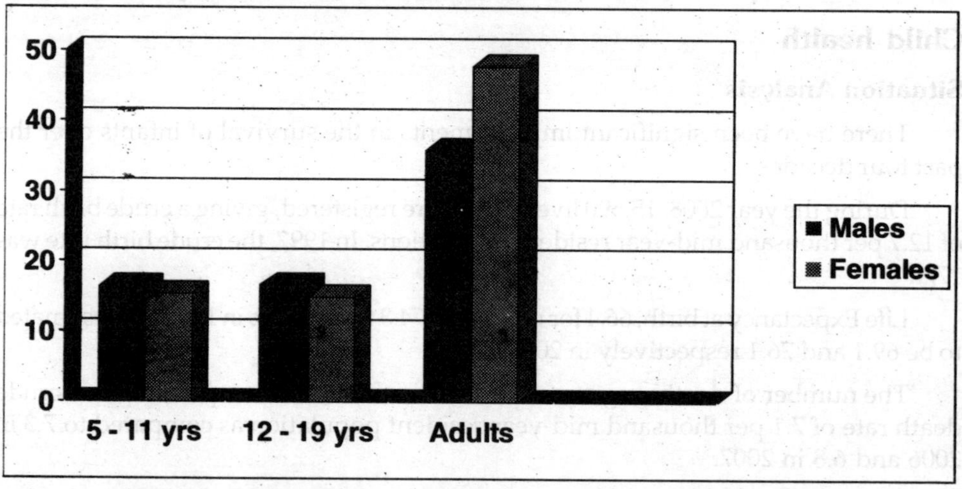

Figure 25.1: Prevalence of Overweight/Obesity in Mauritius - 2004

Child Health Services

The following services form part of the child health programme of the Ministry of Health and Quality of Life:

Newborn Care

- ☆ All infants are examined soon after birth by a Medical Officer.
- ☆ All Regional hospitals are baby-friendly and provide rooming in facilities.

- ☆ Advice is given to mothers to promote and support breastfeeding.
- ☆ Before discharge from hospital, women are given information and counseling on care of the baby, breastfeeding, hygiene, eye care, and how to recognize danger signs of illness.
- ☆ Neo-natal ICUs exist in 2 Regional Hospitals and essential equipment for survival of small and low birth weight babies has been installed in other hospitals.

Growth Monitoring

- ☆ Regular growth monitoring of children is done throughout the island through a network of 134 primary healthcare points. Midwives give appointment for medical check up of the babies at six weeks post partum.
- ☆ The child is weighed every month in the well baby clinic in the first year of life, then once every 2 months during the second year and once every three months during the third year.
- ☆ Babies are referred to the Pediatrician when indicated, and there is a once weekly Pediatrician sessions at AHCs.
- ☆ A cash gift scheme has been implemented since July 1999, whereby children are examined on their first, second and third birthdays, and issued with a cash voucher of Rs 200, which is credited to their post office savings account. The objective is to ensure regular medical examination and follow-up of children in the first three years.

Immunization

- ☆ An effective and well organized Expanded Programme of Immunization (EPI) is in place, with immunization coverage of 90 per cent. Services are offered at all Area and Community Health centers.
- ☆ Haemophilus Influenza Vaccine (Hib) has been included in the EPI package.
- ☆ Polio has been eradicated.
- ☆ No cases of neo-natal tetanus.

Breastfeeding

Mauritius is a Signatory to the International Code of Marketing of Breast Milk Substitutes (WHO, 1981).

- ☆ The Ministry of Health and Quality of Life recommends exclusive breastfeeding up to 6 months.
- ☆ The International Code of Breast Milk Substitutes, adopted by WHO in 1981was enforced in 1989.This Code bans all promotion of bottle feeding and sets out requirements for labeling and information on infant feeding. Any activity which undermines breastfeeding is discouraged. Baby food manufacturers are forbidden to promote their products in hospitals, shops or to the general public, give free samples to mothers or free or substituted

supplies to hospitals or maternity wards, give gifts to health workers or mothers and promote their products to health workers.

- ☆ Government envisages legislating an Infant Food Bill to ensure safe and adequate nutrition for infants by promoting and protecting breastfeeding and by regulating the marketing of certain infant foods and of feeding bottles, teats and pacifiers.
- ☆ Maternity wards of all Regional Hospitals have been designated Baby friendly.
- ☆ There is Breast feeding corners in all Regional Hospitals.
- ☆ Training of staff in counseling for breastfeeding is ongoing.
- ☆ HIEC materials for education of mothers and family members have been prepared and distributed.

Nutritional Surveillance System

- ☆ A Nutritional Surveillance System bulletin based on growth monitoring of children attending vaccination sessions is published quarterly. This bulletin gives timely information about the growth of children aged 0-59 months. The percentage of overweight and underweight children for each region is also provided as well as breastfeeding practices at 14 weeks.

School Health Programmes

The following services are offered for pupils:

- ☆ Screening of all new primary school entrants by Doctors and Community Health Nurses.
- ☆ Screening of pupils in standard five.
- ☆ Screening of pupils in secondary schools.
- ☆ Routine vision check up is done for Std 3, 5 and 6 pupils.
- ☆ Immunization (booster dose) at school entry and school leaving.
- ☆ Health education.
- ☆ Referral for further care at AHC and hospitals.

Some pre-primary schools are also visited by health staff.

There is an ongoing program of health education in all primary and secondary schools by staff from the Ministry of Health. Topics vary according to the age of the pupils and include hygiene, healthy eating habits, physical exercise, smoking and substance abuse, reproductive health issues. Health education forms part of the primary school curriculum.

Some of the Policy Decisions taken by the Ministry of Health

- ☆ In 1999 the levels of saturated fatty acids in most imported food products were regulated through the food regulations fifty eighth schedule, Part B that is Snacks, Cakes, Chocolates and Biscuits amongst others.

- ☆ In 1999 Guidelines for the sale of food in primary and secondary school canteens was established. It was an administrative agreement between the Ministry of Health and the Ministry of Education. A list of foods to be sold was set up. It was agreed that food should not be cooked in school canteens as the canteens did not have the proper facilities for satisfying Regulations 33 of the Food Regulations 1999 concerning "Building and Facilities".

  Since these guidelines did not have a legal framework, there was an abuse in the types of foods sold in school canteens. Most of the foods sold contained high levels of fat, sugar, salt, additives and artificial colors.
- ☆ In 2007, the sale of soft drinks was banned through the Guidelines.

At an *International level*, Standards for meals served in school canteens, that is, cooked lunches have already been introduced in England, USA, Australia, and New Zealand among others.

It is worth noting that in the Mauritian context, all canteens do not provide a main meal as compared to the European countries, except for about six Private schools and a few Catholic schools. In countries where main meals are given to children, 30 per cent of a child's daily caloric requirement should be provided by the lunches. Only a small fraction, that is, 0-5 per cent of calories can be provided from vending machines/tuck shops.

Children are expected to obtain their requirements of nutrients from the main meals and not from the tuck shops. Calories provided by the tuck shops in Mauritius far exceed the children's daily requirement thus increasing their risks of becoming obese.

- ☆ The processes for the legislation on the sale of foods in school canteens were started in 2008. Several consultations were carried out with different stakeholders namely, representatives of the Ministries of Health, of Education, the Private Secondary Schools Association etc.
- ☆ The 'New Regulations on the sale of foods in school canteens' was passed in August 2009. These regulations ban the sale of unhealthy snacks namely: Deep fried foods, foods with high levels of fats especially of the saturated type, sugar and salt. Healthy alternatives rich in complex carbohydrates and fruits which are good sources of vitamins and minerals are allowed for sale. The passing of the legislation has been supported by sensitization campaigns using the mass media as well as the holding of workshops for all stakeholders involved in children's health namely; teachers, canteen holders and representatives of the Parents Teachers Associations.
- ☆ In view of the high prevalence of overweight and obesity in the adult population, a "Know Your Number" campaign for the Republic of Mauritius was launched on World Diabetes Day during the International Conference on Diabetes and Associated diseases held here from 12 to 14 November 2009. The aim of the campaign was to sensitize the adult population about their weight. Tape measures with different cut-offs for males and females were distributed as well as Pamphlets on healthy eating. These tools will be distributed to 100,000 households.

- Re-use oil is a very common practice in Mauritius. Locally, the fried food industry is characterized by multiple, continuous frying over an extended period of time. Frying is quite cheap, rapid and an easy method of food preparation. A study into the trans fatty acids levels and peroxide value of re-used oil was carried out in 2009.
- *National Action Plan for Nutrition 2009-2010* was approved by the cabinet in June 2009. It is a comprehensive document on nutrition, with emphasis on the prevention of Non-Communicable Diseases in Mauritius. It is based on ten theme areas for action, covering the health, social, economic, environmental and foreign policy.

Other Ongoing Activities

Healthy Cooking Demonstrations

Healthy cooking demonstrations as well as Nutrition Talks are carried out at Community level in Social Welfare Centers, Community Centers, Recreational Centers and Youth Clubs. Nutrition talks are also given as part of the Health Promotion Programme of the Ministry in educational institutions as well as in workplaces, In Women Organizations etc.

Healthy cooking demonstrations and food exhibitions are also carried out at the launching of the Mobile Clinics. The Non-Communicable Diseases Mobile service popularly known as the 'Mobile Clinic' is in other words, a ready-to-go "ambulance organization" with an unparalleled service system for the screening and detection of Cardiovascular disease, high blood pressure, elevated blood cholesterol, Diabetes Mellitus, Obesity, Visual problems and Cervical and Breast Cancers. The NCD Mobile service represents an unbroken chain of co-operation between the Community and the team of healthcare providers, comprising of qualified and trained community physicians, community health nurses, community health workers, health educators, community health motivators and members of the Local Health Committee.

Media Campaigns

Daily nutrition messages lasting for 2 minutes each on various topics such as Obesity, Diabetes, cardiovascular diseases, infant nutrition, nutrition during pregnancy, anemia etc. are broadcasted on radio. Nutritionists also participate in various T.V programmes on nutrition. The production of posters, pamphlets and booklets on specific topics of nutrition complements the Radio and T.V programmes whilst also giving consistent nutrition messages.

Dietetic Clinics

These are one to one or group counseling sessions for people suffering from the NCD problems as well as for those who are overweight and obese. The aim is to teach patients suffering from these ailments how to manage their disease through diet. The Dietetic Clinics are carried out in the main hospitals, Area Health Centers and Community Health Centers.

Special Dietetic Clinics have also been set up for people living with HIV/AIDS (PLWHA) where nutritional advice is given to them.

References

1. Ministry of Health and Quality of Life, 2009. Family Planning and Demographic Yearbook 2008.

2. Ministry of Health and Quality of Life, 2009. Health Statistics Report 2008. Island of Mauritius and Island of Rodrigues.

3. Ministry of Health and Quality of Life, 2006. Mauritius Non-Communicable Diseases Survey 2004.

4 Ministry of Health and Quality of Life, 2007. The National Service Framework for Diabetes (NSFD). A ten year programme.